CLINICS IN DEVELOPMENTAL MEDICINE NO. 91

HEADACHES AND MIGRAINE IN CHILDHOOD

To Pat

Clinics in Developmental Medicine No. 91

HEADACHES AND MIGRAINE IN CHILDHOOD

CHARLES F. BARLOW, M.D.
Bronson Crothers Professor of Neurology,
Harvard Medical School;
Neurologist-in-Chief,
Children's Hospital, Boston, MA.

1984
Spastics International Medical Publications
OXFORD: Blackwell Scientific Publications Ltd.
PHILADELPHIA: J. B. Lippincott Co.

© 1984 Spastics International Medical Publications
5a Netherhall Gardens, London NW3 5RN

First published 1984

British Library Cataloguing in Publication Data

Barlow, Charles F.
    Headaches and migraine in childhood—(Clinics in Developmental Medicine No. 91)
    1. Headache.   2. Children—Diseases.
    I. Title   II. Series
    616.92′00472   RJ496.H3

ISBN 0-632-01326-5

Printed in Great Britain at The Lavenham Press Ltd., Lavenham, Suffolk

CONTENTS

FOREWORD

Headache is a common problem in childhood, and yet the index of a famed British textbook of paediatrics has no entry under this heading, while its American rival does rather better producing one page of text. Clearly there is a need for some help for the paediatrician in understanding the problems of children who present with this symptom.

Apart from the importance of identifying the situation where there is an underlying life-threatening cause, the variance of more benign but nevertheless very unpleasant symptoms of the child is substantial. Treading one's way through such diagnostic problems as abdominal epilepsy or abdominal migraine, and the periodic syndrome, has left many a paediatrician confused.

Professor Barlow charts his way clearly through these troubled waters. He emphasizes from the start that diagnosis is a clinical problem, where as yet our technological armentarium gives one little help in diagnosis. Having clearly set out his own experienced view of the different diagnostic entities, he goes on to provide us with clear guidelines for the management of children with this distressing symptom.

The study is based on Professor Barlow's personally ascertained series of cases, and he uses it to increase greatly our knowledge of headache and migraine in children. At the same time, the vivid case histories bring the book to life and show us the sensitive way he handles his young patients and their families. He reminds us again just how much good medical research can still be done by the careful clinician, who uses his personal experience to advance the study of medicine.

Martin C. O. Bax

PREFACE

The subject of headache and related clinical problems in children has been relatively neglected in the medical literature. One reason for this is the fact that headache is merely a symptom, one that reflects many etiologic entities, most of which are benign and relatively inconsequential in the scheme of things in pediatric medicine, whereas the usual textbook presentation centers about disease entities. Yet most patients present themselves with a symptomatic complaint such as headache, and it is only after the complaint is analyzed and a diagnosis made that the student or practitioner can exploit his accumulated clinical experience, go to the appropriate section of a textbook, select the relevant subject monograph, or proceed to the archive literature of original papers. Analysis of the symptom is therefore the first step in the clinical diagnostic process and the cornerstone of the clinical method. This book may help in that process.

Headache is a relatively common complaint in childhood. It is a frequent secondary symptom of the acute and recurring infectious disorders that comprise the bulk of pediatric practice. These acute monophasic headaches are comfortably managed and require little discussion in this monograph. On the other hand, injuries also account for a sizeable fraction of pediatric encounters. In a prepaid health plan that enrolled approximately 2500 individuals between birth and 17 years of age, 80 per cent of all enrolled children were seen for this reason during a six-year period (Starfield *et al.* 1984). A significant fraction of childhood injury involves the head, and I found it particularly interesting and informative to put together the data from my own experience and those of others in Chapter 10.

The same study (Starfield *et al.* 1984) points out that chronic morbidity is a less frequent aspect of pediatric practice, amounting to 11.2 per cent of children, 12.5 per cent of whom had migraine, second in frequency only to obesity. This accounting did not include the 17.3 per cent of children who were categorized as having 'psychosomatic' complaints, where headaches (41 per cent) and abdominal pain (33.5 per cent) led the list. Both of these symptoms involve juvenile migraine in their differential diagnosis. In fact, I suspect that in the headaches regarded as psychosomatic, there may have been a significant number I would consider to be migraine albeit aggravated by psychologic factors.

Juvenile migraine in its various manifestations is the central feature of the book. This inherited pathophysiologic reaction is heavily influenced by psychologic factors, thereby causing diagnostic confusion with psychogenic headache. The distinction between migraine and psychogenic headache has been useful conceptually and therapeutically in my own practice. Migraine is by far the commonest cause of headache in the pre-pubertal child, but headache is not the only manifestation. It figures prominently in the causation of periodic abdominal pain, cyclic vomiting and other aspects of 'the periodic syndrome', as well as in the differential diagnosis of vertigo and the less frequent clinical syndromes of complex migraine such as confusional states, ophthalmoplegia and hemiplegia. The manifestations of migraine in adults are much better recognized than in children, and although there are several excellent brief reviews of the subject as it relates to childhood, there has been no in-depth treatise since Bille's 1962 monograph. My first thought was to confine the monograph to the subject of juvenile migraine. However, the margins of the subject proved difficult to contain, particularly from the perspective of diagnostic implications, and in the end I decided to allow the text to extend into areas that may seem unnatural and arbitrary to some. In particular, discussion of the important organic causes of headache and related syndromes became necessary, including those of metabolic, infectious, and of structural cranial and intracranial origin.

In contrast with the customary impersonal perspective of a textbook, it is perhaps defensible to make a monograph of this type something of a personal statement. It is very much based upon my own experience, illustrated primarily by my own patients of the last 20 years. I have learned most of what I know from my patients, and I think that many clinical features are best illustrated by brief case reports.Such reports have been used extensively as an essential part of the text. My 300 migraine patients have also been used as a previously unpublished source of statistical information.

The book also contains elements of my own bias as a practising child neurologist, and undeniably also expresses the limitations of my own background. It will be clear that I am not a psychiatrist, and this limits the detail with which I have dealt with psychodynamic issues as causative factors in psychogenic headache and as the leading aggravating factor in migraine.

My brief experience as a pediatric generalist is now 30 years behind me and my insecurity when dealing with the full differential diagnosis of such subjects as periodic abdominal pain or vomiting will be obvious to the experts. My personal experience with these syndromes is based upon referral of occasional patients by perplexed pediatricians, with the thought that they may have abdominal migraine or abdominal epilepsy. Often the basis of referral is the finding of an EEG abnormality. I have limited personal perspective of the frequency of migraine as the basis of these complaints and am likely to see them only after considerable initial appraisal and sorting by others. This bias of selection has surely affected my concept of these symptoms, but it would seem that migraine is a significant cause of the syndrome of cyclic vomiting and a reasonably common cause of periodic abdominal pain in children as well.

The final responsibility of the preface is to thank those who have made a significant contribution to the effort. Dr. Roy Strand made an essential contribution to the selection and interpretation of the neuroradiologic studies. Dr. Giuseppe Erba played a similar rôle with regard to the EEGs. Those colleagues who contributed illustrative cases are mentioned in the text. Ms. Rosalyn Vogel contributed her skills in typing and in the mysteries of the word-processor, and somehow managed this job along with her usual work. My family gave up the dining-room table and were patient and understanding during the process of writing and revisions. Finally, I would like to express my appreciation to Dr. Martin Bax for his most helpful and conscientious editing.

1
INTRODUCTION

Headache in childhood

Headache is the commonest indisposition of mankind. It must be the exceptional individual who has not experienced the symptom at some time. Population surveys on the occurrence of complaints support this contention, but other conditions such as upper respiratory infection are more frequently brought to medical attention. Perhaps this is the first lesson. Headache is accepted by most adults as a part of life, a transient affair that is a relatively acceptable concomitant of the common cold, fever, influenza, or the excesses of life whether it be a hangover or a bad day at work. The sale of aspirin and other analgesics over the counter is a testimonial to the frequency of headache, as well as to the fact that it is customary to cope with the problem without medical assistance.

Headache in childhood is different. It is less common over-all, taken somewhat more seriously by the parents, and usually occurs in the context of an intercurrent illness that correctly becomes the focus of attention. It also carries the implication of an 'acceptable' symptom that is relatively inconsequential, and indeed this is usually the case. Even recurring headaches, if not frequent or particularly severe, are often accepted by both parents and physician as an indication of a 'nervous temperament' and of little consequence.

These attitudes may account for the rather surprising lack of attention to headache in childhood in the pediatric literature. Although not as common as in adults, chronic or recurring headache is nevertheless a high-frequency complaint in childhood and even more prominent in adolescence. Adult headache clinics have been established which serve as a base for clinical research, and provide expert patient-care as well. Much of the experience with adults is directly applicable to children, but there are also significant differences, which will be brought out in this monograph.

The extensive literature on adult headache problems is not regarded by pediatricians as of any particular relevance to their own practice and is consequently not read. Textbooks of pediatrics have not given much attention to the problem, in part because the usual presentation in texts is based upon disease entities and not upon a symptomatic presentation such as headache. Seizure disorders are a notable exception to this rule. There are considerable similarities between headache and this other common symptomatic manifestation of disease. Both relate to the nervous system, the expression is paroxysmal, and either may be symptomatic of serious underlying neurological disease such as brain tumor. They both have an 'idiopathic' expression that occupies a central place in the problem. In the case of convulsive disorder, it is idiopathic 'epilepsy', and migraine occupies a comparable position with headache.

One obvious difference between these two common childhood problems is the fact that seizures are more serious and frightening and demand attention and

1

therapy, while over the years migraine has not been fully appreciated as a significant illness of childhood. The work of Bille (1962) was highly significant in calling attention to migraine as a frequent disorder in childhood, but his study was not as widely appreciated as was warranted. Physicians working with children have tended to reserve this diagnosis for the syndromes of classic migraine with characteristic visual aura, while less dramatic expressions such as common migraine have frequently been interpreted as a symptom of nervous tension.

Other relatively common migraine expressions such as 'cyclic vomiting' and the 'periodic syndrome' have been given separate identities. At the same time, physicians with a particular interest in neurologic disease have become preoccupied with concepts of 'abdominal epilepsy' and 'convulsive headache'. Both phenomena are closely linked to the subject of migraine. On the basis of frequency alone, migraine is much more likely to be the cause of both.

For whatever reasons, the subject of headache in childhood and of juvenile migraine in particular has been relatively neglected. Even as excellent a textbook as that of Menkes (1980) has given only three pages to migraine, compared with 42 pages on convulsive disorders. In addition to Bille's monograph, there are several excellent reviews in the literature on the general subject of headache in chilhood (Friedman and Harms 1967, Rothner 1978) as well as those which deal more specifically with migraine in childhood (Holguin and Fenichel 1967, Prensky 1976, Brown 1977, Barlow 1978, Congdon and Forsythe 1979, Shinnar and D'Souza 1981).

It is probably time to bring the subject of juvenile migraine and other headaches in childhood into focus. Pediatric medicine has advanced to the point where some of the less threatening problems have assumed importance. Certainly this would seem to be the case with headache and especially with juvenile migraine, which now accounts for 20 to 30 per cent of my own referral practice in pediatric neurology. This indicates that pediatricians are sufficiently nervous about the symptom to want advice on diagnosis and management.

Differential diagnosis
Patients present themselves to the doctor with a symptom or a complex of symptoms, traditionally designated as the 'chief complaint'. It is the task of the physician to analyze the symptom with two principal objectives in view. The first is to establish an accurate diagnosis using the history, physical examination and appropriate laboratory procedures so that a rational therapy can be instituted. In this effort, the primary goal is to detect specifically remediable disease, however rare. It is also important to detect such disease as early as possible. The second goal is to analyze the pathogenesis of the symptom so that rational symptomatic therapy can be designed. The chief complaint of headache lends itself admirably to this set of goals and objectives (Table I).

In contrast with many other symptomatic presentations, headache is distinguished by being so frequently benign from the point of view of serious organic illness that there is a danger of being lulled into a false sense of security. On the other hand, it is also possible to overreact to the symptom and end up

TABLE I
Differential Diagnosis of Headache in Childhood

	Vascular	*Psychogenic*	*Organic**
Occurrence	Periodic	Continuous	Either periodic or continuous Nocturnal or early a.m. (50% of tumors)
Quality	Throbbing	Pressure Aching Tightness	Throbbing, pressure, aching, tightness, sometimes localized.
Associated symptoms	G.I. — *Anorexia* *Nausea* *Vomiting* *Abdominal pain* Visual— *Photophobia* *Blurred vision* *Scotomata* Other— *Vertigo* *Syncope* *Convulsions (rare)* *Fever (rare)*	Anxiety Depression	May include any symptoms listed under vascular or psychogenic headings, or evidence of infection as in sinusitis.
Family history	Yes, 90% of children	Variable	Variable
Associated signs	Pallor Visual field defects Confusion-amnesia Hemisyndromes-aphasia Ophthalmic sympathoparesis 3rd nerve palsy Brainstem ('basilar')	None	Any transient or persistent neuro- logical signs including signs of elevated pressure. Neurological abnormalities will be found in 95% of tumors in the first 4–6 months of headaches.

*Headaches related to systemic infectious, toxic or metabolic disease as well as cranial (including sinusitis) and intracranial disorders. The features listed under this heading apply especially to arterio-venous malformations, tumor and other mass lesions, hydrocephalus and pseudotumor cerebri.

communicating undue concern to the parents and child as well as ordering an excess of laboratory examinations, particularly computerized tomography (CT) scans. Fortunately headache is particularly well-suited to a systematic clinical assessment, if certain clinical guidelines are used. These are the basis of the synopsis presented in Table I. These clinical features are briefly described in the remainder of this section, and considered in more detail later.

The principal divisions of headache in childhood, as well as in adults, consist of: (i) vascular (usually synonymous with migraine), (ii) psychogenic (usually synonymous with tension headache), and (iii) organic (in which the headache is based upon structural cranial or intracranial disease or is a reflection of systemic metabolic or infectious processes). There may be initial ambiguity as to which category is most appropriate in an individual headache problem. Usually the passage of time and reconsideration of the original premise based on new developments or additional history will clarify the issue. For example, any new headache problem may be only tentatively assigned to either the vascular or

3

psychogenic category for at least the first four to six months pending re-examination for the possible development of neurological signs. To some extent, this proviso should continue indefinitely. Also it is common to become increasingly aware of psychological factors after several visits.

The principal variables that form the basis of the symptomatic diagnosis of headache are occurrence (periodic *vs.* continuous), the quality of painful discomfort, and associated symptoms. To this short list can be added the presence of persistent neurological signs—the principal indicator of the likelihood of intracranial structural lesions.

Occurrence

Apart from those occurring with acute upper respiratory infections, by far the majority of headaches in childhood will be found to be vascular, *i.e.* juvenile migraine (the terms are almost interchangeable). The headache is periodic in its occurrence and this—together with its usual throbbing quality and associated symptoms—is the chief clinical characteristic. The periodic interval and duration may vary greatly. The real meaning of the term is that the headache is either present or absent and there is no ambiguity about it. This feature is so characteristic of vascular headaches that it would be entirely appropriate for them to be designated 'periodic headaches'. In contrast, the usual psychogenic headache as it is presented to the physician is continuously present. It may wax and wane, but head discomfort at some level is almost always present.

Quality

Although not quite as constant a feature as periodicity, the quality of pulsation or throbbing has a very high incidence of expression in vascular headache. Occasionally the pain is so sharp and excruciating that the throbbing quality is lost. In some patients with milder headache, the best description that can be elicited is an aching sensation. The more commonly used descriptive words in psychogenic or tension headaches are sensations of frontal or occipital pressure or tightness, although the term 'aching' is also used with reasonable frequency.

Associated symptoms

The symptoms associated with the headache are also important clinical features. In migraine there is often nausea and sometimes vomiting. The minimal expression of a gastro-intestinal upset is anorexia. Abdominal pain is also common. Visual symptoms such as an aura of scintillating scotomata are not especially common in children but can be distinctive, while photophobia is very frequently mentioned. Light-headedness and vertigo are frequent associated symptoms, and pallor is usually recognized by the parents. A highly characteristic attribute of migraine is that the parents can see that the child is ill, because of obvious changes in behavior as well as pallor. The various neurologically complex associated symptoms and signs are summarized in Table I, and will be discussed in greater detail later.

The symptoms associated with psychogenic headache are those related to the

4

anxiety or depression which forms the basis of the psychiatric disorder. Symptoms are usually behavioral in children, although somatic expression in other organ systems can occur. Cyclic depression is a significant problem in children, and proves to be the basis of an appreciable number of headache problems. Recognition of childhood depression is not only important from a diagnostic perspective, but has therapeutic implications as well. The first clue may come in the depressive demeanor and sad facies of the child, although non-specific behavioral symptoms such as irritability, apathy and outbursts of temper are the usual presenting complaint. A depressive facies can be deceptive in adolescents, many of whom seem to be glum and resentful in the company of their parents. Discussion with the patient alone is necessary to see more of the true personality and to have a somewhat less inhibited discussion. These comments relating to the personality disorder and psychologic stress factors in psychogenic headache apply equally well to the much more common issue of psychological probems as an aggravating factor in the expression of juvenile migraine. This important and common relationship will be discussed in greater detail in the section on precipitating factors in juvenile migraine (Chapter 2).

Family history
About 90 per cent of children with migraine have a family history of vascular headaches. It is therefore a highly significant aspect of the diagnosis, and it is worth examining the history of parental headache in order to make an independent judgement of their nature rather than accept the parents' interpretation and their own self-diagnosis. Family history is equally important as a clue to the diagnosis of childhood depression. The incidence of depression in parents or close relatives is highly significant. It is important to emphasize that a positive family history of migraine or depression does not exclude organic disease. A negative family history is a cause for diagnostic unease, and it may be useful principally for that reason.

Organic headaches
Organic headaches have not been mentioned in the above discussion. This is because headaches with clinical characteristics of both vascular and psychogenic disorders may be directly or indirectly related to systemic, cranial (including sinusitis) or neurological disease. In fact, the overwhelming majority of the occasional headaches of childhood occur in the setting of acute infectious diseases. Organic, systemic and neurologic disease may trigger headaches of either major benign type. This is particularly the case with migraine, leading to the clinical concept of an inherited threshold of neurovascular reactivity that can be exceeded by many precipitating circumstances, including organic intracranial disease. There are several clinical clues to the possibility of intracranial mass lesions. These include frequent occurrence at night or in the early morning, and precipitation by coughing (see Chapter 12). The main point is the fact that neurological signs on examination are the chief factor in the separation of organic causation from the more benign varieties of headache.

5

Epidemiology of headache in childhood

Most epidemiologic studies of headache have been conducted on adult populations. These have been well summarized by Leviton (1978). Several points of interest were made in Leviton's review, including the high prevalence of the complaint in adults (roughly 70 to 80 per cent), the lesser frequency with which it is presented to the physician as a chief complaint, the problems with the dichotomy of nosology into vascular headache and psychogenic headache, and a review of the status of information on the various general risk factors such as heredity, psychologic issues and hormonal factors. A particularly interesting point was quoted with regard to Waters's questionnaire to British physicians: 'Only 28% of men and 50% of women who had unilateral headaches associated with nausea identified their headaches as migraine'. If these highly suggestive criteria of migraine are not so interpreted by physicians, it is no surprise that the non-medical population is also difficult to survey on the subject. As presented in Bruyn's review of the literature (1983), the reported incidence of migraine in adults varies considerably. The data collected by Waters (1974) is probably as accurate as any general population survey. This study gives an over-all prevalence in women of 23.2 per cent and in men of 14.9 per cent. This is in reasonable agreement with the study of Dalsgaard-Neilsen *et al.* (1970) where the data were obtained by personal interview. These authors calculated an adult incidence of 18.8 per cent in women and 11.2 per cent in men.

The literature on the prevalence of headache in childhood populations is by contrast quite easy to review in that it consists of very few studies. The classic reference is that of Bille (1962). The basic data were derived from a questionnaire given to 9059 schoolchildren between ages seven and 15 in Uppsala, Sweden during 1955 with 99.3 per cent replies. Analysis of the sample indicated that 41.3 per cent had never had headaches, 47.9 per cent had 'infrequent non-migrainous headache', 6.8 per cent had 'frequent non-migrainous headaches' (of which 22.5 per cent were 'paroxysmal'), and 3.9 per cent had migraine as defined by the criteria of Vahlquist (1955) *i.e.* 'paroxysmal headaches separated by free intervals, and at least two of the following four: one-sided pain, nausea, visual aura and family heredity in parents or siblings'.

It should be pointed out that the Vahlquist criteria do not include throbbing quality of the pain, or other criteria which might be regarded as specific for migraine, such as some of the more complex auras. One wonders how many additional patients with migraine were relegated to the non-migraine group by the restricted definition. Bille's data probably underestimates the frequency of vascular headaches in childhood; yet the group of patients that were identified as having juvenile migraine can be confidently said to represent the disorder.

On the basis of this data, it was concluded that the prevalence of migraine was 3.9 per cent in the full sample of seven to 15 year olds. In the seven to nine age-group, frequency was 2.5 per cent for boys and 2.4 per cent for girls; at 10 to 12 years it was 3.9 per cent for boys and 5.4 per cent for girls; and in the 13 to 15 year age-group it was 4.0 per cent for boys and 6.4 per cent for girls.

There is little information on headaches in the child under age five. No population studies have been done. In my own migraine sample (see Table IV) only approximately 9 per cent were under age five when first seen. Psychogenic headache in this age-group must be most unusual, and I cannot remember making this diagnosis. On the other hand, the incidence of organic intracranial disease as a cause of headache under age six is higher than at any other time of life.

Bille did not make an effort to ascertain the incidence of psychogenic headache *per se*. His aim was to study the prevalence of migraine, and the residual children with headache were not separated into those whose headaches occurred in association with incidental diseases of childhood and those in whom the basis may have been psychogenic in origin. Perhaps the closest implication of a psychogenic basis is in the 5.2 per cent who 'frequently had non-paroxysmal headaches'.

An especially useful aspect of the Bille monograph reports an intensive personal study of 73 children between the ages of nine and 15, with at least one attack of unequivocal migraine per month, as compared with 73 children in a control group in which the children had 'neither migraine nor other frequent headache'. In addition to the frequency criteria, patients were selected on the basis of duration and severity. Duration of more than one hour was required and the headache had to be of sufficient severity that the patient was unable to carry on usual activities and preferred to lie down and rest. Controls were matched for age, sex and social group. These patients will be frequently mentioned later, and will be identified as Bille's personally interviewed group of patients. Despite the small numbers, they give insight into the frquency and variety of symptoms in the clinically significant migraine syndromes in children, as well as the frequency of associated disorders such as cyclic vomiting. Unlike almost all other studies, the Bille personally interviewed series has the advantage of simultaneously collected comparative control data.

More recently Sillanpää (1983) found that over-all headache prevalence increased from 37 per cent to 69 per cent between age seven and 14 years in a population survey of 2941 Finnish schoolchildren. Migraine, which was defined by the Vahlquist (1955) criteria, was found to increase from 2.7 per cent at seven years to 10.6 per cent at 14 years. At age seven, migraine was slightly more prevalent in boys (2.9 per cent) than in girls (2.5 per cent), and at age 14 boys had increased to 6.4 per cent while 14.8 per cent of girls were affected. With minor exceptions, these data are very close to those compiled by Bille and are probably a reasonably accurate representation of the true state of affairs.

Another population prevalence study is now becoming available as the data are being analyzed from the United Kingdom, *i.e.* the National Child Development Study. The report of Kurtz *et al.* (1984) is derived from this study which provides data on all children born in one week in March 1958 in England, Scotland and Wales. Parental interviews and supplemental examinations by school medical officers provide details about health-related issues at seven, 11, 16 and 23 years of age. At age 16 and 23 years, the subjects were individually interviewed as well.

The questionnaire index query was 'Has the child had attacks of migraine or recurrent sick headaches in the past 12 months?' If positive, a detailed description of the headache was developed. At age seven and 11, inquiry also related to 'headache, vomiting and bilious attacks, travel sickness and periodic abdominal

TABLE II

Selected Studies on the Prevalence of Headache in Childhood Including the Age and Sex Incidence of Migraine.*

Author	No. of patients	Survey method[†]	Headache of all types	Childhood migraine	Adolescent migraine
Bille (1962)	8993	Parent questionnaire Ascertainment—all past years	58.7% (age 7–14)	Male 2.5% Female 2.4% (age 7–9)	Male 4.0% Female 6.4% (age 13–15)
Dalsgaard-Neilsen et al. (1970)	2027	Patient and parent interview by author Ascertainment—all past years.	Data not given	Male 3.1% Female 2.8% (age 7–9)	Male 8.4% Female 9.5% (age 15–17)
Deubner (1977)	600	Patient and parent interview Ascertainment—previous year	Male 74% Female 85% (age 10–20)	Male 14% Female 20% (age 10–12)	Male 18% Female 23% (age 13–15)
Sillanpää (1982)	2921	Pupil questionnaire Ascertainment—previous year	37.0% (age 7) 69% (age 14)	Male 2.9% Female 2.5% (age 7)	Male 6.4% Female 14.8% (age 14)

*See Table III for criteria of migraine used by the above authors.
†Note that Bille (1962) and Dalsgaard-Neilsen et al. (1970) recorded headache experience during the lifetime of the patient, while the Deubner (1977) and Sillanpää (1982) data relate to prevalence in the one year prior to assessment.

8

pain'. At age 16, of 11,228 respondents, 10,046 had had no headaches in the previous year. Of those who indicated that they had experienced headache, 319 had definite migraine (2.8 per cent of the entire cohort), 783 (6.9 per cent) had 'sick headache' and 80 (0.8 per cent) had other headache types. 'Sick headache' applied to children with headache plus anorexia or nausea. If vomiting or specific visual disturbance occurred, the headaches were categorized as 'definite migraine'. The authors found that those diagnosed as 'definite migraine' corresponded to the approximate incidence of classic migraine in other studies in childhood. It was thought that the incidence of 'sick headache' in their series probably corresponded to the prevalence of common migraine.

The greatest discrepancy was in the category of 'any' headache which was much lower than in the Bille (1962) and Sillanpää (1983) studies where over 50 per cent of the total sample had had some variety of headache. The explanation probably lies in the methods of ascertainment in which emphasis was placed on headache with migrainic features, and also to some extent in the request for information from the previous year only. The issue is not of great relevance because the point of particular interest is the frequency of medically significant headache and the type of headache, rather than concern about the occasional expression of the symptom.

The authors of the United Kingdom report express unease about attempting a sharp separation of migraine from headache of other varieties in epidemiological studies. This issue was also addressed by Leviton (1978), and others have been concerned with this problem as well (Friedman et al. 1954, Cohen 1978). It is informative that the children classified as having 'sick headaches' showed about double the incidence of emotional disturbance at ages seven, 11, and 16 years as compared with controls. This does not necessarily challenge the nosologic dichotomy, but does point out the importance of emotional factors in the expression of juvenile migraine.

Deubner (1977) has reported a survey based on 600 responses to a questionnaire that was sent to 780 subjects 10 to 20 years of age chosen at random from people who had attended schools in Cardiff, South Wales. Data were obtained by interview and questionnaire. Migraine was defined as headache with two of three features: unilaterality, nausea or neurologic manifestations. The over-all occurrence of headache was 82 per cent in females and 74 per cent in males of whom 21.1 per cent of females and 15.5 per cent of males had migraine by the above definition. There was no correlation of migraine with travel sickness, or cyclic vomiting, although there was correlation with abdominal pain. The familial incidence of migraine did not reach statistical significance in these patients. The major differences in these findings, such as the higher prevalence of headache in this sample and the lack of family history in the migrainics, are significantly different from other studies. Perhaps the small number of patients, and the extension of the sample to age 20, the method of data collection and the criteria for the diagnosis of migraine are to some extent accountable for the differences. Deubner (1977) made no effort to identify psychogenic headache in this study nor to estimate its prevalence.

Dalsgaard-Neilsen *et al.* (1970) directed their prevalence study to the issue of juvenile migraine, using the Ad Hoc Committee criteria for 'vascular headaches of the migraine type' (Friedman *et al.* 1962*a*). These criteria are presented in narrative form and leave much to the individual judgement of the physician. The patients were identified from a sample of 2027 schoolchildren aged between seven and 18, who were selected on the basis of personal interview. These investigators found an incidence of migraine of 3.1 per cent in males and 2.8 per cent in females between seven and nine years, and in the 15 to 17 year group the incidence was 8.4 per cent in males and 9.5 per cent in females. This study focuses on migraine and gives no data on over-all incidence of headache in children. The migraine data in younger children are consistent with the Bille (1962) and Sillanpää (1983) reports. With regard to the older group, however, the finding of only 9.5 per cent in females may be an underestimate.

In summarizing epidemiologic studies on headache, one must begin by recognizing the problems and strengths of the method, and the objectives that might be attained. With regard to headache, the epidemiologic method can give one a general indication of the prevalence. Data from population studies indicate that it is a common complaint in childhood, and that 60 to 70 per cent of children will have had headache in some context by age 15 years (Table II).

It seems unlikely that epidemiologic surveys will bring us closer to an understanding of the basic causation of either vascular or psychogenic headache, nor can they be expected to do so given the problems in the epidemiologic method alluded to above. In this one must agree with Leviton (1978) who states: 'In the history of the epidemiology of any disorder, the use of manifestational entity as an outcome is a primitive forerunner to the use of the results of a specific biochemical or physiologic test. Thus major advances in headache epidemiology may be expected to occur when migraine is defined by a laboratory finding'.

Problems of differentiation
The problem of a generally acceptable clinical definition of migraine *vs.* psychogenic headache in epidemiologic studies, and therefore an indication of relative prevalence of either type, has been almost insurmountable. Most studies have been content to attempt to identify migraine and to leave the issue of psychogenic headache ambiguous.

Separation of the two major headache categories is poorly adaptable to questionnaire presentation, which is the only practical method of obtaining a large population sample. Moreover, there is a body of opinion which implies that the two major forms of headache cannot be separated, and there is an element of truth in this contention. Table III illustrates the criteria that have been used by a selected group of authors who have addressed themselves to separating migraine from other headaches. The criteria of Prensky (1976) have the advantage of including classic and common migraine, and they reflect a wider concept of the syndrome. It is my belief that Prensky's criteria are the most satisfactory, principally because they include consideration of throbbing quality and a positive family history, both of which are of high incidence and are relatively specific migraine indicators. The

TABLE III
Criteria for the Diagnosis of Migraine

	Essential criteria	Necessary symptoms
1. Vahlquist (1955) Bille (1962) Sillanpää (1982)	Periodic, plus	3 of the following: aura nausea vomiting family history
2. Prensky (1976) Jay and Tomasi (1980)	Recurrent with symptom-free intervals, plus	3 of the following: abdominal pain or nausea or vomiting unilateral throbbing relief after sleep aura (visual, sensory, motor) family history
3. Deubner (1977)	Periodic, plus	2 of the following: unilateral nausea with or without vomiting neurologic symptoms (scotomata scintillations, paresthesias)
4. Congdon and Forsythe (1979)	Periodic, plus	3 of the following: aura nausea vomiting family history
5. Kurtz et al. (1984)	Recurrent with anorexia or nausea, plus	1 of the following: vomiting specific visual disturbance

criteria used by Vahlquist (1955), Deubner (1977), and Congdon and Forsythe (1979) can be expected to emphasize classic migraine, at the expense of leaving out a number of patients with common migraine. The Kurtz et al. (1984) criteria are more difficult to analyze. Certainly the migraine category is relatively solid, and the 'sick headache' group are probably mostly migraine. On the basis of the more inclusive criteria of Kurtz et al. (1984) and including both the 'sick headache' and 'migraine' group to indicate mostly vascular headache patients, together with the data of Sillanpää (1983), the prevalence of migraine may very well be about 10 per cent by age 15 years.

Epidemiologic studies have tended to confirm the important influence of emotional issues in the genesis of headache in childhood. However, assuming that most childhood headaches can be differentiated into psychogenic and migraine, there is no good prevalence data on the psychogenic group.

Personal series of juvenile migraine patients
In setting out to write this monograph, I decided to review my office notes on patients with headache. These records began in July 1963 upon my move to Boston,

TABLE IV

Age, Sex and Family History
(Personal Series of 300 Patients)

	Under 5 years	5–10 years	11–15 years	15–18 years	Total
Male	15 (53.6%)	96 (73.8%)	44 (44.4%)	8	163 (54.4%)
Female	13 (46.4%)	64 (25.2%)	55 (55.6%)	5	137 (45.6%)
Total	28 (9.3%)	160 (53.3%)	99 (33.3%)	13	300 (100%)
Positive family history	26 (93%)	138 (86%)	87 (88%)	11 (85%)	262 (89.7%)*

*Less 8 adopted children.

TABLE V

Characteristics of Juvenile Migraine
(Personal Series of 300 Patients)

Family history	89.7%
Headache	
Throbbing quality	66%
Hemicranial distribution	22%
Associated G.I. symptoms	
Nausea and/or vomiting	62%
Anorexia alone	12%
Total	74%
Aura	
Visual (teichopsia, scotomata)	5%
Numbness (face, hands, usually bilateral)	0.5%
Other factors	
Associated vertigo or light-headedness*	19%
Nocturnal occurrence (occasional)**	9%
A.M. awakening (occasional)**	4%

*During aura or headache.
**The majority of headaches in these patients occurred during the daytime hours in contrast with some patients with mass lesions or hydrocephalus where headaches customarily occurred at night or upon awakening.

when my consulting work became almost exclusively a practice of child neurology. Prior to that time, clinical work in Chicago was about equally divided between adults and children. The experience with migraine in Chicago also included adult patients, an experience that had an important influence on my views on migraine in childhood.

The Boston records were most helpful in reviewing a personal experience that consisted of private initial consultation in all cases and varying follow-up visits. In some patients only initial consultation was provided, but in many cases it has been possible to maintain contact over a number of years. The migraine series consisted of 300 consecutive patients. The final patient was added in August 1983. Clinical data were not collected with this monograph in mind, and are frustratingly incomplete on a number of points of history that a prospective plan might have remedied. For example, data on handedness would have been very interesting in view of Geschwind and Behan's (1982) recent data on the disproportion of left-handedness among people suffering from migraine. Even more obvious issues such as the association of motion sickness were not mentioned in many records. On the other hand, age, sex, and the principal characteristics of the headache and associated symptoms are quite complete, as is the family history.

The breakdown by age and sex are documented in Table IV. It will be noted that there are relatively few patients above age 15, which is a dramatic expression of the bias of referral. Boys predominate under age 11. The history of other members of the family with migraine is approximately the same in each five-year period.

Personal criteria for the diagnosis of juvenile migraine are consistent with those used by other authors, and especially those of Prensky (1976) and the Ad Hoc Committee on the Classification of Headache (Friedman *et al.* 1962*a*), but in the final analysis they represent a personal clinical impression. No apology is made for this.

All headaches categorized as juvenile migraine have been paroxysmal. Rigid criteria, such as the usual formula of paroxysmal headache plus 'three or more of the following', are important in setting the stage for a formal study and are reasonably accurate. However, in practice they may overlook the occasional individual who does not fit the pattern. The physician must retain the flexibility of individual judgement. Diagnosis by formula is appropriate to groups of patients and formal studies. It is not appropriate to the practice of medicine.

The most consistent other features have been throbbing (67 per cent), family history of headache consistent with migraine (89.7 per cent), associated symptoms of gastro-intestinal disturbance, usually nausea or nausea and vomiting (62.3 per cent), aura of visual disturbance, vertigo or light-headedness or peri-oral or upper-extremity numbness (43 per cent). Certain less frequent symptoms, such as hemicrania (22 per cent) and scintillating scotomata (5 per cent), were given special weight because of their highly characteristic diagnostic relevance (Table V).

2
THE SUBSTRATE AND PATHOLOGY OF MIGRAINE

Introduction

Migraine is the commonest basis of recurring headache in childhood. The cause of migraine is not known, although it almost certainly reflects an inherited predisposition. It is possible that there is a family of closely related disorders of differing genotype with similar phenotypic expression. The symptoms are the result of a pathophysiologic reaction in which painful involvement of the extracranial and cerebral vasculature occurs as a prominent feature. The vasculature of other parts of the body such as the gastro-intestinal system may also be vulnerable in some individuals. Other symptoms in the spectrum of migraine have a clear neurologic component, and perhaps it is best regarded as a neurovascular syndrome that leads to a generalized vasomotor instability and vulnerability to multiple extraneous factors. These precipitating factors will be considered later.

The vasomotor instability of migraine is reminiscent of the neuronal instability of seizure disorders. Like reflex epilepsy, the apparent precipitating factors may be the exclusive event leading to decompensation of the system. However, usually an unknown confluence of events is responsible for the paroxysm in both epilepsy and migraine. Migraine has a greater tendency to be precipitated by definable external events than seizures, particularly if one considers the adverse influence of psychologic tensions on the frequency and severity of attacks. In some ways, what is more mysterious is how stability is maintained in the system most of the time.

The migrainic patient has therefore inherited a neurovascular system that is less stable than in the majority of people. However, the abnormality is not unique and the clinical phenomenology of vascular headache can be reproduced in almost any individual if there is sufficient provocation. The vascular headache of febrile illness or of influenza is a sufficient reminder that we are all vulnerable. What distinguishes the migrainic would seem to be the threshold of response that may be variable depending upon age, sex and other factors. It follows that the inherited defect in migraine is likely to be an issue of regulatory control of a responsive system. It is also possible that the patient with clinically significant manifest migraine represents the 10 to 20 per cent of the population who occupy the extreme of a multifactorial bell-shaped curve dealing with the regulation of human vasomotor reactivity. The abnormality need not reside in the blood-vessel wall nor its intimate innervation, but could be a response to a circulating humoral factor released by other tissues in the body. It could also represent a metabolic defect in a system of cells that are widely distributed in many tissues of the body.

The substrate of migraine

If the basic issue in migraine is an inhertied disorder leading to neurovascular

14

instability, what are the features of its inheritance, and what are its other manifestations beyond the customary clinically important syndromes?

Genetics

There is general agreement that there is a significant hereditary factor or factors in the clinical expression of most vasomotor headaches and related syndromes. This is especially apparent in juvenile migraine. In my own series of 300 patients (less eight adopted children) the frequency of a positive family history is 89.7 per cent (Table IV). It may be somewhat higher because the family history was less aggressively sought in the earlier period of data collection. This incidence includes positives in parents, siblings, grandparents and occasionally aunts and uncles related by blood. Aunts or uncles were rarely the only affected relative. Most often the affected relative was the mother or father, and quite frequently both. Where possible, the diagnosis of vascular headaches in relatives was based upon direct history, usually from the parents.

The history in relatives fulfilled my own clinical criteria for migraine, *i.e.* paroxysmal headache, usually throbbing in quality with appropriate associated features to round out the diagnosis. I have collected no series of comparable controls, a defect that is almost universal in the reported studies on the incidence of migraine in families. Certainly in a comparable number of seizure patients, for example, family history of headache has not been pursued with the diligence applied to juvenile headache patients. These data reinforce the utility of a positive family history as a significant point in the diagnostic process. It contributes nothing to the needed scientific genetic studies on migraine.

There are a number of reports in the literature on the family history of childhood migraine. These data were collated by Prensky (1976), who records an average incidence of 72 per cent with a range of 44 to 87 per cent in the nine reports sampled. The family incidence in Bille's (1962) series of 347 questionnaire cases was 78.1 per cent. In his personally interviewed group of 73 patients, the incidence was 79.5 per cent as compared with his group of controls where the incidence was 17.8 per cent. This difference was highly significant. The series of 300 patients reported more recently by Congdon and Forsythe (1979) revealed an incidence of 88 per cent. In a somewhat different approach, Allan (1930) reported a migraine incidence of 83 per cent in the children of families in which both mother and father had migraine.

There is little advantage to be gained by a further review of the literature of familial factors in migraine. The comments expressed by Ziegler (1977), although directed to the subject of the genetics of migraine in general, apply equally well to the subject as it relates to children. He points out that: '(1) varying criteria for the diagnosis of migraine have been used, and only rarely did the definition include the life history of headache over an extended period. (2) The information on relatives varied markedly in completeness, and even in the best studies was obtained second-hand from probands, not from direct interviews'. He also pointed out that there are few studies using controls for comparison.

As indicated in Ziegler's editorial, the status of the genetics of migraine from

15

the adult perspective also leaves much to be desired. Perhaps it is sufficient for our purposes to cite Prensky's (1976) tabulation which indicates a family incidence in adult migraine of 71 per cent, a figure compiled from four reported adult series. It should be noted that in at least one report of personal cases by Dalsgaard-Neilsen (1965) the family incidence was 90 per cent in a group of female patients with ocular symptoms.

The mode of inheritance of migraine is uncertain. Suggestions have ranged from somatic recessive with a 70 per cent rate of penetrance (Goodell *et al.* 1954) to a dominant mode of inheritance. Modern genetic concepts would suggest that multifactorial inheritance involving several genes is a more likely explanation of the available data (Dalessio 1980).

Hemiplegic migraine has a high familial incidence. Instances are recorded in which members of three and four generations have suffered from hemiplegic migraine (Blau and Whitty 1955, Glista *et al.* 1975), and there are a number of reports where family involvement is less extensive (see section on hemisyndromes). In a review of 36 patients, Bradshaw and Parsons (1965) found that approximately half of these patients had relatives who also had hemiplegic migraine.

On the other hand, it is unusual for cluster headache (migrainous neuralgia) to occur in more than one person of a family, and the incidence of other varieties of vascular headache in families of these patients is also low, 15 per cent in Ekbom's (1970) series. The strong male predominance, the usual later age of onset, and certain biochemical features in this variety of headache also sets it apart from other vascular headache syndromes.

There is little question that vulnerability to vascular headaches is usually an inherited trait. The genetic issues are not clear, but polygenic multifactorial inheritance is probably the best hypothesis at the present time. There may be several fundamental pathophysiologic entities accountable for the basic anomaly. Until one or more are identified and suitable easily measured markers defined, the exact genetics will remain a problem. Certain clinical syndromes such as cluster headache are sufficiently distinctive to set them apart, but there may be other pathophysiologically defined groups yet to be determined.

The expression of migraine in adults is more frequent in women than in men. Prevalence rates vary somewhat, but the studies of Waters (1970, 1974) that are summarized in Waters and O'Connor (1975) can be used as a representative indication of the data. These studies dealt with people 21 years and over, and report a population prevalence of 23 to 29 per cent in women and 15 to 20 per cent in men.

The situation in children is quite different. Over-all population prevalence is lower, but the particular point of interest is the reversal of the male/female differences before puberty. Prensky's (1976) compilation of eight published series of juvenile migraine gives an incidence of approximately 60 per cent in males. In my own series of patients in the five to 10 year age-group, the male incidence was also 60 per cent. In the Congdon and Forsythe (1979) series the male incidence was 58.5 per cent in the 268 children under age 10. In Bille's (1962) questionnaire sample, boys predominate over girls until age 10. At this point the relative incidence in girls increases sharply both relatively and absolutely, and at age 11 and 12 girls represent 7 per cent of the total sample, while boys remain around 4 per cent. It can be presumed that the trend continues and the adult prevalence is reached by age 21. In the study of Dalsgaard-Neilsen *et al.* (1970), the interesting point was made that the maximum onset of migraine in males was age 10 years while in females it was 14 years, and that there was minimal onset of migraine in males after age 30 years while this was not the case in women. There is no data available that addresses the question of father to son inheritance in boys who manifest migraine at an early age.

Hormonal factors
Although other factors may play a confounding rôle, the conclusion is inescapable that the hormonal changes of puberty have a significant impact on the clinical expression of migraine. This statement can be reinforced by a number of additional clinical observations that speak to the same point, such as the tendency to occurrence at the time of menses, aggravation of frequency and severity of headache associated with the use of birth-control pills, amelioration during the second and third trimester of pregnancy especially in women who have a history of migraine related to menstrual periods (Lance and Anthony 1966), and the amelioration of menstrual migraine by progesterone prophylaxis (Somerville 1971). Some women experience their migraine headaches exclusively in relation to menstrual periods, while many will have an increased frequency and severity at this time. Another aspect of the hormonal relationship to the expression of migraine is the possibility that androgen may have a suppressive effect, in part accountable for the lesser expression in adult males.

The clear trend to the slight male predominance in the pre-pubertal children is difficult to explain. One possibility relates to psychological factors that may operate to male disadvantage such as greater parental expectations, less natural aptitudes than girls in the early school years and a higher incidence of dyslexia and school learning disabilities. The data on sex-related expression of migraine in which boys predominate by a small margin in pre-pubertal children, as compared with the striking female preponderance in adults, may support the concept that the basic inborn trait is equally distributed between the sexes. The age-related sexual variability is perhaps an epiphenomenon that expreses a significant additional genetic factor, *i.e.* hormonal influences, and is a prime indication of at least a bifactorial representation in the postulated 'multifactorial' inheritance.

Personality
Saper (1983) indicates that the migraine patient has been described as having a personality with 'compulsive, perfectionistic, rigid, and achievement driven elements, often accompanied by internalized anger and excessive self control' and goes on to say 'this emphasis may not be warranted', in support of which a number of references are cited. The concept of a migraine personality is probably more traditional than factual. The features ascribed to it occur with sufficient frequency

17

in the non-migrainic population that little can be made of it. Certainly many migrainics do not conform to the formula and present with widely varying personalities. Yet the clinician perhaps correctly persists in the impression of a disproportionate number of somewhat obsessive perfectionistic goal-oriented people among migrainic patients.

Data dealing with personality factors in childhood migraine are principally dependent upon Bille's survey of his group of 73 personally interviewed patients with control comparison (Bille 1962). Parental ratings indicated that the child with juvenile migraine was more sensitive, more tidy, less physically enduring and more vulnerable to frustration than controls. All of these features reached statistical significance. There was no difference in such behavioral symptoms as 'tics, nailbiting, finger-sucking, enuresis and stuttering' and only a slight difference in temper tantrums. General intelligence was not different in the two groups.

There is little data to support the concept of a 'migraine personality', and children with symptomatic expression of this disorder represent a reasonable cross-section of pediatric patients in terms of intelligence and personality characteristics. Because of the strong adverse influence of psychological tensions in symptomatic expression, there is a somewhat higher representation of those with situational and other adjustment problems. There is perhaps a bias which works to the disadvantage of the conscientious child, because of the tendency to set high goals and internalize their tensions rather than display them to the world. If they have inherited a reactive vasomotor system, vascular headaches are likely to become the symptomatic focus of the problem.

Other symptoms and signs of vasomotor instability
If the inherited substrate of migraine is a metabolic disorder or disorders that leads to an unstable and excessively reactive neurovasomotor system, then there should be other manifestations of this state beyond the more overt clinical expressions such as classic and common migraine, 'cyclic vomiting' and the 'periodic syndrome'. This would seem to be the case.

Motion sickness
One of the more troublesome of these symptoms is motion sickness. It is often an early manifestation, may occur by age two or younger and persists throughout an individual lifetime, although usually the tendency lessens after early childhood and greater provocation is necessary as time goes on. The symptom is not exclusively a precursor of migraine, and like so many of the symptoms of vasomotor instability it may occur in almost anyone if there is sufficient provocation. Expression may be an issue of the threshold of response.

That there is a higher than expected incidence in migrainics is illustrated by Bille's (1962) study in which there was a 54.8 per cent incidence in the interviewed migraine group as opposed to 31. 5 per cent in the controls, a disparity of moderate significance. However, if severe degrees of motion sickness were considered, then 49.3 per cent of migrainic children were counted, as contrasted with only 9.6 per cent of controls, a highly significant difference. Holguin and Fenichel (1967) also commented on the frequency of motion sickness in migrainic children and found 23 per cent in their series of 55 patients. Congdon and Forsythe (1979) found an over-all incidence of 38 per cent in their 300 migrainic children of whom 34.7 per cent were in the classic migraine group and 40 per cent were in the group with common migraine.

A most convincing and useful report on the association of motion sickness with juvenile migraine is that of Barabas *et al.* (1983*b*). These authors directed their attention specifically to this issue in a series of 60 migraine patients between five and 19 years, 45 per cent of whom had three or more episodes of motion sickness. This was contrasted with a group of 162 control patients made up of approximately equal numbers of patients with seizure disorder, non-migraine headaches, and learning disability where the incidence was 6.6 per cent, 7.1 per cent and 5.0 per cent respectively. The authors suggest that motion sickness is found with sufficient frequency that it can be regarded as a 'minor diagnostic criteria for migraine' (Barabas *et al.* 1983*b*). In a similar study of five- to 18-year-old patients, Lanzi *et al.* (1983) found 61 per cent of 100 migrainics had motion sickness, as compared with 13 per cent in 100 with seizure disorder and a 17 per cent incidence in 100 control patients.

My own series of patients contributes nothing to the issue of motion sickness and migraine. Systematic and regular inquiry was not made and my notes are incomplete on this issue. It is my impression that the figures presented by Congdon and Forsythe (1979), Barabas *et al.* (1983*b*) and the data presented by Bille (1962) dealing with more severe degrees of motion sickness are close to the mark. Positive responses will be elicited in about 40 per cent of juvenile migraine patients if direct inquiry is made, and the point has value as an ancillary support for the diagnosis.

Somnambulism
Bille (1962) reported a 46.6 per cent incidence of sleep disturbances in the personally interviewed group of 73 patients *vs.* a control incidence of 16.4 per cent. These statistics included night terrors, somnambulism, head-banging and uneasy sleep. Somnambulism occurred in three migrainic children and one control. Barabas *et al* (1983*a*) reported an incidence of 30 per cent in their 60 patients with migraine, as compared with an incidence of 4.8 to 6.6 per cent in a control series that consisted of comparable numbers in each group of patients with non-migraine headaches, seizure disorders and learning disabilities. They thought that there was sufficient frequency to warrant inclusion of somnambulism as a 'minor diagnostic criterion'.

Orthostatic circulatory insufficiency
As Bille (1962) has pointed out, based on his personally interviewed patients, 28.8 per cent of these children experienced orthostatic circulatory insufficiency (syncope) symptoms as compared with 8.2 per cent of the control group. Only about a third of the affected patients actually had syncope in this context.

Raskin and Knittle (1976) have investigated the issue of orthostatic symptoms in adults. While 8 per cent of controls had symptoms, usually brief light-headedness or vertigo with rapid shifts of posture, 68 per cent of the migrainics interviewed had

19

these symptoms. Three-quarters of the migrainics also reported scintillating scotomata as an associated symptom during the orthostatically provoked episode. In some migrainics, headache was also provoked by the maneuver, and in one of the 108 migrainic patients syncope had occurred. The issue of syncope and migraine will be discussed further in Chapter 7.

Orthostatic symptomatology is frequent in adolescent patients, especially boys during the growth spurt. The point of a significant difference between migrainics as compared with others is of interest in rounding out the concept of a basic vasomotor instability in these patients.

Miscellaneous symptoms

The migraine patient usually has the coldest feet in the family, often with a tendency to cold sweaty hands as well. This is more apparent in adult practice when one can use the non-migrainic marital partner as a control. It is less obvious in children, although the observation of violaceous mottling of distal extremities is reasonably common. The frequency of relatively striking dermatographism is also noteworthy although this point has not been put to the test of a standard stimulus and comparison with controls.

Geschwind and Behan (1982) have called attention to the disproportionate number of strongly left-handed people with migraine. Exactly how this observation fits into the consideration of the substrate of migraine is difficult to assess at this point. It may relate to the greater frequency of dyslexia among the left-handed and the greater expression of migraine among dyslexic boys. No data are available on handedness in juvenile migraine.

Allergy

Although still subject to argument, there is no convincing evidence that migraine is an allergic disorder. It is therefore inappropriate to include inherited allergic diathesis as part of the 'substrate' of migraine. Yet the issue comes up with sufficient frequency that it requires some attention. Allergic disorders such as asthma, hay fever and urticaria are very common in childhood, and overlap with migraine is hardly surprising. It is not appropriate or rewarding to undertake an extensive discussion of the issue in this monograph. It is sufficient to cite Bille (1962) for a brief review and critique of the literature, as well as to indicate the results of his investigation on the subject. A positive family history of allergy was found in 31. 5 per cent of the migraine group and 21.9 per cent of controls, and an individual history of allergic disorders in 24.7 per cent of children with migraine and in 12.1 per cent of controls. But the sample was small, and neither figure is statistically significant.

There is one significant point that should be made with regard to the relatively common allergy-migraine overlap. The frequency of asthma in the migrainic makes the presence of this disorder an important point to establish in the history of an individual patient. Asthma is a relative contra-indication to the use of propranolol in the prophylactic treatment of migraine because of its established ability to worsen this disorder in many patients.

The pathophysiology of migraine
There are a number of reasons why it is not appropriate to embark on an extensive discussion of the pathogenesis of migraine. The foremost of these is the lack of relevance in what is principally a clinical monograph. Many of the basic concepts remain controversial due to inconsistencies in results, problems with method-ologies, and differences in interpretation. There is little that is definitive, and many questions are wide open. But it is worth stating some of the problems, and setting down information that is fairly well established as a basis for a better concept of the clinical problem. Although vascular phenomena remain a central feature of migraine, there has been a shift of interest to what may be more fundamental issues, such as the rôle of serotonin and other vaso-active amines, and consideration of the rôle of platelets as will be discussed later in the chapter.

The discussion that follows will be centered on three issues:
(1) The inherited basic defect
(2) The pathophysiology of the paroxysm
(3) The pathophysiology of complex neurological symptoms and signs in 'compli-cated migraine', and in migraine associated with stroke.

The inherited basic defect
The evidence for the genetic basis of migraine would seem to be overwhelming, and is generally accepted. There is really no information that would indicate what the nature of that basic defect may be, or whether the poorly regulated excitatory-inhibitory system resides in the nervous system, vascular system, or whether it involves a humoral factor or blood platelets. It could be a metabolic disorder that has the potential for expression in many systems including all of the above and perhaps other tissues as well. For want of a more precise definition, the convenient term 'neurovasomotor instability' can be tentatively used to refer to the basic pathophysiologic state. As we have seen, patients with the disorder have other paroxysmal symptoms as well as vascular headache, and many of these symptoms can be attributed to a vascular pathophysiology. Many patients have more subtle continuing indications that they are a bit different as discussed in the section on the 'substrate' of migraine.

There are a number of confounding problems in the search for a basic defect. There may be more than one genotype, with a similar phenotypic expression. A good example in which this is likely to be the case is cluster headache (migrainous neuralgia). It has a characteristic clinical expression, different genetic implications, age of onset and sexual predilection. It is quite possible that the phenotypic expression of the more standard migraine syndromes is based on more than one fundamental type of 'neurovasomotor instability'.

Also, as mentioned earlier in the chapter, we may be dealing with a threshold of responsiveness, and the underlying mechanism of the clinically important reaction is no more than an inherited difference that places an individual at one pole of the curve of biologic variation. Continually adjusted and fine-tuned vasoreactivity is a characteristic of mammalian physiology. With sufficient stimulus, it is possible to provoke symptoms such as vascular headache in anyone.

Pathogenesis of the paroxysm

More is known about the pathophysiology of the individual migraine episode, although we are still far from a reasonable understanding of the problem.

The headache

The best understood aspect of migraine is probably the headache itself. Pulsating and presumably dilated extracranial arteries account for this predominant complaint of most migraine patients. The intensity of headache correlates with the pulsation amplitude of extracranial arteries (Graham and Wolff 1938). The intracranial arteries also contribute, and are the sole source of the pain in a significant number of patients (Drummond and Lance 1983). As the headache continues, the fronto-temporal region sometimes becomes tender to palpitation and the overlying skin may become sensitive. Occasionally arteries can be seen to pulsate. Compression may lead to transient relief, and occasionally patients can abort the headache by firm massage of the temples during the aura.

At the same time, vasoconstriction or shunting occurs in the subcutaneous arterioles to account for the frequently observable facial pallor. This change has been documented by measurement of decreased skin temperature by thermography (Lance and Anthony 1971).

Cerebral blood-flow studies during the headache indicate great variability among patients and are probably irrelevant to the headache itself. It is unchanged in common migraine, and the oligemia of the aura frequently persists into the headache phase in classic migraine. When hyperperfusion then supervenes in classic migraine it frequently persists for many hours after the headache has subsided. Hyperperfusion usually occurs during cluster headache (migrainous neuralgia) and returns to normal at the end of the paroxysm (Edmeads 1979).

Vasodilatation does not fully explain the throbbing pain inasmuch as vasodilatation brought about by other methods is not necessarily painful. This led Chapman and his colleagues to examine tissue fluid in the region of painful vessels. This fluid was found to be capable of lowering the pain threshold when injected elsewhere in the body. The substance or substances responsible for the painful sterile inflammation have never been fully characterized beyond presumptive identification as a polypeptide (Chapman *et al.* 1960).

Recently substance P, a vasodilating polypeptide, has been proposed as a highly interesting candidate for the hypothetical substance that is released by nerve endings in migraine. Its presence has been documented in the trigeminal vasa nervorum of experimental animals, and its physiological properties are consistent with the observed painful vascular phenomena of the headache phase of migraine (Moskowitz *et al.* 1979, Moskowitz 1984).

The aura

The visual and other complex symptoms of the minutes that precede the headache are a less common aspect of the paroxysm in the majority of patients, and in those patients who have 'common migraine' they do not occur at all. The pathophysiology of the aura is more complex and less well understood. The symptoms

22

have been attributed to retinal or cerebral ischemia secondary to either vasospasm or arteriolar shunting (Walsh and Hoyt 1969).

It is postulated that the vascular reactions of the aura may occur as the first phase in common migraine as well, but in common migraine vasospasm or arteriovenous shunting occurs extracranially and is therefore asymptomatic (Edmeads 1979).

Demonstration of spasm of large arteries documented by sequential arteriograms is the subject of a case report by Dukes and Vieth (1964). It is perhaps the only fully documented instance of arteriography before, during and after the aura. Normal cerebral vasculature was visualized before and after, the latter at the time of a typical headache. During the aura there was almost no visualization of intracranial carotid, although the posterior cerebral artery did fill. The patient had classic visual symptoms at this point, and therefore the spasm was inconsistent with the principal area of abnormality. With few exceptions, arteriography even during an attack of complicated migraine is normal.

Most human studies of regional cerebral blood-flow show reduced flow during the aura. However, in some studies, it does not correlate well with the neurologic phenomena in CNS localization or in timing, and may persist beyond the aura into the headache phase (Edmeads 1979).

It is likely that although spasm of larger vessels may occur it is not an adequate explanation of the pathophysiology of the aura, nor is simple oligemia on the basis of arteriolar spasm or shunting a totally satisfactory answer. There are too many inconsistencies, both clinical and in the results from blood-flow studies. An indication of the inconsistencies with regard to blood-flow has been described above, and the smooth clinical evolution of the aura from visual centers (posterior cerebral artery territory) anteriorly into somatosensory and motor centers (middle cerebral artery territory) is so often observed that a different conceptualization is probably required.

Leão's spreading depression
Since Milner's (1958) brief note that called attention to the similarity between the rate of progression of the scotomata of the aura of migraine and the rate of progression of the 'spreading depression of Leão' (1944a), migraine theorists have been fascinated by the possible relationship between these phenomena. Leão (1944a) described a decrease in electrical activity that occurred in rabbit brain shortly after weak faradic or mechanical stimulation. The depression of electrical activity then slowly spread in all directions and in three to six minutes it had encompassed the entire hemisphere. Recovery in a given area required five to 10 minutes, while the front of depression could still be advancing in other areas of cortex.

In a paper that appears in the same issue of the journal, Leão (1944b) described a wave of visible vasodilatation that accompanied the front of electrophysiologic depression. Olesen *et al.* (1982) in regional blood-flow studies in the human found that brief focal or perifocal hyperemia concomitant with the aura was characteristic of some patients with classic migraine. The hyperemia was rapidly followed by more persistent oligemia. Lauritzen *et al.* (1982) have shown that a persistent oligemia lasting as long as an hour follows in the wake of the front of spreading depression in the rat. In a subsequent paper dealing with regional cerebral blood-flow studies in human migraine, Lauritzen *et al.* (1983*b*) found that the time course of the oligemic phase did not correlate with the spread of the aura, and persisted well beyond the clinical manifestations. The authors concluded that the focal symptoms of the aura were not secondary to oligemia. Rather they propose that it is a spreading inhibitory phenomena akin to Leão's spreading depression that is accountable for the aura and that a metabolic event in the cortex is more likely to be the initial reaction in migraine.

If the spreading depression hypothesis is correct, one is still left with the question of what the basic event may be that triggers the reaction that then leads to an advancing front of electrophysiologic inhibition and its secondary blood-flow changes. Leão produced spreading depression by mechanical and electrical stimulation, and a brief application of a 1M.KCl is also effective. The initial event in the clinical problem could be the action of a local, locally elaborated or blood-bourne humoral factor. It is also possible that a brief episode of vasospasm or a platelet thrombus too transient to be detectable in regional blood-flow studies is the inciting stimulus. In the final analysis, the triggering stimulus is a total mystery.

Systemic humoral factors
The possibility of a systemically elaborated vaso-active humoral factor as a central feature of migraine has been a subject that has excited considerable interest. This concept was perhaps stimulated by the belief that histamine was implicated in the pathogenesis of cluster headaches, and that histamine 'desensitization was an effective treatment' (Horton 1941). Although the histamine treatment program did not endure, there is evidence that whole blood histamine increases during cluster headache, and some abnormality of histamine release remains a viable theory in this variety of vascular headache (Anthony and Lance 1971).

Exogenous factors
The observation that certain physiologically active amines contained in foods are capable of precipitating headache has supported the humoral hypothesis. Only susceptible patients respond with headache, and they are not necessarily those with other evidence of symptomatic migraine. The Chinese restaurant syndrome of monosodium glutamate-induced headache is well documented (Schaumburg *et al.* 1969). The 'hot dog headache' due to nitrates in frankfurters and other processed meats represents a similar problem for susceptible people (Henderson and Raskin 1972). Alcohol as a trigger in cluster headache has been frequently observed and is generally recognized. Alcohol may also act as a trigger in migraine but with lesser regularity. The incidence of alcoholic hangover headache, a headache that has vascular characteristics, must be almost universal if sufficient stimulus is provided.

The rôle of tyramine is controversial. It has been tentatively identified as the provocative amine contained in chocolate, cheeses, sour cream, chopped liver, herring, *etc.* However, reports of the effect of administering tyramine itself are about equally divided. Some migrainics seem to be tyramine sensitive, others are not (Kohlenberg 1982). Phenylethylamine has also been implicated as the offender in chocolate. It is apparent that substances in certain foods can occasionally precipitate headache in migrainics, and some substances such as nitrate and glutamate can also have an effect in non-migrainic individuals who apparently have special susceptibility.

Endogenous factors
Serotonin has been the most intensively studied and best substantiated humoral factor in migraine. The serotonin story in migraine dates to the observation that urinary excretion of its end metabolite 5H/AA (5 hydroxy indol acetic acid) is increased during migraine episodes (Kangasniemi *et al.* 1972). Moreover, serotonin measurements in plasma, whole blood and platelets reveal a statistically significant modest decrease during the attack in most patients (Curran *et al.* 1965, Anthony and Lance 1971, Rydzewski 1976, Mück-Seler *et al.* 1979). There may be a transient increase in plasma serotonin at the beginning of the headache (Dalessio 1976).

These observations have drawn attention to platelets, which contain 98 per cent of blood serotonin. Platelet serotonin may be released upon appropriate stimulus. There is evidence that a 'platelet releasing factor' is present in the plasma of migrainic patients during the episode (Mück-Seler *et al.* 1979), and the search for this releasing factor takes us into the murky area of the prostaglandins, free fatty acids as a stimulus to prostaglandin synthesis, *etc.* (Anthony 1976). The platelet will be considered again when we deal with the pathogenesis of complicated migraine; only at that point the issue will relate to hyperaggregability.

These observations may represent the beginning of a cellular and biochemical description of the basic phenomenology of the migraine attack. The serotonin changes, although they cannot be demonstrated in all migrainics, are convincing and may be at the core of the problem in the majority of patients. These changes could also be an epiphenomenon that happens to parallel the main event, and at best is secondary to the more basic question of what initiates the release reaction. Serotonin has definite vasomotor effects, and is attractive for this reason (Hardebo *et al.* 1978). It is also present in brain and other tissues. In those patients who do not show changes in serotonin, a search for other vaso-active substances may be in order.

The interest in platelets is an important development, and platelets probably play a rôle in some aspects of the migraine problem. However, the selective focal vascular and neurologic clinical phenomena must also be considered. It is possible that some of the biochemical events characterized in platelets are also occurring in other tissue, especially in cells of selected vessel walls and perhaps in the brain itself. The mast cells of cerebral blood-vessels with their packets of serotonin, leukotrienes, histamine and substance P is an interesting candidate for this rôle (Theoharides 1983).

The commonly associated gastro-intestinal symptoms of the migraine attack, which in children may so predominate the clinical presentation as to warrant the terms 'cyclic vomiting', or when painful 'abdominal migraine', have not been

25

studied. It is not known whether these symptoms relate to local gastro-intestinal involvement or reflect CNS mechanisms. Either or both possibilities may be correct, although it is perhaps more likely that the biochemical mediators of migraine are operative locally.

The pathophysiology of complicated migraine
The designation 'complicated migraine' is used by most authors to refer to focal neurological signs that persist as much as 24 hours *beyond* the headache phase (Dalessio 1980). Others include signs that occur during the headache and then subside *coincident* with the resolution of the headache and associated symptoms of the paroxysm (Saper 1983).

Pathogenesis
The pathogenesis of the process probably represents a continuum, the important feature of which is the presence of neurological signs that do not subside with the aura. At the end of the spectrum are those patients with 'complicated migraine' whose focal neurologic defect persists for several days or longer, and infarction of tissue can be proved or surmised. When this occurs, the designation of migraine with stroke is more appropriate.

It is a well-known observation that the extracranial vessels involved in the migraine paroxysm not only visibly pulsate in some individuals, but may occasionally thicken slightly and become tender as the headache proceeds. Sensitivity and thickening may persist beyond the headache for a number of hours. Wolff in particular has pointed out that edema may develop in the tissue adjacent to the affected vessels as well as in the arterial wall, and even local ecchymosis has been observed on rare occasions (Wolff 1955). It has been suggested that it is the pressure of pulsating thickened edematous arteries of the circle of Willis on the adjacent oculomotor nerve that accounts for ophthalmoplegic migraine. A similar pathogenesis may account for the sympathoparesis that develops in patients with cluster headache, only in this case the internal carotid artery is the site of abnormality.

There is some arteriographic support for the concept of edematous pulsating arteries exerting local pressure palsy in ophthalmoplegic migraine, although the evidence is indirect and based upon arteriographic observation of arterial narrowing in some patients during the event with the presumption that the observed constriction was due to swelling of the wall rather than vasospasm (Walsh and O'Doherty 1960, Bickerstaff 1964a). Most arteriographic studies of ophthalmoplegic patients have shown no detectable abnormality. However, the proposal remains an attractive hypothesis to account for oculomotor or symphoparesis in the course of migraine. Swelling of the arterial wall need not lead to narrowing of the lumen, and the traumatic effect of pulsation cannot be measured in the artierogram.

Parenchymal symptoms that develop in the course of headaches, whether in carotid or vertebral-basilar territories, are more complex. A point to be made at the outset is that evidence of focal parenchymal dysfunction as reflected in the EEG,

CT scan, or based upon blood-flow studies may not be concordant with expected cerebral localization as predicted from the symptoms. Changes in these laboratory parameters are frequently multifocal or diffuse. The process is more widespread in brain than the overt symptoms.

Persistent signs of the paroxysm

The more persistent signs of the paroxysm itself, as opposed to the aura, could be due to neurologically active materials that enter from blood due to abnormally permeable vessels or substances that are elaborated locally, perhaps in the vessel walls themselves. It is the local effect of these materials on neuronal function that is more likely to be accountable than increased tissue water *per se*. Edema must be relatively massive to account for symptoms by itself, and edema to this degree must be exceptional in migraine. The CT demonstration of unexpected regions of lucency even in migraine patients without focal symptoms is supportive of the position that areas of abnormal permeability may develop in the course of severe migraine attacks (Mathew *et al.* 1977).

A frequently proposed possibility is that transient ischemia is the cause of focal cerebral symptoms. This could be secondary to prolonged shunting or vasospasm of small arterioles, or to platelet emboli or thrombin that are too small or fragile to cause permanent infarction under most circumstances (see discussion below). Also, Blau and Davis (1970) have recorded their observation of intravascular erythrocyte aggregation as observed in conjunctival blood vessels during migraine paroxysm in 35 of 35 patients. Although this issue has attracted much less attention than the issue of platelet aggregation, it is of interest and possible relevance to the subject of complicated migraine.

Alternatively, arterial walls may become edematous and temporarily insufficient. As mentioned above there is arteriographic evidence of segmental narrowing in a few cases, and edematous vessel walls may be a preferable explanation to persistent vasospasm. It is recognized that areas of low blood-flow, whatever the basis, may persist into the headache phase. But there is still much to be learned about the pathogenesis of neurologically complicated migraine.

Hyperaggregability

It is appropriate to return to a consideration of the blood platelet in a discussion of complicated migraine, and in particular to deal with another aspect of platelet abnormality than its serotonin content and release, *i.e.* the issue of hyperaggregability. This was first demonstrated by Hilton and Cumings (1972) and subsequently studied by others (Kalendovsky and Austin 1975, Couch and Hassanein 1977, Deshmukh and Meyer 1977, Jones R. J. *et al.* 1982). The change is not found in all migrainics, is more marked during a paroxysm, and it can also be demonstrated during headache-free intervals. There may be some correlation of this phenomenon with complicated migraine (Kalendovsky and Austin 1975) particularly in young patients who have both migraine and stroke. The paper by Kalendovsky *et al.* (1975) is of particular interest because three of the four patients who had platelet abnormality had had classic migraine, and one of these patients

27

developed an infarct in the context of a typical headache. The phenomenon is probably not part of the central pathophysiology of the headache itself, as would seem to be the case with serotonin release, but could be of importance in complicated migraine and the occasional occurrence of stroke in young migrainics. Parenthetically, serotonin has been shown to induce platelet aggregation. A number of other substances will also induce the reaction such as adenosine diphosphate from disrupted tissue, epinephrine and thrombin.

Migraine and stroke
Thrombotic or embolic stroke in children is not particularly common. Among the patients with stroke, one encounters occasional children who also have juvenile migraine. In some patients the infarct develops in the context of a migraine headache while in others this is not the case. However, there are a number of convincing reports in which migraine is clearly implicated in thrombotic or embolic stroke (see Chapter 7). The rôle of platelet hyperaggregability (see discussion above) as a factor in the pathogenesis of stroke in migraine is uncertain. However, the possibility that platelet thrombin or emboli may be the fundamental lesion in stroke associated with migraine is an attractive hypothesis. Alternatively infarction resulting from prolonged vasospasm or luminal restriction resulting from edema of the vessel wall has been implicated, but proof for this hypothesis is also lacking. Perhaps both combine to provide the critical convergence of factors that lead to this rare complication.

Some patients have an additional anatomical lesion that is also associated with stroke such as prolapsed mitral valve (Litman and Friedman 1978, Barnett *et al.* 1980, Rice *et al.* 1980, Jones H. R. *et al.* 1982). Case 17 is illustrative of this association (see Chapter 7), and the report of Conomy *et al.* (1982) also addresses this issue. Mitral valve prolapse is a frequent abnormality, especially in the female where 6 per cent have the lesion (Procacci *et al.* 1976). The likelihood of chance overlap with migraine is appreciable, but the risk of stroke in patients who have both migraine and prolapsed mitral valve may be greater than a chance association (Litman and Friedman 1978, Conomy *et al.* 1982). The same potential for enhanced jeopardy may apply to other anatomical lesions of the heart and great vessels as in case 35 (see Chapter 7) who had Marfan's Syndrome and a redundant aorta.

Mettinger and Ericson (1982) found that of their 37 patients with fibro-muscular dysplasia, 12 had had recurrent unilateral vascular headaches before infarction and six had had migraine since childhood. One could interpret this association as an indication that either periodic vascular headache is a frequent symptomatic expression of fibromuscular dysplasia, or that migraine plus fibro-muscular dysplasia increases the risk of stroke. Another possibility is that medications frequently used by migrainic patients play a rôle in the causation of fibromuscular dysplasia.

Finally, if migrainics are at increased risk of stroke if they also have prolapsed mitral valve and other anatomical vascular risk factors, what is the relationship to other risk factors of thrombotic or embolic stroke in childhood such as sickle cell disease, antithrombin III deficiency, trauma and all of the other disorders that have been associated with stroke in childhood? Epidemiologic studies are clearly needed to resolve these questions.

With available medication such as aspirin and persantin which act to prevent platelet aggregation, the therapeutic implications of the association of migraine, stroke and anatomical lesions of the heart or arteries as well as other risk factors of stroke in children become apparent.

3
PRECIPITATING FACTORS OF THE MIGRAINE ATTACK

Introduction

Any paroxysmal process is characterized by prolonged periods of latency which represent the steady state of a susceptible patient's lifetime. This applies to all etiologic varieties of paroxysmal disorder including epilepsy, many metabolic events, cardiac arrhythmias and transient ischemic attacks as well as migraine. In all of them, the ictus must be triggered by a convergence of factors at a point in time. In most instances the crucial event or events are unknown, but in migraine a sizeable list of relatively specific factors can be compiled (Table VI).

In a few patients the expression of migraine only occurs with a relatively specific precipitating factor. More commonly, most migrainic episodes are apparently spontaneous, and only occasionally may the identified trigger be responsible for an attack. In either circumstance, recognition of these factors is of value in that preventive measures and avoidance can sometimes be employed.

Psychologic factors

There is essentially no argument with the fact that psychologic stresses and strains are the commonest factor relating to the frequency and severity of vascular headache at any age.

At times a stressful incident or series of incidents may be directly correlated with a vascular headache. This association may easily be made by the patient or family, and the basically correct conclusion is reached that the headache relates to nervous tension even if the headache itself has throbbing quality associated with nausea, pallor and photophobia. Such headaches are often discounted by the parent, and may be accepted and managed without medical help. This may be unfortunate for the child whose headache may be regarded as psychogenic and appropriate symptomatic treatment is not prescribed.

Leviton et al. (1984) have examined the issue of psychologic precipitating factors by means of a computerized interview program in 69 school-age children and young adults to age 22 years. The subjects were asked to relate their headaches to various events on either the day of the headache or the immediately preceding day. It was found that 33 per cent of 11 and 12 year olds were able to relate their headache to an especially hard day (whether at school, work or at home) while this was identified in 65 per cent of the 17 to 21 year age group. Similar incidence could be related to such factors an an 'unpleasant emotional situation', and 'unexpected excitement or pressure'. Younger children were less able to correlate their headaches with such incidents, especially those under age 10 years.

Similar findings have been reported by others such as Bille (1962) who found that 31 per cent of his personally interviewed patients were able to identify

TABLE VI

Precipitating Factors Identified in 300 Personal Juvenile Migraine Patients*

Factor	Frequency
Psychologic factors	Common—incidence not recorded
Food factors	Low—incidence not recorded
Lactose intolerance	3
URI and sinusitis	13
Hypoglycemia	2
Physical exertion	7
Trauma	32

*No data on other factors such as sleep deprivation, excess of sleep, sunglare, heat and other climate factors, motion, *etc.* as a trigger.

schoolwork, especially examinations, as a factor in their headaches. Others, such as Vahlquist (1955) and Maratos and Wilkinson (1982), found that over 80 per cent were precipitated by emotional upset.

Continuing anxiety or depression (Ling *et al.* 1970) has a lower profile, but nevertheless serves to aggravate the frequency and severity of headache. At times this is recognized by the patient, parents, or physician, and it is incorrectly concluded that the problem relates to psychogenic factors alone. The variety of situational factors that may be important range widely, but prominently include issues such as stress at home due to parental marital difficulties as well as difficulties in school. This aspect of the subject is more extensively discussed in Chapter 9.

The Leviton *et al.* (1984) study also provides insight into the issue of the frequency of an adverse emotional substrate to headache incidence as perceived by the patient. Young children again had less insight or were less affected by such factors as 'worrying a lot', 'tension' or 'feeling sad'. The perceived relationship was uncommon in children under 13 years, but was acknowledged by 25 per cent of those older than 16 years. The stressful circumstances may be exceptional and susceptible to remedy, and these manipulations may be sufficient to relieve the problem. More frequently the level of stress is well tolerated by others, but the child with juvenile migraine becomes symptomatic. This results in even more anxiety or depression, and a vicious circle is established.

These observations relate directly to the close relationship of migraine frequency and severity to the school year. It is unusual for a migraine patient to present during the summer holiday months of July and August. The first patients begin to present in September, often old friends returning. By October and November, juvenile migraine, both new and returning patients, has become a significant part of my work and this continues until June. Most of these children are doing well in school, some undertake a disproportionate amount of extra-curricular activity, and many seem unusually conscientious about their work. However they are paying a price in headache which their equally busy schoolmates do not pay.

A significant group, usually boys, are faced with the burden of some variety and degree of learning disability. Whether this is disproportionate to the frequency in the general population is not known. A systematic study has not been done, but the general impression that learning disability is more common in boys with manifest migraine than expected by coincidence is held by many including myself. Specific inquiry on this issue may reveal a source of difficulty which may have been previously overlooked. When present as a tension-producing factor, proper attention to the learning disability is necessary as a most important contributor in the manifestation of migraine.

In most respects the issue of psychologic factors in juvenile migraine is not significantly different from the issues relating to psychogenic headache and will be considered further in that context.

Food factors
In some individuals the intake of specific foods has a clear association with headache. In children the most common offender is chocolate. Other foods include certain cheeses (often macaroni and cheese), nuts and Chinese restaurant food (where the offending substance is glutamate, used to enhance flavor). Red wine has also been identified as a precipitating factor of migraine, but is not a serious consideration in childhood.

These observations have given rise to a commonly held belief that migraine is an allergic disorder. More likely there is a direct biochemical reaction between vaso-active amines or peptides in the food and the receptors which initiate the migrainic reaction. In addition to glutamate in Chinese food, tyramine and other vaso-active amines have been implicated. Other food factors have been identified such as nitrate used as a food preservative ('hot dog headache' in the USA) and the caffeine in coca cola (universal distribution). There are certainly more offenders to be identified in the future.

If one mentions the possibility of food-precipitated headache, the association will sometimes be made by the parents or child. Frequently it is presented as part of the initial history. I have not found it rewarding to embark on an extensive search of food factors more than to mention the common offenders. If a substance such as chocolate is identified, avoidance is useful, but this usually accounts for a minor fraction of the total number of headaches. In fact, systematic studies indicate the relative unimportance of the ingestion of chocolate in 25 migrainic adults (Moffet *et al.* 1974) which revealed that only two responded consistently to chocolate. In another study Medina and Diamond (1978) found only occasional headaches were 'time-locked' to specific food, and the impression was gained that dietary factors do not 'increase the frequency of headaches but may precipitate them earlier. In general, diet appears to be relatively unimportant in migraine'.

There are several other studies that deal with children and reflect the continuing controversy over food factors in migraine. The computerized interview program of Leviton *et al.* (1975) found that chocolate was the only food or beverage identified as a headache antecedent in 69 young people. Chocolate was identified in 18 per cent of children under 12 years and in 10 per cent of adolescents. Food factors were identified in 24 per cent in Bille's (1962) report and the same percentage was identified by Maratos and Wilkinson (1982), while Vahlquist reported food as a trigger in only 1.6 per cent of 186 patients.

On the other hand Egger *et al.* (1983) have recently reported the spectacular recovery of 93 per cent of 88 migrainic children in a double blind study using an 'oligoantigenic' diet. After the baseline restricted diet was established over a period of three to four weeks, other foods were gradually added. It will be of great interest to learn of the results of a similar effort by other investigators. It is my own guess that the dietary approach to the treatment of juvenile migraine may prove to be useful for a hard core of patients in whom simpler measures, such as the benign group of pharmacotherapeutic agents or behavioral therapies fail. Perhaps it will become possible to identify patients who are good candidates for this therapeutic approach on the basis of the clinical history.

The management of the dietary approach can only be difficult. It requires the dedicated and somewhat compulsive collaboration of child, mother and nutritional therapist. This is evidenced by the 10 per cent dropout rate in this well-organized study (Egger *et al.* 1983). The children usually reacted to multiple foods, which compounds the problem of long-term management.

Although the 93 per cent rate of cure is very impressive, it is appropriate to question whether the patients studied represent a cross-section of juvenile migraine as it usually presents to the generalist or consultant. In many respects they do not. The patients had had headache at least once per week for six months (about time for a natural remission particularly if the end of the school year is near). Although the number who were taking drugs was not given, presumably at least those patients whose medication was continued represent drug failures, already a relatively small (10 to 20 per cent) residual of juvenile migraine. Of other features, 7 per cent had residual neurologic signs secondary to migraine (complicated migraine), 14 per cent had 'fits' (perhaps seizures or syncope) and almost 50 per cent had principally hyperkinetic behavior disturbance as well as migraine. 54 per cent had a history of allergic disorder and 70 per cent had abdominal pain, diarrhea and flatulence. All of these clinical features are distinctly higher in this sample than in the usual cross-section of children with migraine headaches.

It is of interest that over 50 foods were implicated, and that multiple foods were responsible in many patients. Chocolate was identified in 22 patients and other frequently identified foods were eggs (24 patients), orange (21 patients), wheat (21 patients), cheese (13 patients) and tomato (13 patients). The most frequently identified food was cow's milk in 27 patients (30 per cent). This observation, in conjunction with the frequency of the symptoms of abdominal pain, diarrhea and flatulence in these patients, is of special interest in view of the next section in which lactose intolerance as a trigger of migraine is discussed.

Lactose intolerance
Juvenile migraine is occasionally aggravated by the intake of usual or somewhat excessive quantities of milk, *i.e.* the 'milk migraine' of the experienced pediatrician (Berenberg 1983). The association became particularly interesting to me in conjunction with several of my patients who were found to have demonstrable lactose intolerance and whose migrainic symptoms were significantly alleviated by

restriction of the intake of milk and milk products.

Initial interest in the possibility came about as a result of concern about the differentiation of abdominal migraine from other causes of abdominal pain. It was in this context that the relatively recent literature on lactose intolerance was reviewed. The clinical description of a number of these patients conformed reasonably well to that of abdominal migraine. Many of these patients did not have diarrhea, a relatively uncommon manifestation of the usual juvenile migraine syndromes (Bayless and Huang 1971).

Information accumulated in the decade of the seventies which indicated that intestinal lactase declined with age, beginning in the pre-school period. This leads to decreasing inability of the intestine to metabolize the disaccharide lactose. Bacterial action on the unabsorbed lactose produce gases, short-chain organic acids and perhaps other products. These substances may cause localized abdominal pain, distention, flatus and diarrhea due to local intestinal effect. It seemed reasonable that certain of these bacterial products when absorbed could act as triggers of vasomotor reaction, especially in susceptible individuals. The availability of the 'lactose-breath-hydrogen test' (Perman et al. 1978) and the knowledge of a high incidence of abnormality (40 per cent) in a prospective study of patients with abdominal pain syndrome (Barr et al. 1979), resulted in testing and the indentification of four patients where lactose intolerance seemed to play an important rôle in the expression of their migraine. Moreover, restriction of the intake of milk and milk products resulted in significant alleviation of symptoms, although adjunctive treatment with migraine pharmacotherapy was also useful and sometimes necessary in these patients.

The migraine patients who were selected for lactose tolerance testing were identified on the basis of clinical symptoms of abdominal pain, flatus and abdominal distention either as part of the paroxysms of headache or occurring independently. There was an admixture of vasomotor symptoms with abdominal complaints in these patients and it is not at all clear which symptoms were attributable to lactose intolerance or to migraine. Further study is clearly necessary.

In the meantime it is appropriate to hypothesize that these patients have an inborn tendency to migrainic reactivity and that symptoms are to a significant extent triggered by absorbed products of bacterial action on the excess intestinal lactose that has resulted from age-related decline in intestinal lactase function.

In addition to the beneficial effect of the restriction or elimination of milk products including cheese and ice-cream in these patients, oral administration of the enzyme can also be useful. Lactase tablets can be administered on a regular basis or milk can be pre-treated with lactase before use.

Lactose intolerance

CASE 1 The patient was age seven and a half when first seen. He had been having headaches for about two years. The headaches consisted of a sensation of 'a hammer pounding' centering about the left eye although sometimes they would occur on the right. This was associated with abdominal pain about

34

50 per cent of the time, and he was occasionally nauseated but had never vomited. In addition he had generalized abdominal pain that occurred independent of the headaches. Episodes of either variety occurred three to four times per week and were of about 30 minutes duration. His other mentioned that he was quite 'gassy' and passed frequent flatus. These symptoms were particularly marked during episodes of headache or abdominal distress. He had had a gastro-intestinal work-up that included an upper GI series, examinations of his blood and stools, and none of these were abnormal.

The family history indicated that both father and paternal grandmother had migraine and an 11-year-old brother was subject to periodic headaches that were throbbing in quality and were probably juvenile migraine.

He had developed normally in all respects, and was doing excellent work in the second grade.

Physical examination revealed no abnormalities.

A lactose breath test was positive at 61 parts per million hydrogen gas, with a normal of less than 10.

A modified lactose-free diet was instituted which resulted in considerable improvement in the severity of his symptomatology and reduction of frequency to one or two brief episodes of headache or abdominal pain per week. Improvement was sufficient that no migrainic pharmacotherapy was necessary.

Comment: This boy, with a strong family history of migraine, had periodic headache and periodic abdominal pain, both of which responded to a lactose restricted diet.

Upper respiratory infection and sinusitis
It is not widely appreciated that a series of vascular headaches may be initiated by acute sinusitis and other upper respiratory infections. Several authors have remarked on this relationship, especially in patients with migrainous neuralgia or 'cluster headache' (Horton 1956, Sjaastad and Dale 1976). This was noteworthy in 13 of the patients in my series where the circumstances were sufficiently obvious to be noted in the diagnostic formulation, although only one had the migrainous neuralgia syndrome. The URI either precipitated the initial series of headaches or seemed to be responsible for exacerbation of a chronic problem. On several occasions documented acute sinusitis was the initial infection. Vascular headaches then developed and accounted for a recurring series of headaches that were clinically different from the initial pain due to the acute sinus infection. The persistence of headache prompted referral with concern centered about 'chronic sinusitis', or some more serious intracranial extension of the original infection (see Chapter 12 for a discussion of the clinical features of headache related to sinus infection).

Vascular headaches of this variety tend to respond to customary anti-migraine pharmacotherapy.

35

'Cluster' of juvenile migraine headaches

CASE 2 This nine-year-old girl had had occasional periodic headaches over one to two years. They were bitemporal in location and had a throbbing quality. During the headaches she had photophobia and looked pale and wan. The headache usually was of less than one hour in duration. With the more severe headaches she would lie down. They were occasionally relieved by acetaminophen.

Two weeks prior to admission she had a febrile illness associated with nausea and diarrhea sufficient to require hospitalization for four days. During this period she had two severe headaches accompanied by persistent vomiting that awakened her in the middle of the night. Subsequent to her recovery in the week and a half prior to visit she was having headaches of about two hours duration that would awaken her every night. They had the usual bitemporal location with throbbing quality, but were more severe and invariably accompanied by repeated vomiting.

A maternal aunt had classic migraine. Her mother had relatively mild periodic headaches. Occasionally she had severe throbbing headaches associated with nausea and vomiting.

On examination there were no general physical or neurological abnormalities. x-ray of the skull including the paranasal sinuses revealed no abnormalities.

She was treated with phenobarbital 30 mg b.i.d. and given one Cafergot tablet at night. With this regimen she had had one headache on telephone report two weeks later. When seen one month later, she had had no subsequent headaches. Medication was discontinued and there has been no follow-up contact.

Comment: A one-and-a-half-week history of frequent and severe nocturnal headaches was triggered by a flu-like illness in this nine-year-old girl who had had occasional mild migraine for the previous two years.

Migrainous neuralgia precipitated by sinusitis

CASE 3 This 11-year-old boy developed pain over the region of the right maxillary sinus and x-rays demonstrated sinusitis four months prior to his visit. The pain was continuous and of sufficient severity to require propoxyphene. It subsided after four to five days with ampicillin therapy. Within approximately one week he developed increasingly frequent paroxysmal episodes of face pain that occurred approximately twice a day, usually in the later afternoon or early evening. The pain was continuous and boring in character and was of 15 to 20 minutes in duration. He was entirely well between paroxysms. During the episodes his face became flushed and there was some swelling. Pain was located in the right mid-face. Repeat x-rays showed no continuing evidence of the sinusitis.

The family history revealed that a 16-year-old brother had occasional throbbing headaches as did his mother and maternal grandmother.

Examination revealed him to be well developed and comfortable at the time of the examination. There was no sinus tenderness. Hearing was good. There was no evidence of cranial nerve dysfunction although there was some mild edema of the right cheek which tended to displace the angle of the mouth downward slightly. (This observation concerned the referring pediatrician with the question of an incipient facial nerve palsy.)

In the day or so prior to his visit he was having distinctly less trouble, so no treatment was initiated. A follow-up call indicated that he had had no subsequent trouble.

Comment: Subsequent to x-ray-proved sinusitis that was successfully treated with antibiotics, this 11-year-old boy developed paroxysmal face pain with local flushing that had the characteristics of migrainous neuralgia. After a three-and-a-half-month course it subsided spontaneously.

Physical exertion (effort headache)

Unusual physical exertion is recognized as a precipitating cause of migraine (Rooke 1968). The headache may be exclusively related to physical activity, or the patient may be subject to juvenile migraine, and exertion is implicated as a triggering factor only on some occasions. The responsible physical activity varies widely, and may be relatively specific for a given patient. The effort is usually sustained, physically stressful, and associated with exhaustion. Examples of reported activities include running (Massey 1982), football, bowling, weight-lifting, dancing and digging (Diamond 1982). Headaches related to sexual intercourse (Lance 1976) are another rather special variety of exertional headache that is inappropriate for further consideration in a monograph on headaches in childhood.

Contributory factors include heat and high humidity, either of which may occasionally trigger incidents. Headaches may also be precipitated by high altitude (Appenzeller 1972) where unaccustomed physical exertion probably plays a significant rôle.

As a factor in juvenile headaches, the chief incidence is among boys, usually in relation to competitive sports and endurance contests. In a few instances the duration of activity required to produce a headache is relatively predictable, as for example in case 4 reported below. In some patients there is sufficient warning to enable the patient to forestall the headache by discontinuing the activity. Physical exertion was identified as a precipitating factor in children by Vahlquist and Hackzell (1949), and Bille (1962) found that it could be identified as a factor in 24 per cent of his personally interviewed series. In my series it was sufficient to be noteworthy as an occasional or exclusive factor in the headache problem of only seven patients.

The quality of headache in the young is characteristically vascular, with throbbing pain, which occasionally may be unilateral and associated with nausea, *etc.* In my own experience, a disproportionate number of patients have had complex symptomatology (see cases 2, 4 and 6 below). Usually the headache induced by physical exertion is more severe than the customary headache the patient may have.

The duration of headache is from 10 minutes to a number of hours. In contrast with the brief paroxysm of 'cough headache' (see Chapter 11), there does not seem to be a greater incidence of structural abnormality in this group of patients.

The genesis of the pathophysiologic factors that induce vascular headache in relation to physical exertion is not known. It is quite possible that they may vary with the individual patient. Issues such as the outpouring of vaso-active chemicals, or vascular response to altered carbon dioxide have been proposed. Another possible factor could be exercise-induced hypoglycemia, which then precipitates the vasomotor reaction and headache. Exercise to exhaustion has been demonstrated to induce hypoglycemia to levels of less than 45 mg/100 ml in some subjects (Felig *et al.* 1982).

Management of vascular headache triggered by exertion is hardly different from the usual treatment of migraine, with the exception of recommendation to avoid or moderate the precipitating exercise. In some this may be sufficient, but in others continuous pharmacotherapy is required, especially if non-exertional headaches are frequent. Diamond (1982) has pointed out that daily indomethacin in doses of 25 to 100 mg has a special therapeutic advantage in this group of patients.

Hemiplegic migraine related to physical exertion

CASE 4 This 14-year-old boy had three episodes over the previous six months. On each occasion he had been playing basketball longer than usual. The episode began with a feeling of light-headedness, then double vision, followed by a frontal throbbing headache. After the headache had lasted about 30 minutes, his left arm developed a sensation of pins and needles. There was accompanying weakness of the arm such that he could 'barely move it'. He then became somewhat disoriented and shortly thereafter went to sleep. The following day he was normal. A similar episode occurred during the stress of a prolonged basketball practice about three months later. The headache was less severe but had the same quality as before. His entire left arm and leg became numb and were noticeably weak. On this occasion, a skull x-ray was normal. A third episode occurred several months later but the only symptomatology consisted of a severe throbbing headache. He learned that each time he indulged in heavy physical exertion for approximately three hours he would begin to feel a headache at which time he would rest. This was successful in aborting further symptomatology.

Family history was negative with the exception of a maternal aunt who had migraine.

Examination revealed no abnormalities. An EEG showed no abnormality other than unusual responsiveness to overventilation.

The only treatment was to advise him to rest when he felt a headache coming on. This has apparently been successful inasmuch as he has not returned for further consultation.

Comment: This boy developed migraine with hemisensory and hemiparetic episodes only after over three hours of exertion.

Migraine related to physical exertion

This 15-year-old boy had been subject to headaches for one and a half **CASE** years. They began subsequent to an accident after which he had had **5** headaches about three times per week for a period of six months. Although less frequent in summer, they recently occurred about once a week. They often seemed to be precipitated by physical exercise. They were frontal in location and throbbing in quality; he would become noticeably pale and slightly nauseated but would not vomit. Duration varied from one hour to almost the entire day.

On a recent occasion, about one hour after doing an unusual number of sit-ups, he found that he could not see because of blurred vision. He was dysarthric, confused, and could not hold objects in his left hand. This lasted for an hour, followed by a throbbing headache of several hours duration. An EEG and a CT scan were normal.

The family history revealed no individual with migraine or vascular headaches.

Past history indicated that on three occasions, after mild head trauma, he had developed throbbing headaches accompanied by nausea and vomiting over a two- to three-day period.

General physical and neurological examination were entirely normal.

He was returned to the care of his referring physician with the suggestion that he be given either phenytoin or propranolol. No follow-up information is available.

Comment: This patient first developed periodic headaches after trauma, many of which seemed to be related to physical exertion. On one occasion he had an exertion-related complex migrainic episode marked by confusion and hemiparesis.

Migraine related to physical exertion

This 13-year-old boy had had four similar episodes in the previous 18 **CASE** months. All occurred after strenuous exercise, either baseball or basket- **6** ball. Onset of the episode was marked by what was described as 'blurred vision' after which his gums, hand and forearm became numb. His speech became garbled, and he found that he was unco-ordinated when he attempted to write. These symptoms were followed by throbbing headache and irritability that lasted several hours or until he was able to sleep.

Family history revealed that his mother had classic migraine through-out her life. Up to the age of four or five years the boy was subject to motion sickness.

He was believed to have migraine precipitated by physical stress. The episodes were sufficiently infrequent that no treatment was prescribed. No neurodiagnostic studies were recommended because of the alternating laterality of the phenomenology.

Comment: This boy had four complex migrainic episodes in a period of 18 months all related to strenuous exercise.

Hypoglycemia

Hypoglycemia has long been recognized as a trigger of migraine (Critchley and Ferguson 1933). Headache is only occsionally a part of the usual syndrome of symptomatic hypoglycemia which in most people induces diaphoresis, light-headedness, confusion, convulsions or coma. In patients with migraine, vascular headache may supervene at an early stage. It may occur with degrees of hypoglycemia that are otherwise asymptomatic.

Whether low-grade hypoglycemia is responsible for the 25 per cent incidence of young people who relate their migraine to 'skipping a meal' (Leviton *et al.* 1984) is not known. Other factors certainly enter into the equation in many if not most of these patients. The response was commonest in the 13 to 16 year age-group, which will not surprise many whose children have exceeded that age and are therefore familiar with the habits of adolescents. Maratos and Wilkinson (1982) reported that a 'hunger feeling' preceded headache in 35 per cent of their patients, while Bille (1962) recorded 'hunger' as a factor in 18 per cent. Probably the commonest clinical circumstances in which documented hypoglycemia occurs is in diabetics and in individuals with reactive hypoglycemia. Prolonged fasting can also be responsible, but this circumstance is unusual. Children may be more prone to a hypoglycemic trigger than adults (Critchley and Ferguson 1933).

The best clinical clue that hypoglycemia may be a factor is the occurrence of headaches associated with diaphoresis, especially if they occur in mid-morning or mid-afternoon. this may be confirmed by the demonstration of blood sugar below 65 mg per cent or a drop of 75 mg per cent in one hour during a prolonged five-hour glucose tolerance test, especially if a typical headache ensues. A more convenient and less cumbersome approach is a therapeutic trial of sugar or orange juice shortly after the onset of symptoms.

The juvenile diabetic is at special risk for hypoglycemia and if the child has also inherited the migrainic diathesis, expression of even relatively mild hypoglycemia may include migrainic symptomatology. There is no data on the incidence of simultaneous occurrence of the two disorders. Moreover, the distinction between symptoms related to migraine and what may be attributable to hypoglycemia *per se* is difficult to define (see case 7 below).

Treatment with dietary management alone may be sufficient. Aside from the technique of frequent feeding, it is appropriate to emphasize protein as well as to maintain normal caloric intake. With this regimen, studies of patients with vascular headache induced by reactive hypoglycemia indicate that 75 per cent were significantly improved (Dexter *et al.* 1978). This study also indicated the relatively high incidence of reactive hypoglycemia as a contributory factor in migraine generally. See Chapter 8 for a discussion of the relative contra-indication of propanolol in diabetics.

At times complex symptomatology such as hemiparesis (case 7) may be provoked by hypoglycemia (Ravid 1928, Montgomery and Pinner 1964). This raises the question as to whether the focal signs that occasionally develop in the course of hypoglycemia may not in some instances occur in patients with a migrainic diathesis, with focal vasoreaction triggered by hypoglycemia.

Low blood sugar would seem to be the basic metabolic event in the process of hypoglycemia-triggered migraine, but other factors such as adrenergic output induced by the hypoglycemic insult could play a more specific rôle in the pathogenesis of the vascular reaction.

Hemiplegic migraine triggered by hypoglycemia
This child was four and a half when first seen, and was known to have had CASE diabetes mellitus for the previous two years. In general, her diabetes was 7 considered to be under good control with insulin. She came for neurologic consultation because of episodes beginning at age three and a half that occurred every six to eight weeks on the average.

She had had a total of about 10 episodes. They all occurred in the early morning. She usually awakened her parents by crying, was found to be conscious but unable to speak and her comprehension was impaired. In addition, there was overt weakness of the right lower face, arm and leg. The weakness lasted up to an hour and was followed by a severe headache associated with nausea, lethargy and vomiting that was of several hours duration.

On several occasions there was an effort to give her orange juice or other sugar-containing foods, but this was never accomplished during the prodrome of neurologic signs. When given later during the headache she would invariably vomit. In addition she had had several episodes that were considered to be insulin reactions. They tended to occur in late morning when she became irritable and confused but there was no diaphoresis. Administration of sugar would successfully abort this type of episode. Treatment of her diabetes consisted of nine units of NPH and four units of regular insulin given at 9.00 a.m.

The family history revealed that her father had classic migraine. Her mother had had occasional headaches and a maternal grandmother had migraine. Past history was uneventful and her development was normal.

An EEG showed no abnormalities, and her physical examination was entirely normal.

Parents were advised to administer concentrated sugar paste at the very earliest point in the episode, and on the next occasion she awakened at 6.00 a.m., was unable to speak and there was slight weakness of her right arm. She was given sugar and after 10 minutes she was neurologically normal. Although she remained sleepy for an hour there was no subsequent development of headache or vomiting. On two additional occasions she awakened at 4.00 a.m., explained that she was 'dreaming', was given glucose and there was no further development. Subsequently insulin dosage was adjusted, and she has had only rare minor hypoglycemic episodes since that time.

Comment: It is well known that focal neurologic signs including hemiparesis can be the symptomatic expression of hypoglycemia in occasional patients. The pathogenesis of such focal symptomatology is

41

unknown, although in some otherwise asymptomatic patients, compromised circulation (such as from atherosclerosis) can be the presumptive
cause.

This patient raises the possibility of hypoglycemia-triggered migrainic
vasoreaction in certain of these patients. The subsequent vascular
headache with nausea and vomiting, and the strong family history of
migraine, are indications that this may indeed be the case in patient 7.

Hormonal factors
Menstrual migraine
The occurrence of vascular headache coincident with menstrual periods is common
in adult experience. Some women experience all or almost all of their migraine at
this time. In others menstrual-associated migraine is only a part of their headache
experience. All headaches during menses are not migraine, but the menstrual
headache frequently has a vascular component, often without associated
symptomatology such as nausea and vomiting. In others the headache has the
quality of a tension headache or the headache may be even less specific. Menstrual
headache is probably multifactorial in pathogenesis, with hormonal shifts, water
balance and psychologic stress factors playing variable rôles. If the individual has
inherited the migrainic diathesis, then the changes of menstruation presumably
trigger the characteristic neurovasomotor reaction. It may result in classic,
common, and rarely complex migraine. The general subject of menstrual headache
other than migraine will not be further discussed.

The most significant hormonal factor in menstrual migraine would seem to be
estrogen withdrawal (Somerville 1975), although administration of estrogenic
substances in the pre-menstrual phase was not therapeutically useful in preventing
headache. The migraine attack is not associated with change in progesterone levels
(Somerville 1971).

One might expect that menarche-associated menstrual migraine would be
common in adolescent girls. Although there is certainly a general increase in
frequency and onset of migraine during this period of life and a general trend
toward a female predominance that is moving toward the adult male/female
distribution, the complaint of migraine associated with menstruation in this group
of patients has been relatively uncommon in my own experience. Perhaps this is a
reflection of self selection, and the symptoms experienced during periods are
accepted as part of menstruation.

Vahlquist (1955) found menstruation to be a significant factor in 2.5 per cent of
patients in the 16 to 19 age-group, while Bille (1962) recorded the association in
nine of 20 menstruating girls in his series of personally interviewed patients. The
relationship may be useful in establishing a family history, and a mother's
menstrual migraine may need to be ferreted out by directed questioning.

Management of this problem is based on the general principles of pharmacotherapy of vascular headache and depends upon frequency and severity.
Anticipatory treatment just before, or during the prodromal symptoms of
menstruation may be useful if the headaches are severe and of regular occurrence.

Migraine related to birth-control medication

This is not an issue that requires extensive discussion in a monograph on childhood headache. However, many girls of college years and some in high school suppress menstruation by regular use of progesterone-estrogen medication, and many retain a pediatric orientation in terms of medical care. The relationship to a new or aggravated headache problem may not be appreciated by the patient. The physician must ask the question although it is wise to be discrete.

There is little doubt that use of birth-control pills can initiate or aggravate vascular headaches in some patients (Whitty *et al.* 1966). Moreover it would seem that it is this group in whom there is greater risk of thrombo-embolic phenomena. It is probably another example of enhanced risk of stroke in patients with a migraine diathesis, when neither factor, *i.e.* migraine or progesterone-estrogen medication, carries a very significant burden of risk alone. Young women who develop periodic headache while on birth-control pills should be advised to discontinue this medication and adopt other means of avoiding pregnancy.

Miscellaneous factors

Exposure to sun

Sun exposure has been implicated as a factor in precipitation of migraine by Vijayan *et al.* (1980). Based on a questionnaire in 263 patients with various types of headache, these authors indicate that exposure to sun was a factor in 30 per cent of patients with classic and common migraine and only 7 per cent of patients with muscle contraction headache. Dependable data could not be assembled regarding the duration of exposure or height of temperature, although it was stated that duration of exposure was usually 30 to 60 minutes or more and that the sun 'had to be bright'. Use of dark glasses was only occasionally useful as a preventative measure.

Sun exposure has only occasionally been implicated in my own series of juvenile migraine patients although it could easily have been overlooked because questioning along these lines has not been routine. Leviton *et al.* (1984) have found sun glare to be a recognized factor in about 20 per cent of their patients between 11 and 17 years of age. The fact that summer headaches are not commonly a problem amongst the school-age child would seem to argue against this factor being very significant in the over-all incidence in the young. It does however raise some interesting questions relating biochemical factors and skin vasomotor reactions to sun exposure in the pathogenesis of an attack. The obvious advice to avoid sun may not be acceptable to the young in the sun-worshiping cultures of much of the world.

Visual factors

'Eyestrain' is a popular putative cause of headache according to popular wisdom. Refractive errors and the possible need for glasses is often the first thought of many parents. The results of the visit to the opthalmologist is usually not productive, although lenses may be prescribed for minor refractive errors and used without relief of the child's headache.

On the other hand, various artificial and natural visual stimuli are quite frequently encountered in surveys of precipitating factors. Bille (1962) found that visual stimuli were significant in 79 per cent of his series. This included sun reflections from sea or snow and sitting too near movie or television screens. Maratos and Wilkinson (1982) found 'light' to be a factor in 56 per cent of their patients.

Sleep and fatigue
A well-regulated life is good advice for anyone, but many patients with migraine pay the price of headache when excesses occur. Excess physical exertion and the general effect of psychologic stress have been mentioned above. Many times these factors are combined in the effort to prepare for examinations, periods of highly-concentrated social life, and the convergence of a heavy schedule of extra-curricular activities. These excesses will lead to 'exhaustion', even with the apparently limitless energy of the young. In particular, the adolescent appetite for periodically rising with exuberant activity from their seeming torpor is note-worthy.

These periods of excess can lead to a single event of vascular headache, or set off a train of headaches. The headache may occur at the time exhaustion is finally acknowledged, or may come in the period shortly after the pressure is off, the 'let-down' or 'weekend' headache of adults (Graham 1956). It should be remembered that the weekend is often the period of action in the adolescent or young adult and the let-down may be deferred to Monday morning.

Closely related to the general subject of fatigue is the relationship of sleep to migraine. Lack of sleep and an unaccustomed long and exciting day can be a factor, especially in the younger child. The opposite side of the coin, *i.e.* prolonged sleep into the late morning hours, can also be a significant and identifiable issue on occasion in some individuals, especially adolescents (Leviton *et al.* 1984).

An additional factor relating to sleep and migraine is the onset of headache during sleep. It is relatively uncommon in juveniles, amounting to 26 patients in my series in whom this history was obtained and nine more who awakened with headache. Cluster headaches quite characteristically and frequently have nocturnal occurrence. The most important point to remember, however, is the frequent incidence of tumor headaches which awaken the patient from sleep or are present on arising (Honig and Charney 1982).

Motion sickness
The frequency of motion sickness in migrainics has been mentioned earlier. It is commonly the earliest manifestation of the migrainic diathesis. The motion of auto or boat may act as the trigger of a common or classic migrainic episode. Bille (1962) found it to be significant in 14 per cent of his patients. In the very young child it produces only nausea and vomiting, comparable to a brief episode of cyclic vomiting. In the older child, throbbing headache with nausea is a more likely manifestation. The tendency lessens with age as a rule, but in some migrainic patients it may be a persistent problem.

Trauma

Head and other trauma may trigger an episode of common, classic or complicated migraine in susceptible individuals. The trauma may be quite mild and certainly need not be sufficient to be designated as concussion. The problem is reasonably common, especially in children. Head trauma may also be the factor responsible for a periodic vascular headache syndrome that extends over a period of weeks and months. Both issues are discussed in greater depth in Chapter 10.

4
THE EXPRESSION OF CHILDHOOD MIGRAINE

Introduction
Migraine is a pathophysiologic state that may present with several symptomatic clinical syndromes. All clinically important presentations are paroxysmal or periodic. The most frequent manifestation is headache, either 'common' or 'classic'. Other relatively frequent manifestations include episodic abdominal pain, cyclic vomiting, and less commonly vertigo.

Periodic or paroxysmal expression
The outstanding feature of migraine in any of its manifestations is its paroxysmal or periodic occurrence. This refers to the almost invariable tendency to return to baseline with resulting symptom-free intervals. One could say that without periodicity it is not migraine. It is the hallmark of the disorder, and all authors agree on his point. Most epidemiologic studies correctly use periodicity as the primary feature of ascertainment.

The frequency of expression is highly variable from several attacks per day to several per year. There may be none at all during the course of a number of years. The usual incidence of paroxysms in patients who present for consultation and advice ranges from one per month to two or three times per week. As discussed in the section on precipitating events, there is a high correlation of frequency with the school year, usually followed by summer remission. Perhaps this is in part accountable for the observation of Prensky and Sommer (1979) that the usual course of a sequence of headaches in children was approximately six months. As Bille (1962) has observed, the most frequent onset of a given episode of childhood migraine is during or immediately after school, and attacks are most frequent and severe during the spring term which is a period of particular stress.

The periodicity can sometimes be explained by recurring precipitating factors or a continuing substrate of emotional distress. These factors are more fully considered in the section on precipitating factors, but include most commonly psychological stress-factors the day before or the day of the headache (Leviton *et al.* 1984). It is relatively uncommon for children to experience 'let-down' or 'weekend' headaches. This refers to headache occurrence on the first quiet day following several days of stress. However, adolescent patients may make this observation. The association is more common in adults (Graham 1956).

Age of onset
Age of onset of the headache syndrome in prepubertal patients has a peak incidence between the ages of six and 10, when boys tend to predominate slightly (Burke and Peters 1956, Holguin and Fenichel 1967, Dalsgaard-Neilsen *et al.* 1970,

Prensky and Sommer 1979). Of particular interest is onset in very young children. Vahlquist and Hackzell (1949) were able to report 31 cases with onset between one and four years of age. In my own series the youngest patient was 18 months at onset, and there were three additional patients with onset around age two.

It is a common experience in pre-adolescent patients that from the year of onset there will be three to six consecutive years of recurrent symptoms and then total remission for an indefinite number of years. Congdon and Forsythe (1979) pointed out that about 70 per cent of their children with sufficient follow-up had a remission between nine and 16 years of age. 29 per cent had obtained an eight-year remission, but if headaches persisted to 18 years of age, remission did not occur. Bille (1962) has indicated that 35 to 50 per cent of his patients had become symptom-free by the teenage period.

Headache may then recur later in life when a confluence of exogenous and endogenous factors may produce an exacerbation. Graham (1955) has been particularly eloquent in relating exacerbation of migraine to life events in the longitudinal natural history of the disorder.

Classic migraine
Classic migraine is defined by the aura of symptoms that precede the headache. It is therefore a somewhat arbitrary separation from common migraine which consists only of headache and associated symptoms. When a characteristic visual aura is present, there is usually little diagnostic difficulty and there is no ambiguity in the separation from psychogenic headache, however important psychologic factors may be in the frequency or severity of headache in the individual migraine patient. There may be some difficulty in distinguishing structural intracranial lesions on rare occasions (see Chapter 12).

Frequency of a visual aura in children
A characteristic visual aura, and its unequivocal acceptance as diagnostic of migraine, is unfortunately present in a minority of patients with migraine. It is more common in adult patients than in children. Lance and Anthony (1966) found fortification spectra in 10.2 per cent of their 500 adult patients and photopsia (scintillating speckles of light) in 26 per cent. This is in contrast with a much lesser incidence of these phenomena in children.

My own series indicates an incidence of visual manifestations in 5 per cent of the total group (Table VI). Separate tabulation of photopsia and fortification spectra was not done, and other manifestations such as micropsia, negative scotomata and colored patches of light were included. Blurred vision was treated separately, and if included would roughly double the incidence of visual symptoms.

The incidence of classic migrainic visual aura in my series of children is lower than indicated by most authors. Prensky (1976) records an incidence of visual aura varying from 10 to 50 per cent in eight reported series. In several more recently-reported series of patients, the values are also higher: for example Congdon and Forsythe (1979) where it was 30 per cent. Prensky and Sommer (1979) found 32 per cent, while in the patients reported by Jay and Tomasi (1981) the incidence was just 9 per cent.

The Jay and Tomasi (1981) series consisted of 54 patients of whom five had a visual aura that was described in more detail. They included one patient with each of the following characteristics: 'blurred vision solely; blurred vision and dizziness; blurred vision and a negative scotoma; negative scotomas solely; and one with fortification phenomena'. Only three of these patients would have been included in my personal series. Blurred vision is more common in migraine but less distinctive than scotomata or photopsia. Moreover, like photophobia, it is more frequently a manifestation of the headache itself than the aura.

The higher incidence of visual aura in most reported series of cases is probably a reflection of several factors. The history of characteristic migrainic visual phenomena is somewhat difficult to elicit in younger children and reflects the enthusiasm and vigor with which it is sought. It occurs usually in only a small proportion of headaches in a given individual, and is quite easily forgotten. These reasons may account for some portion of the lower incidence in my personal series of cases. Also the relative percentage will be higher when more restrictive criteria for the diagnosis of vascular headaches are used. The status of blurred vision as a component of the headache *vs.* the aura may also be a factor. These several factors probably account for the disparity between my own and almost all reported series.

The issue is worth laboring because it may come close to the heart of the matter of the general impression of the infrequency of migraine in childhood. If one expects to hear the classic migrainic visual phenomena described in a high percentage of cases, then the diagnosis of migraine may not be entertained in a significant number of children who actually experience vascular headaches.

Common symptoms of the aura
What are the diagnostic visual phenomena of the aura in classic migraine? They consist of both positive hallucinations and negative scotoma, as well as other visual symptoms that are especially well described in great detail by Walsh and Hoyt (1969). Negative phenomena may be described as a greyish patch in any area of the field of vision in either eye, or it may consist of a cut-out of a portion of images with smooth or ragged edges. The scotoma may also be hemianopsic, quadrantic, or consist of a concentric constriction of the field of vision. Total blindness occurs only rarely, and central scotomata are very unusual. Scotomata may be surrounded by rings of color and be filled by scintillating flashes of light or by other positive phenomena.

Positive phenomena occur more frequently without obvious scotoma, although effective vision is usually reduced when they are actively present, and they may leave a negative scotoma in their wake. Photopsia is probably the commonest, defined as tiny intermittent flashes of light. 'Fortification spectra' are another very characteristic visual symptom. This refers to zig-zag lines of brilliant white, often surrounded by a rainbow of colors.

Both the positive and negative scotomata may have either retinal or cortical localization. If the symptoms involve one eye, retinal localization is likely. If bilateral, the localization may be ambiguous. If hemianopsic, the cortical origin is clear. It is also characteristic of cortical location that the visual abnormality evolves in a deliberate slow march requiring a major fraction of a minute to several minutes to proceed to completion.

Less frequently the visual disturbance is more complex and consists of illusions of micropsia, macropsia or irregular distortion of objects reminiscent of the images produced by the distorting mirrors of the amusement park. The history of several young patients with complex visual disorders is recorded in Bille's monograph (1962). The complexity of these esoteric visual symptoms usually exceeds the scope of the vocabulary of the younger children, and one must frequently supply the words in order to get an accurate picture. The best start is usually to ask if something 'funny happens to your eyesight' before the headache. If the answer is affirmative, one can proceed to extract a more complete description. A description of blurred vision may be the only clue—a clue which, if possible, should be followed by a more concise description. Sometimes a child will not remember a visual aura, but has informed a parent at the time of the incident. Occasionally when the mother recalls the incident she is unable to prompt the child to remember, and it is still denied. The young child is apparently quite threatened by visual aberration and may overtly deny total blindness on occasion whatever the cause. Perhaps this is a contributory factor to the difficulty of obtaining a positive history of visual abnormality during the aura.

A common area of symptomatology during the aura is light-headedness and vertigo. These symptoms have a greater predilection to extend into the headache phase than the classic migrainic visual aura, and share this characteristic with visual blurring. They may occur only after the headache is established. Light-headedness is more common than true rotatory vertigo, and perhaps one should distinguish between the two phenomena since vertigo is a much more definitive symptom of focal neurologic involvement. In a number of instances vertigo and light-headedness are combined with visual blurring or true diplopia. There is conceptual overlap between these relatively frequent symptoms of migraine and the broader concept of basilar artery migraine as enunciated by Lapkin and Golden (1978). This issue is further discussed in Chapter 6. Both central visual and vestibular symptoms are related to the vascular territory of the vertebral-basilar system. This has given rise to the quite reasonable point of view that classic migraine is in fact basilar artery migraine in most instances, *i.e.* except when the visual disturbance has a retinal origin.

Other sensory symptoms may occur, either alone, or more commonly in association with a visual aura. Sensations of tingling or numbness are occasionally mentioned. The distribution may be the most characteristic feature. There is a tendency to bilateral perioral involvement, often combined with numbness of both hands and lower arms. These features were mentioned by 15 young people in my personal series of 300 patients (Table V). In one adolescent it was accompanied by mild carpal spasm and was quite evidently related to hyperventilation, but this was an isolated example. In most instances there is no obvious basis for the numbness and it is a matter of speculation whether it is localized to the periphery or to some difficult-to-define cortical topography.

Less commonly the numbness is confined to one side of the body and slowly extends from its origin in the hand or face in the typical deliberate march of migrainic phenomenology. The leg is less commonly involved although an entire half of the body may be encompassed. There may be slight weakness or clumsiness of the ipsilateral hand, and slight confusion or word-finding problems. This brings us to the subject of 'complex' migraine (see Chapter 5).

Other senses may be affected. Auditory symptoms are unusual, although tinnitus may occur. Heightened sensitivity to sound is frequently mentioned as part of the phenomenology of the headache, but occasionally may begin during the pre-headache phase. Olfactory aura are rare, but do occur. There are two such patients in my series. In these and other recorded instances, the smell experienced is usually foul and unpleasant and comparable in all respects to the uncinate aura of temporal lobe seizures (Wolberg and Ziegler 1982). If the olfactory aura occurs in the midst of other more typical migrainic phenomena and followed by headache, it is diagnostically reassuring. However, the unease engendered by the symptom, compounded by the knowledge that in seizures an olfactory aura is correlated with a higher incidence of neoplasm, is sufficient to warrant a CT scan in these patients (see discussion of the patient in Mitchell *et al.* (1983) in Chapter 5).

Fascinating and possibly frightening distortions of body image may occur in some patients. Lippman (1952) has pointed out that they are 'peculiar to migraine'. He describes patients in which neck, ear, hip or flank 'balloon out', or the head enlarges and seems to float to the ceiling. He also describes illusions of shrinking or becoming very tall, and one patient in whom one side of the body seemed to enlarge and then grow smaller. All of this is reminiscent of Alice in Wonderland whose author 'Lewis Carroll' (Charles L. Dodgson) suffered from migraine (Todd 1955). Golden (1979) reported two 11-year-old patients with migraine who had complex distortions of body image and time sense that occurred as discrete episodes, as well as in an aura that preceded the headache.

Golden's (1979) patients illustrate the occasional observation that the aura in classic migraine may occur alone, and is not followed by either headache, adbominal pain, or nausea and vomiting. Most frequently the occurrence is occasional in a patient who most of the time experiences the classic sequence of aura followed by headache. In the unusual patient, the aura may be the only manifestation in a given epoch of the total migraine experience. This situation leads to a more vigorous differential diagnosis *vis à vis* seizure disorder. Consciousness is usually significantly impaired in seizures and not in migraine; migraine is of longer duration, and periodic vascular headache has a positive family history. The slow evolution of migraine is also characteristic, as compared to the sharp onset of seizures in time. The frequency of EEG changes in migrainics does not allow this procedure to occupy a key rôle in the distinction, although it can be helpful in some instances (see Chapter 7 for a more complete discussion). In the final analysis, the distinction is based on clinical grounds.

In the typical case, the headache and associated symptoms follow the aura. Apart from a somewhat higher incidence of hemicranial involvement, the headache and other symptoms are not significantly different from those of common migraine and will be discussed below. Usually hemicranial throbbing pain is on the side opposite to lateralized hemispheric symptoms and ipsilateral to the involved hemisphere. The majority of children with aura seem to have bilateral headache.

Prodrome
Both classic and common migraine may be preceded by a symptomatic prodrome which lasts several hours or a day (Dalessio 1980, Saper 1983). The phenomenon is distinctly less commonly reported in prepubertal children than in adolescents or adults. Blau (1980) has studied the symptomatology of the prodromal period in 50 consecutive adult patients, of whom 17 gave a positive response. The symptoms of the prodrome varied from elation and high spirits, restless overactivity and wakefulness (which are more common than malaise), loss of appetite, depression and sleepiness. Visceral symptoms such as frequent urination, constipation or diarrhea also occur.

Common migraine
The designation 'common migraine' was included in the Ad Hoc Committee Classification (Friedman *et al.* 1962a) and has gained general acceptance in North America. It is useful in that it includes vascular headaches without prodrome or aura, although the purist may prefer to restrict the term migraine to refer to the classic syndrome, and consider the remainder as 'vascular headaches'. A patient may have only occasional headaches with an aura, while the majority are without. A child with common migraine will frequently have a family history of relatives with classic migraine. In the present state of our information, there is an advantage in maintaining a unified concept of the clinical syndrome. Certainly the management of common and classic migraine is much the same.

The headache of classic and common migraine
The migraine headache of children is similar to that of adults. The chief differences are in the lower frequency of hemicranial distribution and the lesser duration of headache in children. Hemicranial headache was described by 22 per cent of my personal series of patients (Table V). Usually this did not amount to more than the occasional headache amongst many that were bilateral. Fronto-temporal distribution was the rule, and posterior localization was uncommon. The Prensky (1976) review indicates an incidence of hemicranial headache in 25 to 66 per cent of patients in nine pediatric series, and in 75 to 91 per cent in four series of adults.

Duration of headache was not tabulated in my series of patients, but the impression of relative brevity as compared with adults is definite. The pain may last only five to 10 minutes or be sustained over many hours although rarely for more than a day. The usual duration is one to three hours. Duration is not specified in most juvenile migraine reports, but the relative brevity is mentioned beginning with Vahlquist (1955). Holguin and Fenichel (1967) gave attention to this point and reported that in 45 per cent of their cases the duration of the episode was one to two hours with a range from '10 minutes to one or two days'.

The outstanding feature of the pain in vascular headache is pulsation that is synchronous with the heartbeat. Throbbing is perhaps the most descriptive word used, but children may be more familiar with words like hammering, pounding and beating. Augmentation of words by gesture is sometimes necessary and always useful to communicate the concept of a pulsating pain. It is usually necessary to supply a selection of descriptive words supplemented by gesture to elicit the quality of throbbing. There is some danger of playing upon the natural suggestibility of children by this effort. The incidence of throbbing pain in my personal series was 66 per cent (Table V). This is lower than I would have guessed, but it is consistent with other series such as that of Holguin and Fenichel (1967) where it was 60 per cent, Bille (1962) who found 68 per cent in his personally interviewed series, and Prensky and Sommer (1979) where it was 52.4 per cent.

Other descriptions of the quality of pain are less characteristic of the vascular nature of the headache, but are consistent with it. Some indicate intensity such as 'splitting' or 'vice-like', words more often used by older children and adolescents to carry an implication of severity as well as quality of pain. In a number of instances 'ache' or 'hurt' are the best description one can develop and it is necessary to depend on other symptoms to build the case for migraine.

Observable concomitants may be quite dramatic in expressing the significant discomfort of the child during a paroxysm. They are perhaps more common and certainly more useful in the clinical assessment in the younger children. It is always worth inquiring of the parent if they can determine whether the child is having a headache without asking. In migraine the answer is frequently 'yes'. This response is common in migraine or organic headaches, uncommon in the psychogenic syndrome. Noteworthy change in facial appearance is frequently observed: usually pallor, but occasionally flushing. Parents will also describe 'dark circles' under the eyes, but this observation is difficult to assess. In more severe headaches, the child acts ill, and may spontaneously retreat from play, lie down and seek quiet and subdued light. Photophobia is very common and sensitivity to sound occurs as well. Irritability and lethargy in varying mixtures are the usual behavioral concomitants.

Sleep is the most effective measure to relieve a vascular headache, and this is often part of the history. However, daytime sleep or an early bedtime is resisted by many children except when the headache is quite severe. At times sleep is neither convenient nor possible.

Migraine may awaken the child at night or appear upon awakening. Either is less frequent than with adult patients. It is an important issue in differentiating headache due to tumor where nocturnal awakening or early morning onset is common (see Chapter 12). Only 9 per cent of my personal series of migraine patients were awakened at night and about half that number experienced headache upon awakening (Table V). Even more significant, these events were very uncommon in the total number of headaches in a given child, and it was an unusual occurrence in the total headache history.

Associated gastro-intestinal symptoms
Nausea, sometimes with vomiting, is the associated symptom that occurs most frequently in childhood migraine. Anorexia is the least common expression of

gastro-intestinal upset but is more difficult to ascertain, partly because of the shorter duration of attack which may not extend to mealtime, and also because of the relatively capricious appetite of children in general. In my personal series, 62 per cent had nausea or nausea plus vomiting (Table V). In the Prensky (1976) compilation of eight reported series, the incidence of nausea and/or vomiting is given as ranging from 70 to 100 per cent, while in his own subsequently reported series (Prensky and Sommer 1979) the incidence was 65.5 per cent. When these symptoms are present, they tend to occur with most headaches, and there is a trend in most patients for these associated symptoms to be positively correlated with severity. Sometimes, especially in the younger group, nausea and vomiting may dominate the clinical expression. This presentation blends almost imperceptibly into the subject of the syndrome of cyclic vomiting (see Chapter 5). In many patients the occurrence of vomiting may afford some relief of headache.

Abdominal pain may accompany the headache, especially in younger children. It is also frequent as a manifestation of the aura (4 per cent in the Congdon and Forsythe series), or has occurred in episodes without headache in the prior history of about the same number of children (Congdon and Forsythe 1979). For further discussion see the section on abdominal migraine.

In occasional patients, diarrhea may occur alone or be combined with nausea and/or vomiting. The incidence has not been recorded in reports of juvenile patients although it occurs in 1 to 2 per cent of adult series (Lance and Anthony 1966).

Other associated symptoms
The relatively frequent occurrence of vertigo and light-headedness during their course of the headache has been mentioned above in discussion of the aura. Next to gastro-intestinal symptoms, it is probably the commonest associated phenomena. Bille (1962) records 'giddiness' in 47 per cent of his personally interviewed series, while only 19 per cent of the Prensky and Sommer (1979) patients were described as having 'dizziness', a frequency that is comparable to my own series (Table V). The more specific observation of true vertigo was recorded in almost 20 per cent of the 286 patients described by Watson and Steele (1974). Blurred vision and photophobia during the attack is also frequently mentioned, as indicated above. Fever, although it occurs, is rare but disproportionately troublesome in differential diagnostic considerations. Occasional patients will have syncope during occasional episodes. At times migraine will apparently trigger major convulsions (see Chapter 7).

Family history
It should be possible to obtain a positive family history of migraine in at least 90 per cent of children who have the disorder. It is the commonest feature of the syndrome with the possible exception of headache. Consequently the occurrence of migraine in other members of the family is a highly significant factor in the diagnosis, and without it one should be uneasy.

A small minority of parents will volunteer their migraine history and I would estimate that this is increased to 50 to 60 per cent by the direct inquiry as to the presence of migraine or 'sick headaches' in the family, especially father and mother. At this point the physician must go to work and extend inquiry to include information about grandparents, siblings and aunts and uncles who are blood relatives of father and mother.

At some point I often confront the mother and/or father with the request, 'Now tell me about your headaches'. A frequent answer is, 'I just have ordinary headaches' or 'sinus headaches'. At this point it is wise to elicit a proper history of periodicity, quality and associated symptoms and make one's own diagnosis. The diagnosis will often be common migraine. The available parent can then be instructed in the proper questions for other members of the family who are not available for direct discussion. It is not usually necessary to extend the inquiry beyond the parents. On occasion psychogenic headaches may also have familial expression, and when this occurs it is usually a mother's headache that is expressed by the child. The clinical features of occurrence, quality and associated features in the history are the critical factors in distinguishing this relatively uncommon situation from migraine. The process of developing the family history is not only diagnostically useful but can be reassuring to parents and child that the problem is fundamentally benign. It is surprising how many people do not appreciate that migraine is also a disorder of childhood.

A final caveat is the cautionary reminder that the family history does not settle the issue. Vascular headaches in childhood can be symptomatic of structural intracranial disease. In fact the child who has inherited 'neurovasomotor instability' is probably more likely to react with vascular headache to tumor or other lesions than those who are not susceptible.

Status migrainicus
A state of almost continuous expression of migrainic symptoms, usually headache, is uncommon at any age, especially in childhood. The designation is reminiscent of the phenomenon of status epilepticus and has the same implication, *i.e.* repeated episodic headaches with little or no relief between. It is appropriate to employ the term if repeated headaches continue for a period of three days or more.

On the other hand, extended duration is relatively common in the migrainic cyclic vomiting syndrome in children. In these instances the relatively trivial question might be raised as to whether one is dealing with a series of paroxysms as opposed to a single prolonged event.

The clinical problem of continuous migraine headaches in the pediatric age group is almost exclusively encountered in adolescent girls. In some measure this may relate to the hormonal influences of puberty. More important in most cases is the influence of psychologic distress which is then compounded by the secondary gain achieved, such as the solicitation of parents, boyfriend, *etc.* or the relief and pleasure of missing school.

The factors associated with the conversion of periodic to continuous migraine in adults have been examined by Couch and Diamond (1983) and Mathew *et al.* (1982). The Couch and Diamond study was based on physician responses to a questionnaire, while the report of Mathew *et al.* was based on a personal study of 80 patients, 54 per cent of whom had had menstrual migraine in the past. In both studies the results were similar. Identifiable emotional stress accountd for 67 per cent of the precipitating incidents. Abuse of medication, such as caffeine, narcotic analgesics and ergot, was accountable for about 30 per cent over-all. These investigators found that birth-control pills or estrogen replacement was associated with a smaller fraction, between 10 to 15 per cent. Precipitating factors could not be identified in 5 to 10 per cent of patients. In some, a convergence of several factors could be cited.

In many patients with continuous or daily headaches it may be quite difficult to draw the line between status migrainicus and mixed psychogenic and migraine headaches. The designation is of much less importance than recognition of the psychodynamic issues, and appropriate attention to the anxiety state or depression that may be the basic cause.

In younger children, either very frequent headaches or status migrainicus may be triggered by head trauma or paranasal sinus infection. These issues are discussed in Chapters 3 and 10.

The management of status migrainicus may require hospitalization, especially if vomiting and dehydration are severe. The treatment program is necessarily individualized, to take into account the pathophysiologic and psychologic factors. These may include parenteral fluids, anti-emetics, sedation and parenteral dihydro-ergotamine. Several of my own patients have responded to a loading dose of phenytoin in amounts similar to that used for status epilepticus, *i.e.* 10 to 15 mg/kg administered intravenously at a rate no greater than 50 mg per minute followed by oral maintenance. The management issue is not dissimilar to status epilepticus, and the immediate objective is to break the repeating cycle of headaches and vomiting.

If other approaches fail, treatment with IM dexamethasone in dosage comparable to its use in cerebral edema has been empirically useful. Rationale is based upon the anti-inflammatory effect of the preparation and the presumed clinical inflammation of blood-vessel walls that occurs in migraine. Whatever is done pharmacologically, the major issue in the management of status migrainicus is to ascertain the precipitating psychodynamic factors and initiate relevant therapy.

Cluster headache

Definition

This distinctive vascular headache was first described in the English literature by Wilfred Harris (1937), repeatedly confirmed, and the clinical description extended by others (Symonds 1956a, Bickerstaff 1959, Nieman and Hurwitz 1961, Ekbom 1970, Pearce 1980). The chief clinical features are: a very severe boring pain, centering about one eye, associated with ipsilateral conjunctival injection; lacrimation; and often nasal congestion as well. The episodes are typically relatively brief (10 to 60 minutes), and cluster in a series of single or multiple daily episodes over a period of several weeks. Nocturnal occurrence is common, and there is little if any nausea. Males are predominantly affected at all ages, and the family incidence is much lower than in migraine. It is a vascular headache, but it should be set apart from classic and common migraine.

In the context of a discussion of cluster headache, it should be mentioned that the tendency for other vascular headaches to recur in series in young patients may be quite prominent. This tendency is well recognized and has sometimes been designated 'cluster migraine'. In childhood this is often correlated with external events such as head trauma, or upper respiratory and other incidental infections, especially sinusitis. It is therefore inappropriate to use clustering as the only diagnostic criteria, a point that favors use of the terminology more popular in the United Kingdom, *i.e.* migrainous neuralgia. For the sake of variety, the terms will be used interchangeably in this monograph.

Epidemiology
The prevalence of cluster headache is unknown but has been said to affect from a half million to two million people in the United States (Kudrow 1980). It is rare in childhood; in my own series of 300 patients there were four sufferers, age seven, eight, 11 and 15. In one patient it was precipitated by maxillary sinusitis (see case 3 in Chapter 3), and another developed frequent severe episodes of migrainous neuralgia that responded to IV followed by oral phenytoin in the setting of an infectious mononucleosis-like illness.

Cluster headache is significantly different from most migraine syndromes in that males predominate at all ages. This is most dramatic in the adult but is true in children as well. The typical age of onset is 20 to 40 years, but approximately 10 per cent of patients of a reasonably large series were age 10 to 19 years and all were males (Pearce 1980). Although not stated, it can be assumed that very few were at the lower end of the 10 to 19 decade. Onset under age 10 years is quite unusual. My youngest patient was age seven (see case 8 at the end of this section). Symonds's (1956*a*) youngest patient was 14 years, and Bickerstaff's (1959) youngest was 11 years.

Family history of cluster headache is unusual, in striking contrast with other vascular headaches of childhood. A family history of common and classic migraine in patients with cluster headache is also low, reported at 15 per cent in Ekbom's series of 105 patients (Ekbom 1970). It is not particularly unusual, however, for cluster headache patients themselves to have either common or classic migraine in their life history of headache. The 11-year patient reported by Bickerstaff (1959) had cluster headache over a two-year period, and then at age 14 years he began to have ordinary migraine. One of Symonds's patients (1956*a*) had isolated migrainic visual scotomata unassociated with headache between bouts of cluster headache.

Differential diagnosis
This characteristic, dramatic, and extremely painful headache syndrome is so uncommon in childhood that those who work with children are generally unfamiliar with it. The nocturnal occurrence of headache is highly suspicious of tumor or AVM under ordinary circumstances, and the severity of the pain is provocative.

Age and sex are important features in the diagnosis of true migrainous neuralgia. Any patient with this syndrome in the pediatric age group should be suspected of anatomical pathology such as tumor, vascular malformation or even slow and otherwise aysmptomatic major vessel occlusion.

Vannucci *et al.* (1974) have reported a patient of three and a half years who had bouts of right facial pain, orbital erythema, injected conjunctiva and lacrimation in bouts lasting two to six hours. For the previous year, headaches had occurred nightly over a one or two week period, followed by remission for several months. The physical examination was negative except for cutaneous evidence of neurofibromatosis, as was CSF and a radio-isotope scan. Angiography showed an occluded right carotid above the ophthalmic artery, with narrowing below.

Arteriovenous malformation has also been recorded as a symptomatic expression of cluster-type headaches (Herzeberg *et al.* 1975, Mani and Deetor 1982). See Chapter 13 (page 222) for a discussion of this.

The possibility of symptomatic trigeminal pain is a consideration in the differential diagnosis. In the young, trigeminal nerve involvement is usually due to tumor, demyelinating disease or mastoiditis at the apex of the petrous bone. There are a number of points of clinical distinction. Trigeminal neuralgia characteristically produces lancinating 'flashes' of pain, often is precipitated by eating and talking, and may be induced by facial touch trigger points. The periodicity and duration of paroxysms is also quite different. Paroxysms of trigeminal neuralgia usually last less than a minute and occur many times a day. Moreover, trigeminal pain is not felt deep to the eye which is the typical location of cluster headache. Lacrimation may occur with either, and both may involve upper or lower face. The distribution of trigeminal nerve pain respects the anatomical divisions of the nerve, while vascular face and head pain, whether upper or lower face in its distribution, has only a superficial similarity to fifth nerve anatomy.

Oculosympathetic paresis is a common feature of migrainous neuralgia (Kunkle and Anderson 1961, Nieman and Hurwitz 1961). For the differential diagnosis of this complication as well as a discussion of Raeder's paratrigeminal syndrome (Mokri 1982), the reader is referred to Chapter 6, p. 123.

Intermittent glaucoma is a reasonable differential consideration in adults, but is very rare in children.

Clinical features
The clinical presentation of the cluster headache or migrainous neuralgia is dominated by a characteristic periodicity. The headache may occur once or several times in a 24-hour period, and is more often consistently nocturnal than in any other variety of vascular headache. There is a tendency for headache to recur at the same time of day. The periods of frequent headache usually last four to eight weeks and occur once or twice a year in adults, often in the spring or fall. Experience with children and adolescents is limited, but it is my impression that bouts are likely to be spaced at wider intervals. In children, cluster headache is quite frequently precipitated by sinusitis and other upper respiratory infections. It follows that the pain is attributed to sinusitis, but paroxysmal headache persists after the active infection has been treated effectively. At this point, treatment must be directed to

the vascular headache. In some few adults the expected clustering does not occur, and the problem is one of extended chronicity (Ekbom 1970, Pearce 1980), but this must be extraordinary in children if it occurs at all.

The headache is sharply lateralized and as a rule centers about the eye and forehead, but may include maxilla and jaw. Attacks occur on the same side during a given cluster, but may recur later on the opposite side. Pain is extreme, associated with agitation, but is not usually of throbbing quality. Throbbing may develop as the pain subsides. Older children and adolescents may use such terms as 'boring' with an accompanying twisting gesture of the extended finger which points to the eye. 'Burning' pain is also described. Duration is distinctly shorter than in most juvenile migraine attacks, and is measured in minutes to a portion of an hour, although some have one- to three-hour bouts.

In a significant number of patients (about 30 per cent) pain centers about the lower face, especially the malar region and upper and lower jaw. Often it includes the eye as well, and has a similar incidence of associated symptoms (Pearce 1980). In contrast with migraine, where the patient gets better if he lies quietly in a darkened room, the migrainous neuralgia patient is often restlessly physically active during the painful experience. This activity seems to afford some slight relief.

Where gastro-intestinal symptoms are frequent in most patients with other varieties of vascular headache, they are unusual in cluster headache, and then limited to nausea. The incidence of ipsilateral lacrimation and conjunctival injection is high but not invariable, and nasal congestion occurs during the attack in about 50 per cent of patients.

The only associated neurological sign is Horner's syndrome in about 10 to 20 per cent of adult patients (Kunkle and Anderson 1961, Nieman and Hurwitz 1961). Miosis is the most frequently observed finding, sometimes with mild ptosis. Hyperhidrosis and localized flush may be seen, but anhidrosis does not occur (Nieman and Hurwitz 1961). Ptosis and miosis occurs during the peak of headache and persists for a period of time after the pain has subsided. In a significant number of patients the Horner's syndrome may become permanent, usually after repeated bouts.

There may be a tendency for seasonal change of temperature to set off clusters, and there is general agreement that alcohol acts as a trigger during bouts in most patients. It is not clear whether any of the latter phenomena occur in children.

Pathogenesis
The distinctive clinical features of cluster headache and absence of family history suggest that this variety of headache may have a different basic causation. The vascular basis of the problem is generally accepted, but the fundamental biochemical defect is likely to be different from migraine. This hypothesis is supported by the finding that plasma serotonin and whole blood histamine levels are elevated during cluster headaches (Anthony and Lance 1971), which is generally not the case in migraine.

The frequency of an associated incomplete Horner's syndrome suggests that the involved vessel is the internal carotid artery, at least for this aspect of the syndrome. The development of oculosympathic paresis occurs during the headache or during a cluster of headaches and not as part of a prodromal period. Its timing, therefore, is similar to the development of third nerve palsy in ophthalmoplegic migraine. It is likely that the mechanism is similar and relates to vasodilation or swelling of the vessel wall, and perhaps compression in the bony canal at the base of the skull.

Management
The diagnosis of cluster headache begins with a careful clinical assessment, and attention should be given to the possibility of concurrent sinusitis. Sympathetic paresis may warrant arteriographic investigation of the carotid in some cases. The possibility of AVM or tumor should lead to CT scanning in most instances, and certainly should be done in any young patient in whom the trigeminal nerve is suspected, with special attention to the middle fossa.

Continuous pharmacotherapy is indicated in all patients during a cluster because of the severity and frequency of episodes. A large number of standard treatments for vascular headache have been used, and any may be effective. Often, however, cluster headaches are very resistent to the usual therapeutic approaches. Analgesic or immediate anticipatory therapy has limited value because of the brevity of headache and lack of aura. Inhaled ergotamine can abort attacks, but there are practical limitations in younger children. Methisergide two or three times per day, in appropriate dose for age, is probably the best initial approach for older children and adolescent patients. Ergonovine malleate used in the same way can also be helpful. Symonds (1956*a*) recommended the daily injection of ergotamine tartrate, although the mode of administration has obvious disadvantages. Occasionally an intravenous loading dose of phenytoin can interrupt a cycle of headaches, followed by continuing oral administration. A course of prednisone (Jammes 1975, Couch and Zeigler 1978) and lithium carbonate (Mathew 1978) have been reported to be effective in adults, especially for the unusual patients with chronic presentation. A regimen of high dose chlorpromazine treatment (Caviness and O'Brien 1980) has not been used in children. In chronic cluster headache, also named chronic paroxysmal hemicrania (Sjaastad and Dale 1974), which is probably a variant on the basic theme of cluster headache, daily indomethacin has proved to be useful (Price and Posner 1978).

Cluster headache
This seven-year-old boy complained of headache that had been occurring **CASE** repeatedly over the previous three to four weeks. The headache consisted **8** of a very sharp pain which centered about the right eye and forehead. It usually was of about ten minutes duration, and was associated with ipsilateral conjunctival injection, nasal discharge and light-headedness. The headache was almost invariably nocturnal and awakened him from a sound sleep.

His mother had occasional periodic headaches and a maternal grandfather had classic migraine. A left sixth nerve palsy was noted at the

59

time of birth and had been present throughout his lifetime. No abnormalities were noted in general or neurological examinations except the congenital left abducens palsy.

A skull x-ray was normal. The frontal sinuses were undeveloped and other visualized sinuses were clear. He was treated with phenytoin 50 mg b.i.d. and after about two weeks he had no further headaches. Phenytoin was continued for another two weeks when he had a recurrence of two headaches at which time it was increased to 50 mg in the morning and 100 mg at night. This dosage was continued for the subsequent three months, when it was discontinued. In the subsequent two years he had occasional similar headaches on about three occasions, but no prolonged clusters.

Comment: This seven-year-old boy had typical cluster headache. He is the youngest patient I have seen with this disorder, and perhaps the youngest on record.

See also: case 3 (migrainous neuralgia precipitated by sinusitis) in Chapter 3, and case 53 (atypical face pain caused by brainstem tumor) in Chapter 13.

Vertigo

Definition

Recurring vertigo (abnormal sensation of movement of self or surroundings) is not a common symptom in childhood. It occurs occasionally as part of the aura of migraine, but more often it is part of the associated phenomenology of the headache itself or occurs during episodes of migrainic cyclic vomiting or abdominal pain.

Occasionally vertigo may be a migraine equivalent and occur as a separate event in children who also have juvenile migraine headache, or it may be the first expression of migraine in a younger child who at a later age develops classic or common migraine. This latter circumstance was first recorded by Fenichel (1967) as a possible outcome of the syndrome of 'benign paroxysmal vertigo of childhood' (see below under differential diagnosis).

Epidemiology

Watson and Steele (1974) made a careful study of vertigo in juveniles with particular reference to the frequency of this symptom in migraine. They found 66 children (23 per cent) who had true vertigo, out of 286 who were diagnosed as suffering from the migraine syndrome. Of these, 43 had accompanying vascular headache, and about half of this group had other symptoms or signs that were consistent with basilar artery migraine. The remainder had classic or common migraine. Only 15 of the 43 patients had vertigo prior to the headache, *i.e.* during the aura.

Of particular interest were 23 patients (18 girls and five boys, mean age 5.3 years with a range of two to 10) whose paroxysmal vertigo occurred without headache, three of whom had associated abdominal pain (abdominal migraine). Of the remaining 20 patients whose initial attacks consisted of vertigo alone, the attacks were of less than five minutes duration and accompanied by nausea and vomiting. Several had additional symptoms that were highly suggestive of migraine with basilar artery expression such as paresthesias, transient visual disturbance and unilateral weakness of the extremities. The frequency of attacks was highly variable. Follow-up for three to nine years revealed that nine had developed classic migraine, eight were asymptomatic and one patient had developed a temporal lobe seizure disorder.

Differential diagnosis
There are many possibilities to account for pediatric patients whose cardinal symptom is episodic vertigo. The commonest basis for this symptom is an entity designated 'benign paroxysmal vertigo of childhood' which will be discussed below. Certain disorders such as Menière's disease and what has been called 'vestibular neuronitis' are almost exclusively diseases of adults, although some childhood cases of Menière's disease are known. They conform to the classic description of this disorder with tinnitus and continuing deafness as well as episodic vertigo. Patients whose vertigo is related to acute labyrinthine infection or labyrinthine hemorrhage may have periodic attacks of vertigo in the recovery phase of their illness, but the acute onset and more violent early course set them apart. The same may be said for most traumatic cases, who are also distinguished by the high incidence of deafness and associated signs (Healy 1982).

Trauma may be less conspicuous or absent in the history of patients with perilymphatic fistulas. This disorder is of particular importance because of the possibility of definitive otologic surgical treatment. Rare examples are due to congenital malformation, but appreciation of the rôle of minor trauma in the pathogenesis and the fuller elaboration of the syndrome date to the mid-1970s due to the work of Healy *et al.* (1976) and others (Singleton *et al.* 1978). The commonest basis (50 per cent) of the disorder is head trauma which can be minor, and in the next largest group of these patients (37 per cent) there is no obvious etiology. Swimming, diving, and physical exertion (especially abrupt efforts that implicate the valsalva maneuver) can be identified in some.

Characteristic symptoms are episodic vertigo in most patients, often with accompanying mild to moderate hearing loss and tinnitus. A significant number are slightly ataxic between paroxysms. Vestibular and auditory testing should distinguish this disorder from migraine and other causes of vertigo in childhood. A positive fistula test, when air pressure is applied to ear, plus rapid-onset positional vertigo especially in the head-hanging ear-down position, are the key features of the diagnosis.

Endolymphatic fistulas can also develop in the context of chronic middle-ear infection with or without cholesteatoma. The history of repeated acute infection or chronic otitis media and careful x-ray studies of mastoid and petrous portion of the temporal bone should establish the possibility of this uncommon cause of childhood vertigo, to be confirmed by appropriate otologic studies.

Tumors of brainstem, cerebellar-pontine angle or of the auditory nerve may

TABLE VII
Vertigo of Childhood*

	BPV**	Migraine	Seizures	Perilymphatic fistula
Age of onset	1–4 yrs.	2 yrs, usually older	2 yrs or older	Any age, usually older
Family history	0	++	±	0
Clinical features				
Duration	1–5 min	5 min, usually longer	1–5 min	1–5 min
Altered consciousness	0	±	+++	0
Amnesia	0	±	+++	0
Postictal drowsiness	0	±	++	0
Nystagmus	++	±	±	++
Fear	+++	±	±	+
Pallor	++	++	0	++
Nausea	+	+++	±	+
Vomiting	±	++	0	±
Decreased hearing, tinnitus	0	±	0	++
Laboratory features				
Canal paresis	+++	?	0	+
EEG	0	±	+++	0
Positive fistula test	0	0	0	++
Positional vertigo	?	0	0	+++

*Any patient with persistent episodic vertigo may have a mass lesion of the posterior fossa. The chief features of ascertainment are abnormal cranial nerve or long tract signs, including laboratory evidence of auditory or vestibular abnormalities.
**Benign paroxysmal vertigo of childhood.

produce paroxysmal vertigo as an unusual early sign. Vertigo may be the only symptom at the outset, and persist as such for a number of months. However, the presence of signs of dysfunction of other cranial nerves (especially reduced corneal response), corticospinal and cerebellar signs, and in particular auditory nerve dysfunction will usually provide clues. The presence of cutaneous evidence of neurofibromatosis should be a particular indication for careful study, indicating the possibility of acoustic neurinoma. This tumor is frequently bilateral in this setting and there may be very little visible evidence of neurofibromatosis (café-au-lait spots or subcutaneous tumors) in this sub-group of neurofibromatosis patients (Kanter et al. 1980).

Seizures may present with predominantly vestibular symptomatology. When vertigo occurs in the aura of seizures, there is no diagnostic problem. The clinical distinction of pure vertiginous seizures from benign paroxysmal vertigo and migrainic vertigo may be quite difficult (Table VII). All are characteristically of sudden onset, and duration is measured in a few minutes or less. Certain clinical points are useful, including the observation of nystagmus during episodes, which favors a vestibular origin, and alteration of consciousness during some (but not necessarily all) episodes, which is an almost essential characteristic of seizure disorder. Postictal sleep, although sometimes found in migraine, is also more characteristic of seizures and it has not been described in benign paroxysmal vertigo. Alpers, in his excellent brief review of the subject of vertiginous epilepsy (1960), makes a particular point of the sharp ending to the attack of epileptic vertigo as a strong differential feature. He also emphasizes alteration of consciousness as an important feature in the differential diagnosis. Support for seizures can be gained from normal caloric responses and the finding of a paroxysmal abnormality in the EEG, although migrainic vertigo may show focal and paroxysmal discharges as discussed in the EEG section of this monograph. The EEG of vertiginous epilepsy may be normal. The temporal lobe origin of epileptic vertigo makes a sleep EEG a necessary aspect of the study before it can be regarded as negative.

Benign paroxysmal vertigo of childhood (BPV)
This syndrome is probably predominantly a single entity, but does include the early manifestations of migraine in some young children. It was first described by Basser (1964) who speculated that it was 'a variety of vestibular neuronitis'. Additional cases were reported by Koenigsberger *et al.* (1970) and Dunn and Snyder (1976). Together these reports account for 67 children and document a consistent clinical syndrome.

The symptoms of the disorder are relatively stereotyped. Sexes are equally affected. Onset is predominantly between one and three years of age, with isolated examples occurring after age five. Attacks usually last one to five minutes, seldom longer than 10 minutes and frequently less than one minute. At times parents may note nystagmus during the episode, and ataxia or prostration are frequently observed. The young child is obviously panicked by the sudden loss of control, and it is typical that they cling to the mother during an episode. Even young children will often describe rotational symptoms, but consciousness is unchanged and there is no post-event sleepiness. Pallor and sweating are frequent, and nausea and especially vomiting are less common. Episodes occur on average between one and four times per month and tend to extend over a period of one to two years, thereby running a self-limited course. Hearing is not affected. Unlike the vestibular neuronitis of adults, where mild symptoms are almost continuously present, the child is entirely well between attacks.

Most patients will have depressed or absent vestibular function in one or both ears on caloric testing. Abnormal vestibular function tests are a key feature of the diagnosis, particularly *vis-à-vis* migrainic vertigo. Unfortunately, cold water caloric testing is sometimes uncertain and not always possible in young children, so this feature is sometimes ambiguous.

The EEG is usually normal, as was true of 30 to 33 cases in the Dunn and Snyder (1976) series and 14 of 17 of the original group reported by Basser (1964).

After the disorder has run its natural course, the depressed caloric responses tend to return to normal. Koenigsberger *et al.* (1970) reported beneficial effects in some patients from the use of dimenhydrinate, but neither phenytoin nor phenobarbital are useful in the typical case.

Fenichel was the first to suggest the possibility that the syndrome was an early manifestation of migraine (Fenichel 1967). He reported two siblings with episodic vertigo beginning at about age two years, the older of whom had developed headache as part of the syndrome by age four. Family history was strongly positive for migraine. The episodes as described in the index case were longer in duration than those of typical benign paroxysmal vertigo, and caloric testing was not reported. In the report of Koenigsberger *et al.* (1970) two of their 17 patients had family members with migraine and one child went on to have periodic headaches. One of the 33 patients in the Dunn and Snyder (1976) series developed migraine and two others had a family history of migraine. It is not clear whether those few patients who subsequently developed headache had the characteristic vestibular defect during the period of active attacks of vertigo. Children who have had benign paroxysmal vertigo with associated vestibular defect are no more likely than average to suffer from headache later.

It is my own conclusion that benign paroxysmal vertigo is a distinct nosologic entity. It can perhaps be distinguished from vertiginous migraine in most instances by vestibular testing. There may be ambiguity on this point because subtle vestibular defects have been found in a significant number of migrainic adults (Kuritzky *et al.* 1981) and in children with migraine headaches accompanied by vertigo (Eviatar 1981). The clinical expression is quite similar to migrainic vertigo although attacks are shorter in duration on the average, and it tends to occur in a younger age-group. It is the commonest basis of vertigo in the child under five years. In a minority of patients a clinically identical syndrome may be the first expression of migraine; this group may be distinguishable by normal caloric responses.

The clinical presentation of migrainic vertigo
As mentioned before, vertigo is an occasional part of the aura of migraine and more frequently a part of the paroxysm itself. This section will deal with migrainic vertigo that occurs in separate episodes interspersed between periodic headache, or as the early manifestation of juvenile migraine before headache is identified or prominent. In the latter instance, the child tends to be young, although episodic vertigo may be an expression of migraine at any age (Moretti *et al.* 1980).

The episodes usually consist of true rotational vertigo—sometimes described as seeing the ground weaving, the floor rising up or slanting. Any sensation of movement of self or surroundings is consistent with the definition of vertigo. Frequency is widely variable and duration is usually five to 10 minutes. More prolonged episodes are not too unusual.

Consciousness is not impaired, although the child may be exhausted and want to sleep afterwards, especially if the episode is prolonged. Usually nausea, pallor and sweatiness accompany the paroxysm, and vomiting and abdominal pain are frequent associated symptoms. Occasionally the episode is preceded by a typical migrainic visual aura, or is accompanied by other neurologic signs. Usually these signs are attributable to the basilar artery territory, and when this occurs the syndrome blends imperceptibly into the concept of basilar artery migraine (Lapkin and Golden 1978). Throbbing headache may also occur in some episodes or as an expression of a later evolution of the clinical picture. The development of headache allows for a clear designation of migraine as the basis of the complaint which is otherwise clinically similar to the benign paroxysmal vertigo patients, with the exception of the abnormalities on caloric testing mentioned above. In the Watson and Steele (1974) report of migrainic vertigo, of the six patients who had vestibular function testing in their group of 23 patients with paroxysmal vertigo without headache, two had unilateral canal paresis. It seems likely that these two patients had benign paroxysmal vertigo rather than migraine.

Pathogenesis
No exact answers can be given, but it seems that vertiginous migraine is a fragment of basilar artery migraine and that the restricted symptom of vertigo relates to vasomotor disturbance of labyrinthine vascular supply.

Management
Diagnostic assessment of the pediatric patient with vertigo must include evaluation of hearing by audiogram and labyrinthine function by caloric or rotational testing. This should set the stage for the next phase of the investigation if further testing is necessary at all. CT scan is indicated if there is suspicion of tumor, certainly if auditory as well as vestibular function is depressed or if there are other neurologic signs on examination. An EEG is appropriate in most cases, especially if there is a clinical indication of altered consciousness. If there is a hint of trauma or frequent otitis in the history, otologic consultation should be arranged, with special attention to provocative positional testing and negative pneumatic otoscopy (Healy 1982).

Prophylactic treatment with any of the pharmacologic agents useful in juvenile migraine may be beneficial and they are indicated if the episodes are sufficiently frequent or severe. Phenobarbital or phenytoin may relieve both migraine and seizures, but have no value in benign paroxysmal vertigo. This approach may provide a therapeutic test in ambiguous circumstances. Propranolol or cyproheptadine may be useful if the basis is migraine.

Vertiginous migraine
This nine-year-old girl had had five episodes of vertigo over the six months **CASE** prior to her visit. Vertigo occurred on and off over a period of 30 minutes, **9** and was followed by sleep or occasionally by a headache. This headache was similar in its characteristics to other headaches which she had had for about one year that were not associated with vertigo. They were unilateral, centered about either right or left eye, and lasted between 30 minutes and three hours. The pain was intense but there was no throbbing quality. The headaches were accompanied by nausea. Her mother suffered from classic migraine, and a paternal grandmother, aunt and cousin all had migraine headaches.

Comment: This child had episodes of vertiginous migraine sometimes followed by headache. She also had independent hemicranial headaches consistent with juvenile migraine.

Vertiginous migraine

CASE 10
At age two and a half this boy was evaluated by Dr. Bruce Berg of San Francisco because of an eight-month history of one- to five-minute episodes during which he became 'dizzy' (nystagmus was noted at this time by the parents). During the episode he became unsteady or would fall to the floor. There was no loss of consciousness. CT scan and EEG were normal. Caloric testing could not be done at that point and was not carried out later because the boy had no episodes subsequent to his visit. The diagnosis was benign vertigo of childhood. In the meantime, the family moved to the Boston area.

He then presented at age seven because of a two-month history of weekly headaches that were frontal in location and consisted of a pressing and throbbing sensation, sometimes associated with nausea but no vomiting. Duration was about four to five hours. On occasion dizziness and unsteadiness without rotational sensation accompanied the headache. He was noticeably pale during the episode. In addition he had episodes of dizziness alone that occurred about three times per week during which it was necessary for him to sit down for 15 to 20 minutes. Occasionally there was nausea but no accompanying headache.

Family history indicated that his father had relatively infrequent throbbing headaches during which he preferred to lie down in a darkened room. They were often precipitated by sun and heat. A maternal grandmother and aunt also had periodic headaches.

Examination was negative. He was treated with propranolol 10 mg t.i.d. with good results.

Comment: This boy had episodes of vertigo in early childhood, and an exacerbation of more characteristic migraine syndrome intermixed with episodes of dizziness at age seven. There was good response to propranolol.

EEG and migraine

The EEG is the easily available procedure of choice to assess derangement of neurologic function. As such it is often employed to study patients with juvenile migraine, especially those with complex symptomatology. It is frequently 'abnormal' in patients with juvenile migraine, as might be anticipated given the fact that migraine (whether it be classic, common or complex) has an impact on cerebral function.

It should be emphasized at the outset that the positive diagnosis of migraine, as well as seizure disorder, rests with the clinician and not the EEG. This diagnostic distinction is based upon the given history and less frequently upon direct observation. Although the EEG can be helpful, more often it may be confusing because of the high incidence of what has been regarded as mild to moderate abnormality in young migrainic patients, and the fact that it can be normal in seizure disorder. It should be done whenever seizure or complex symptomatology is an aspect of the clinical problem, but must be regarded as an adjunct to the

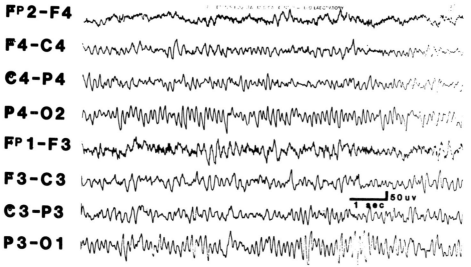

FP2–F4

F4–C4

C4–P4

P4–O2

FP1–F3

F3–C3

C3–P3

P3–O1

Fig. 1. This sixyear-old girl presented with a two-month history of throbbing headaches that began unilaterally and were associated with nausea, irritability and a desire to lie down. They occurred three times per week. A maternal aunt and grandmother had classic migraine and her father had periodic severe throbbing headaches. The EEG demonstrated an asymmetry due to intermittent slower activity in the fronto-parietal regions and was reported as 'abnormal'. This alteration is probably the commonest change in juvenile migraine (parasagittal bipolar, right over left).

investigation and not as a means to achieve an unequivocal diagnosis. An EEG is seldom required in the assessment of the usual patient with vascular headache.

The EEG between paroxysms
There is a fairly extensive literature on the EEG in migraine, dating back to 1941, when Strauss and Selinsky wrote their paper. Most reports deal with an effort to determine the over-all incidence of EEG abnormality in migraine and include all age-groups, with principal emphasis on adults. The incidence ranges from abnormal EEG findings in no more than that expected in the normal population (Boudin *et al.* 1962) or a control group with psychogenic headache (Giel *et al.* 1966) to an over-all incidence of 60 per cent abnormal records in migrainics (Hockaday and Whitty 1969). Intermediate values of 30 per cent are also recorded in a large series by Selby and Lance (1960), and by Goldensohn (1976) who found that 32 per cent of patients with vascular headache show EEG abnormalities as compared with 12 per cent in muscle contraction headache. Towle (1965) called attention to the high incidence of unusually active response to hyperventilation in migraine. This high-voltage slow-wave change is expected in almost all children, but is often particularly striking in juvenile migraine.

Problems common to all studies include the difficulties in defining or selecting the patients to be designated as having migraine as well as ambiguity as to what to regard as EEG abnormality.

A study of 500 children between two and 15 years with recurring headaches,

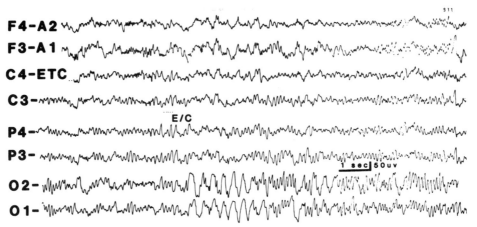

F4-A2

F3-A1

C4-ETC

C3-

E/C

P4-

P3-

1 sec 50uv

O2-

O1-

Fig. 2. This 12-year-old boy had periodic headaches and episodic 'dizzy spells' for about eight months that usually occurred as separate events about two to three times per week. During the month before consultation he had several episodes during which he became confused, couldn't fully understand what was said to him, and blurred vision. During this period he developed a generalized throbbing headache of 45 minutes duration and for the remainder of the day he felt unwell. His EEG showed bursts of posterior high voltage 3 to 4 HZ slowing with eye closure (marked E/C in record) that occurred on either side (parasagittal reference to the ear, right over left).

not associated with organic neurologic disorder including seizures, was reported by Froelich *et al.* (1960). It can be presumed that most of these patients had juvenile migraine, but more precise selection based on the clinical features of headache was not used. Approximately 44 per cent of records were 'disordered', mostly slow or paroxysmal slow, with 22 per cent showing 'spike abnormality'.

A smaller group of 27 children between four and 15 years was studied by Ziegler and Wong (1967). Clinical criteria for selection were more precise and consisted of 'severe, intermittent headache, interfering with school, and in every case accompanied on at least one occasion by nausea and vomiting'. Two of the patients also had *petit mal* seizures and were counted with the nine (33 per cent) who had 'definite paroxysmal abnormality'. The EEGs were performed after 24 hours without sleep, and included activation by photic stimulation and over-ventilation. This resulted in 52 abnormal EEGs in the headache group, and 4 per cent abnormality in 21 age-matched controls, none of whom had paroxysmal abnormality.

Prensky and Sommer (1979) recorded the EEG in 64 of their series of 84 patients. Only 17 (26 per cent) were normal. The majority of 37 patients with abnormality showed either diffuse slowing or slowing with sharp waves. 18 patients had paroxysmal EEGs, although 11 of this group either had seizures (seven) or a family history of seizures.

In a study of 28 patients, Whitehouse *et al.* (1967) called attention to the high incidence (46.4 per cent) of 14 and six cycle/sec. positive spikes in young migrainics as compared with controls where the incidence was 18 per cent. They interpreted this to suggest a 'primary autonomic disturbance' as the basic issue in migraine. The

TABLE VIII
The EEG in Migraine

Study	Patients	Age	Selection	'Abnormality'	
Froelich *et al.* 1960	500	2–15	All headaches	Total	44%
				Paroxysmal	22%
Ziegler and Wong 1967	27	4–15	Severe migraine	Total	52%
				Paroxysmal	30%
Prensky and Sommer 1979	64	1½–14	Migraine	Total	74%
				Paroxysmal	17%
Kinast *et al.* 1982	100	3–15	Migraine	Total	11%
				BFEDC	9%

*Patients who also had seizures not included in percentage calculations.
**Benign focal epileptiform discharges of childhood (Rolandic spikes).

14 and six cycle/sec. finding was also the basis used by Chao and Davis (1964) in one category of patients designated as having 'the convulsive equivalent syndrome of childhood', the symptoms of which reiterated the spectrum of symptoms of juvenile migraine. However, the careful evaluation of the 14 and six positive spike phenomenon by Lombroso *et al.* (1966) and the conclusion that it is essentially a normal pattern with a high incidence during a critical age-period is a convincing alternative point of view. It casts considerable doubt on the validity of any correlation of this phenomenon with disease states including migraine.

A recent paper by Kinast *et al.* (1982) reported a 9 per cent incidence of 'benign focal epileptiform discharges' or 'mid-temporal or Rolandic spikes' in 100 seizure-free children with migraine of age four to 15 as compared with a 1.9 per cent incidence in normal controls.

Table VIII records the results of these several selected studies since 1960. It will be noted that EEG 'abnormalities' have been identified in 40 to 70 per cent of migraine patients in all but the most recent series of Kinast *et al.* (1982). Most of these changes consisted of background alterations in the direction of periodic or continuous temporo-occipital slowing for age, although roughly 20 per cent identify paroxysmal changes. However, as Kinast *et al.* (1982) point out, the concept of abnormality in the juvenile EEG has undergone significant change in the relatively recent past. Certain types of posterior slowing are now believed to be a normal finding by many electroencephalographers, as well as 'hypnogogic hyper-synchromy, six HZ phantom spike and wave, psychomotor variant, and small sharp spikes'. The controversy over the 14 and six HZ positive spike is being recapitulated with regard to other EEG alterations. It is predictable that the concept of what is normal and acceptable will be broadened although the details are currently controversial.

EEG interpretation may be described as being 'in the eye of the beholder'. Perhaps even 'benign focal epileptiform discharges' (Rolandic spikes, see Fig. 6) will be downgraded as an abnormality, although this seems unlikely. Nevertheless, one should probably not totally discount the impression of electroencephal-ographers for the past 20 years. There may be a quantitative alteration in various

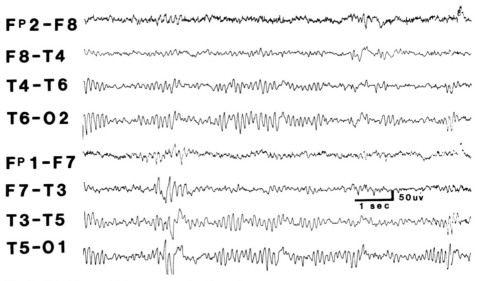

FP2–F8

F8–T4

T4–T6

T6–O2

FP1–F7

F7–T3

T3–T5

T5–O1

50 uv

1 sec

Fig. 3. This 13-year-old boy presented with a three-year history of periodic, usually throbbing, headaches associated with nausea and occasional vomiting. A maternal aunt had classic migraine and mother had rare common migraine headaches. There was no history of seizure disorder in the patient or family. His EEG was read as 'borderline' due to occasional bursts of unilateral shifting sharp theta activity in the temporal regions in the waking record which were seen on the left more than the right. This feature is one of the commoner minor alterations encountered in juvenile migraine patients (bipolar recording, right over left).

unusual parameters of the extremes of normal 'aberration' in migraine that will require computer analysis to define.

At this point it is clear that there is no specificity to the EEG in migraine and the physician needs be wary of the interpretation of what is abnormal in juvenile records. Discharges and spikes will be described with about 10 to 20 per cent frequency in juvenile migraine, and slowing in an even greater number. The final interpretation of 'normal, borderline or abnormal' will be dependent upon the attitude of the electroencephalographer. What was 'correct' in 1960 is probably not acceptable today.

In a significant number of my headache referrals, the leading complaint is an 'abnormal EEG', and the child's head-pain is secondary in the concern of referring physician and parents.

The EEG during the paroxysm
The above discussion is pertinent to the usual use of the EEG as an inter-paroxysm study. There is little or no information that deals with the EEG during a bout of common migraine in childhood. The EEG has been frequently recorded during complex migraine, where symptoms and signs occur during the headache phase. In these instances the frequency of EEG changes in children approaches 100 per cent except perhaps in ophthalmoplegic migraine where the involvement of the nervous system is extra-axial. The usual finding in complex migraine is lateralized or focal

70

high-amplitude slowing in the theta or delta frequency. Less frequently there is focal depression of electrical activity. Discharges are distinctly uncommon in tracings recorded during the event. The focality is usually consistent with the expected cerebral location, as predicted by the clinical signs (Isler 1971). In a number of instances, slow-wave foci are multifocal or diffuse, which implies that disturbed cerebral function may be relatively silent clinically, and can be more widespread than the clinical signs would suggest.

Focal EEG changes subside more or less synchronously with the resolution of clinical signs, perhaps with a delay up to an hour. In some, the changes persist for several hours and in rare instances they may continue for a week or so beyond clinical resolution. Dalessio (1980), in his review of the EEG in migraine in the reprinted and expanded Wolff monograph, proposes that the brief changes correlate with vasospasm, more prolonged slow-wave foci relate to edema and that the rare changes that persist for a week and beyond may represent infarction.

After the migrainic event, the EEG returns to baseline, *i.e.* either normal or showing the spectrum of changes consistent with the basal state of a given patient. In cases in which slow-wave abnormality persists, especially if the delta focus shows polymorphic configuration, there is a strong implication of a focal lesion (Goldensohn 1976; also see case 53 in Chapter 13). Further studies such as CT scan and careful follow-up are clearly indicated in such patients, because polymorphic delta slowing is not found in migraine unless infarction has occurred.

Finally, attention should be drawn to a curious migraine-seizure syndrome that was first described by Camfield *et al.* (1978) in which the interictal EEG showed almost continuous discharges bilaterally over the posterior hemispheres. The discharges were dramatically prominent with eyes closed or in darkness (Panayiotopoulos 1980). This syndrome will be discussed more fully in the section dealing with migraine and seizures.

Summary
Several points are appropriate with regard to the EEG in juvenile migraine:
(1) There is no specific EEG *abnormality* in juvenile migraine.
(2) Incidence of *unusual* EEGs in children is greater than in adults with migraine and greater than in non-migrainic children of comparable age.
(3) The commonest change is slowing or paroxysmal slowing which may be found in 50 to 70 per cent of migrainic children (Figs. 1 and 2). From observations on my personal series, slowing is usually in the theta frequency, sometimes delta, usually over the temporal or occipital regions, and often asymmetrical. The findings often include what would seem to be an unusual build-up with over-ventilation.
(4) Paroxysmal discharges are relatively common (Figs. 3 and 4) especially with photic stimulation (Fig. 5), in juveniles with the migrainic diathesis. Benign mid-temporal or Rolandic spikes (probably in about 10 per cent) are encountered with greater than normal frequency (Fig. 6). It follows that it is inappropriate to use these findings as confirmatory of the 'epileptic' nature of recurring headaches, abdominal pain, vertigo, vomiting or complex symptomatology such as hemi-sensory phenomena or confusional episodes.

FP1-F3
F3-C3
C3-P3
P3-O1
FP2-F4
F4-C4
C4-P4
P4-O2
FP1-F7
F7-T3
T3-T5
T5-O1
FP2-F8
F8-T4
T4-T6
T6-O2

252

CHILDREN'S HOSPITAL, BOSTON, MA.
EEG-PHYSIOLOGY LABORATORY

100 uV

1 SEC

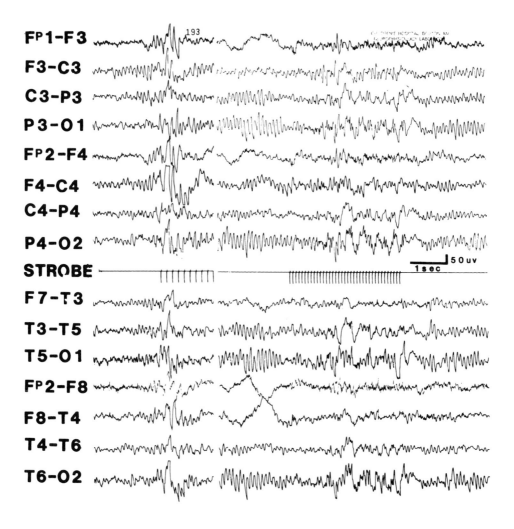

Fig. 4. *(left)* This 12-year-old girl had classic migraine and no personal or family history of seizures. Family history was positive for migraine. Her EEG showed rare generalized bursts of 3 to 4 per second spike and wave discharges during wakefulness, which were more frequent in the period of drowsiness ('hypnogogic bursts').

Fig. 5. *(above)* This 12-year-old girl had had episodic throbbing headaches for two years. They were preceded by visual scotomata and accompanied by nausea and vomiting. Neither family nor patient had had seizure disorder. Both parents had common migraine. The EEG showed a prominent photoconvulsive response (bipolar recording, left over right).

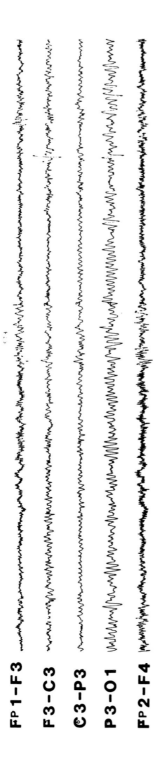

FP1–F3

F3–C3

C3–P3

P3–O1

FP2–F4

F4–C4

C4–P4

P4–O2

1 sec 50uv

Fig. 6. This 12-year-old girl had had periodic throbbing headaches associated with nausea and occasional vomiting during which she was pale, lethargic and complained of photophobia. A maternal aunt had migraine and her mother had had periodic throbbing headaches in her teens. There was no history of seizure disorder on either side of her family. Her EEG showed multifocal independent spike discharges in both parasagittal areas ('Rolandic spikes'), most frequent at C4 (illustrated above), but also at C3 to P3 and F3. In this illustration the abnormality is seen in leads F4 to C4 and C4 to P4 where there are spike reversals. The EEG alteration was the chief reason for referral (bipolar recording, left over right).

74

(5) Both slowing and certain paroxysmal discharges described in (1) and (2) are frequently found in normal children. The prevalence and quantitative expression may be greater in juvenile migraine.

(6) The EEG recording during a complicated migrainic episode is usually abnormally slow with high amplitude, may be asymmetrical or focal, and if focal it is usually but not invariably consistent with the expected cerebral areas of dysfunction. Persistent polymorphic delta is not consistent with benign functional migraine.

Conclusions

In my own work the EEG is not routinely employed in the diagnostic assessment of patients with migraine, and in my view it is not clinically useful except in complex and complicated syndromes. However, there is reason to explore the possibility of a quantiative difference in the EEG of migraines, especially from the perspective of the frequency of normal paroxysmal events of various kinds. Certainly, the nervous system as well as the vascular system participates in the phenomenology of migraine and the EEG is the most useful and available laboratory method of assessing function. The objective of this effort would be to learn more about migraine. The clinical method will probably remain in the forefront of practical diagnosis.

5
THE PERIODIC SYNDROME—CYCLIC VOMITING AND ABDOMINAL MIGRAINE

The periodic syndrome
In 1933 Wyllie and Schlesinger called attention to 'The Periodic Group of Disorders in Childhood'. The concept did not become well established, but has appeared sporadically in British, Australian and Canadian literature over the subsequent years (Kempton 1956). As one reviews the literature, it becomes apparent that Cullen and MacDonald (1963) were correct in their statement that 'juvenile migraine is another name for "periodic syndrome"'. This conclusion can be deduced from the concise expression of the several features of the syndrome as presented by Cullen and MacDonald (1963): 'A child with this condition sometimes presents with typical adult migraine, but more frequently with one or a combination of the following symptoms:
(1) Cyclical vomiting or repeated bilious attacks
(2) Recurrent vague central colicky abdominal pains
(3) Recurrent headaches, sometimes commencing as 'hemicrania'
(4) Dizzy spells
(5) Periodic attacks of fever, sometimes reaching levels of 103° to 104° F (40° C) for several days
(6) Periodic attacks of limb and joint pains or stiffness.'
     The list of symptoms is familiar in the context of juvenile migraine, although the emphasis is not on headache as much as vomiting, abdominal pain and to a lesser extent, dizziness. Less familiar symptoms such as fever are also included, and the mention of periodic limb pain may come as something of a surprise. However, fever is certainly encountered in patients with migraine, especially younger patients, and extremity pain is also known.
     It is likely that the periodic syndrome has tended to focus attention on a generally younger group of patients, with resulting emphasis on the symptoms that predominate at that age. Perhaps it is best to look at the periodic or recurrent syndrome as an incident in the longitudinal history of juvenile migraine. The contribution is valuable in that it helps to incorporate the syndromes of cyclic vomiting and abdominal migraine into the concept of the full expression of juvenile migraine. To equate migraine with headache is clearly an inadequate posture which does not encompass all of its manifestations.
     Because it is preferable to focus on the principal symptom from the perspective of differential diagnosis, and also to some extent in terms of symptomatic management, I prefer to present the issues encompassed by the designation of the periodic or recurrent syndrome in terms of the more traditional and more generally accepted terminology of cyclic vomiting, abdominal migraine and of the several other migraine equivalents such as vertigo. A clean separation is hardly possible in

a number of instances. Any separation is somewhat artificial and as Farquhar (1956) points out, the categories 'merge into the other'.

Cyclic vomiting
Definition
Vomiting is a common symptom of childhood over a wide range of clinical disorders. Moreover, children are especially prone to emesis and have a significantly lower threshold than adults. Yet it is possible to identify a periodic syndrome of childhood in which repeated vomiting is the central feature. The identification of this syndrome is traditionally ascribed to Samuel Gee who reported nine cases of 'fitful vomiting' in 1882.

Epidemiology
A common reason for recurrent episodic vomiting is juvenile migraine. The syndrome itself is not nearly as frequent as periodic headache as a manifestation of migrainic disorder in children. There is no epidemiologic study that separates the syndrome of vomiting without headache from patients where the leading symptom is headache. The epidemiology of the 'periodic syndrome' as reported by Cullen and MacDonald (1963) is really the epidemiology of migraine between age four to 16 years. Although the over-all incidence of vomiting is given as 2.3 per cent of the total of 3440 children surveyed, the overlap between the various symptom categories was presumably great. Therefore, the survey gives little indication of the population frequency of the syndrome of periodic vomiting alone, or of vomiting and abdominal pain without headache.

Some insight into the frequency of the syndrome can be gained from surveys of migrainic children in whom cyclical vomiting is recorded either as separate episodes or as a prelude to the development of the more usual migraine syndrome. Vahlquist and Hackzell (1949), in their report of 31 cases with onset between one and four years) indicated that three of these children had cyclic vomiting at an early phase of the disorder. Burke and Peters (1956) in their review of 92 patients with childhood migraine, recorded three in whom repeated vomiting dominated the clinical picture and was categorized as a migraine variant. Similarly in Bille's (1962) personally interviewed series of 73 patients, three had cyclical vomiting along with their migraine headaches while there were none in the matched controls. Lanzi *et al.* (1983) found that 40 per cent of 100 migraine patients between five and 18 years had cyclic vomiting as compared with 6 per cent in epileptic patients and 11 per cent in controls. The high incidence in this study is surprising in view of the experience of others. The issue was not systematically addressed in my own series of headache patients, but there were a number in whom episodes of unexplained episodic vomiting preceded the development of headache.

Another estimation of the relative frequency of cyclic vomiting as a manifestation of migraine is contained in Farquhar's (1956) report of 112 patients aged 18 months to 15 years whose paroxysmal syndrome consisted of attacks of vomiting (seven patients); headache and vomiting (21 patients); abdominal pain (nine patients); abdominal pain and vomiting (24 patients); abdominal pain and

77

headache (21 patients); abdominal pain, headache and vomiting (30 patients); and headache (nine patients). Periodic attacks of vomiting alone comprised 6 per cent of the total series, all of whom were regarded as having varying expressions of juvenile migraine. On the other hand, in the Lance and Anthony (1966) report of 500 adult patients, 23.2 per cent reported childhood vomiting attacks, as contrasted with 12 per cent of the comparison group with tension headache.

Insight into the incidence of severely affected patients can be gained from Hammond's (1974) report. She examined all the records of admissions to the Hospital for Sick Children in London during a 10-year period, and found 35 cases of cyclical vomiting. It can be presumed that only the most troublesome cases were admitted, and the total number of admissions to the hospital during that period was not given. The primary purpose of this report was to give a long-term follow-up of 12 patients at age 17 to 27 years. Eight of the 12 patients developed migraine headache, and five of these had developed their headaches by the early teens. In a control group of 12 patients who had been admitted to the same hospital during the same period, only one had migraine.

Eight of the patient group on follow-up examination had significant psychological disorders: there were four depressives, three suffered from anxiety, and one had a personality defect and a record of criminal behavior. Abdominal pain persisted into adult life in six cases, and two additional patients had had a recurrence of vomiting and abdominal pain. None had developed structural gastro-intestinal disease or epilepsy. Although the number of cases is small, it is apparent that the incidence of later migraine and significant psychologic disorder is appreciable in severe cyclic vomiting. It is very likely that as yet undefined etiologies may account for a significant number of patients, especially in the group with persistent gastro-intestinal disorder who do not ultimately develop overt migraine headaches.

Differential diagnosis
In recurrent headache, diagnostic concern is focused on intracranial disease: but this is unlikely to be the case when the problem is vomiting. Although vomiting is a prominent symptom of acute and chronic intracranial disease, including brain tumor, it is seldom the leading symptom or sign. An exception is the occasional ependymoma of the fourth ventricle or other tumors of the posterior fossa, where several weeks or months of vomiting may precede symptoms or signs that indicate the unequivocal intracranial site of the disorder.

Cyclic vomiting from lower brainstem tumor
CASE 11 This nine-and-a-half-year-old boy had episodes of vomiting lasting 15 to 60 minutes at monthly intervals beginning 18 months before admission. They gradually increased in frequency and by six months before admission they were occurring weekly. He began to experience dizziness and later true vertigo during the episodes. He was entirely well between attacks, and there was no associated headache. In the ten weeks before admission his voice gradually developed a nasal quality and became lower in volume. In

addition he had episodes of hiccoughs. There was no family history of migraine.

Examination showed nystagmus, left palatal and tongue weakness, very mild intention tremor on the left, and a right extensor plantar response. Gait was normal.

CT scan revealed an asymmetrically enlarged medulla that distorted the fourth ventricle. There was no hydrocephalus. The diagnosis of tumor was followed by radiotherapy.

Comment: This boy had an 18-month history of brief episodes of vomiting accompanied by dizziness and vertigo, during most of which time he was otherwise asymptomatic. He then developed lower brainstem signs and a diagnosis of brainstem tumor was established. The older age of onset and brevity of episodes are both unusual features in migrainic cyclic vomiting.

Organic basis

The organic basis of the clinical problem of episodic vomiting is more likely to be an intermittent obstruction of stomach or intestine from a congenital abnormality such as fibrous bands, intermittent intusseption or a new growth. Nevertheless, these explanations are not commonly the answer. Recurrent infection of the urinary tract must also be given consideration especially if fever is part of the symptom complex.

Episodic metabolic disorders of amino acids, organic acids and the urea cycle are also potential causes of episodic vomiting especially if there is some alteration of consciousness. A more common cause is ketotic hypoglycemia especially if the event culminates in seizures. These conditions are more fully discussed in Chapter 13. Lactose intolerance can also be a basic stimulus to episodes in some, perhaps by acting as a trigger to a migrainic response (see Chapter 3). One such case has come to my attention.

Dysautonomia, the Riley-Day syndrome (Riley *et al.* 1949), should also be considered. Cyclic vomiting is a dramatic aspect of this condition, but other features of the disorder such as hypertension and fever with episodes of indifference to pain, hypotonia with absent reflexes, blotching of skin, emotional instability and lack of tearing, lead one to the correct diagnosis. Stigmata of the disorder are apparent from early infancy, and episodic distress is usually most prominent in the first year of life. Autosomal recessive inheritance and Jewish ancestry are useful background features in the diagnosis. After a stormy infancy many patients have episodic vomiting, fever, *etc.* into childhood.

Psychologic factors are prominent in the pathogenesis of vomiting and may be solely responsible (Green 1967). This is particularly likely to be the case if provocative incidents can be correlated with episodes of vomiting, and especially if there is a relatively regular morning occurrence just before the time to set off for school. Vomiting with or without complaint of abdominal pain is a frequent somatic expression of school phobia. The regular timing in relation to school helps distinguish this etiology from migrainic cyclic vomiting, where more widely spaced episodes of repeated vomiting are the rule. The usual strong influence of general psychological factors that act as a trigger to migrainic events is a significant and important issue in cyclic vomiting, and may lead to ambiguity as to whether the process is purely psychogenic or whether psychologic factors have triggered a pathophysiologic event. This relationship is in no way different from that expressed in many other places in this monograph. The psychologic issues are similar to the issues related to headache and are further discussed in Chapters 3 and 9.

A final cautionary point is worthy of re-emphasis. Where headache in childhood is highly likely to be migraine, cyclic vomiting has a wider range of diagnostic possibilities. Migraine is a relatively common explanation but is not the leading cause.

Seizure disorder has been implicated as the basis of the syndrome of cyclic vomiting in some patients (Millichap *et al.* 1955). The argument was based upon abnormality of the EEG in all of the 33 patients selected. Seven of these patients also had major convulsions or psychomotor seizures. The most frequent EEG abnormalities consisted of atypical spike-wave discharges, paroxysmal high voltage waves and single spike discharges. The clinical expression consisted of repeated attacks of vomiting associated with abdominal pain in 50 per cent, but without loss or impairment of consciousness. The authors reported a therapeutic response to phenytoin prophylaxis. In seven patients, episodic abdominal pain replaced the cyclic vomiting at a later age and five patients developed migraine headaches during the period of observation. The issue of using paroxysmal EEG abnormality and therapeutic response to phenytoin as indicative of seizure disorder will be considered at greater length in the discussion of abdominal migraine *vs.* abdominal epilepsy, where a genuine differential distinction must be made. In cyclic vomiting, epilepsy is usually not a serious differential consideration.

There are a few case reports where vomiting is a leading manifestation of seizure. Mitchell *et al.* (1983) report a boy whose vomiting was initiated by a foul odor, and occurred in attacks that never lasted more than a minute. The first was initiated by *grand mal* seizures and in many, but not all, consciousness was impaired. An episode was recorded electrically with confirmation of seizures. The boy proved to have an astrocytoma of the right temporal lobe. Another patient had EEG-proved 'ictus emeticus', was unresponsive during attacks, and had seizures of several varieties as well (Jacome and Fitzgerald 1982).

The clinical presentation
The central feature of the episode is repeated vomiting. It may begin at any time during the day, but is more likely to begin in the morning. After emesis on several occasions the vomitus contains little food, becomes yellow-green and frothy and reduced in quantity, but nausea, retching and distress continue. The duration of the attack is variable, but usually it lasts at least several hours and in most patients it persists for the remainder of the day. More severe episodes last several days and lead to dehydration, ketosis and acidosis unless fluids and caloric intake are maintained. The odor of acetone may become marked and develop early, as was especially noted in the older literature. This led to speculation that ketosis was the primary factor in the disorder, but the study of Wyllie and Schlesinger (1933) made

it clear that both ketosis and the moderately low levels of blood sugar were secondary to repeated vomiting and inadequate caloric intake. See the section on symptomatic issues (p. 261) for a more complete discussion of the syndrome of ketotic hypoglycemia.

Photophobia is common, and episodes are frequently associated with diffuse abdominal discomfort. When abdominal pain is a later development in the course of an episode, it may be secondary to repeated retching and vomiting. Diarrhea or loose stools are sometimes present. Non-specific, relatively low-grade diffuse headache is mentioned by some children, especially as they grow older and become more articulate. In very rare patients, an aura of visual disturbance may precede the nausea and vomiting.

Pallor is the most common associated sign in the typical case and this is often accompanied by cold clammy skin and sweatiness. The child is in obvious distress and has no desire to be up and about. Both lethargy and irritability are common behavioral accompaniments. Some patients have a low-grade fever, at times as much as 103° to 104° F (40° C). Fever is more frequent in cyclic vomiting than in any other juvenile migrainic syndrome, although it is known to accompany other manifestations of childhood migraine including headache. Syncope may also occur during severe episodes. True convulsions may indicate a metabolic defect, especially ketotic hypoglycemia, although some may be a non-specific response to fever.

A single episode is indistinguishable from many acute gastro-intestinal illnesses, and until several episodes have occurred there is usually no reason to suspect migraine. The periodicity is highly variable. In most patients, the interval between episodes is greater than with headache and varies from one a month to one every three or four months. This is particularly the case with severe and prolonged attacks.

The onset of the cyclic vomiting syndrome is usually the earlier years of childhood, commonly in the third or fourth year (Wyllie and Schlesinger 1933). In the Farquhar (1956) study the mean age of onset in the patients with attacks of vomiting was 2.75 years. In some patients episodes of vomiting have occurred in infancy (Farquhar 1956, Cullen and MacDonald 1963). As the child with migrainic cyclic vomiting grows older, it is typical that headache is mentioned as part of the symptom complex or that episodes of vomiting are interspersed with periodic throbbing headache. It is unusual for episodic vomiting without headache to persist beyond age eight to 10 years, or to begin after age 10.

A family history of migraine is frequent in children with cyclic vomiting although there are no large series that report the approximate incidence. Farquhar (1956) reports that 'four mothers and four fathers' of his seven patients had migraine. A positive family history can be of some value in the diagnostic distinction of the migrainic basis as opposed to other possible causation.

Pathogenesis
For practical purposes, there is no information that gives insight into the pathogenesis of migrainic cyclic vomiting. There is little to suggest that the vascular

system is the basis of the disorder and one must turn to consideration of a central nervous system locus or one involving a systemic metabolic causation.

Management
The alternative diagnostic considerations require x-ray investigation of the upper gastro-intestinal tract, and more prolonged episodes are indication for metabolic studies (preferably at the time of the episode) to include blood ammonia levels, blood and urine amino acids, lactose tolerance tests, blood glucose, urinary ketosis, blood pH, CO_2, electrolytes, and lactate-pyruvate measurements, liver function tests, and possibly estimation of urinary TTP inhibitor. Especially if fever is part of the syndrome, it is necessary to seek sources of infection with particular emphasis on the urinary tract. Assessment of possible psychologic factors is also important, either as triggers to migrainic cyclic vomiting or as the full explanation of episodic vomiting as a symptom. Unusual clinical features and any hint of neurologic abnormality on examination warrants CT scan.

Symptomatic management of an episode is based upon the use of anti-emetic preparations and maintenance of fluid intake and electrolyte balance, as well as parenteral nutrition in the more prolonged episodes. The younger the child, the more important are the issues of fluid balance. Details of fluid and electrolyte replacement therapy must be individualized and further discussion is not germaine to the purpose of this monograph. Blood glucose should be carefully monitored during severe or prolonged attacks.

Anti-emetic medications can be helpful in symptomatic therapy. Oral preparations are seldom useful unless they are employed early. Administration by suppository is more generally valuable, and intramuscular injections may be necessary in some instances. Trimethobenzamide HCl (trade name Tigan) can be used either orally (100 to 200 mg t.i.d.) or by suppository (100 to 200 mg t.i.d.). Major tranquilizers such as chlorpromazine or hydroxyzine also have anti-emetic effect and can be used intramuscularly if necessary. Although I have had no personal experience, it is said that cromalyn by inhalation (20 mg ampule t.i.d. or q.i.d.) can be very effective (Delong 1983).

If the episodes are of sufficient frequency, prophylactic daily therapy may be useful, and phenobarbital, phenytoin, or propranolol are worth a therapeutic trial. The principles of management in this regard are no different from the prophylaxis of migraine headache, but the value of these regimens is less certain in cyclic vomiting.

Migrainic cyclic vomiting

CASE
12
This four-year-old girl had had episodes of nausea and repeated vomiting accompanied by dizziness and unsteadiness since age two. The episodes occurred every three to four months, usually were of two to three hours duration but had occasionally continued for eight hours. As a rule the episodic disturbance occurred sporadically over a two-day period, but had occasionally lasted as long as five days. During the episode, she was lethargic and during the most recent attack she indicated that she also had

a headache. Full gastro-intestinal work-up, EEG and CT scans were normal, as was audiologic testing. Her family history revealed that her mother had 'sinus headache' in childhood and adolescence without remembering much more about them.

Physical examination and neurological examination was negative.

Comment: This child has a typical history of cyclic vomiting complicated by dizziness and slight unsteadiness, which in the most recent episode revealed more of its true nature by the development of headache. The episodes were sufficiently infrequent that continuous medication was not warranted.

Migrainic cyclic vomiting

The history of this 12-year-old boy dates to one year of age when he began **CASE** to have episodes of pallor, trembling, nausea and repeated vomiting that **13** lasted several hours and occurred monthly. At age four he had a prolonged episode that required hospitalization to repair dehydration. Rectal thorazine was helpful in ameliorating the attacks. Between age seven and 11 years, headache was added to the symptom complex. The headache was unilateral, centered about the right eye, and when severe had a throbbing quality. On occasion, he would lose peripheral vision at the peak of the headache. Medication trials with phenobarbital, periactin, amitriptyline and phenytoin were not successful.

The family history indicated that both father and paternal grand-mother had migraine and his mother had scotomata followed by headache during a seven-month period of her teenage years.

Examination showed him to be normal in all respects.

Comment: This patient illustrates the typical evolution of infantile onset cyclic vomiting which developed into typical juvenile migraine in childhood.

Abdominal migraine

Definition

As with cyclic vomiting, it is possible to isolate another common presentation of the periodic syndrome in which the leading symptom is paroxysmal abdominal pain. Although it is a more frequent expression of juvenile migraine than cyclic vomiting, abdominal pain shares the feature of being a common symptom of many disorders of childhood. It is perhaps the commonest expression of psychosomatic illness in this age-group. The hallmark of abdominal migraine is abdominal pain of variable severity. It is paroxysmal in occurrence and may be associated with nausea, occasionally with vomiting. It is often the antecedent of periodic throbbing headache, or occurs in association with headache.

Epidemiology

Recurrent abdominal pain is a high-incidence symptom of childhood. Apley and Naish (1958) have estimated that it occurs in one of 10 children of school age. There is no indication of the frequency of migraine as the causal basis. The Apley and Naish (1958) series of 1000 schoolchildren revealed 108 individuals with periodic abdominal pain, about equally divided between boys and girls. The incidence in boys fell by age 14, while in girls there was a sharp increase at age nine. Associated symptoms of pallor (38 per cent), headache (23 per cent), and vomiting (22 per cent) were appreciable, and 14 per cent of these patients also had separate episodes of periodic headache. These suggestive symptoms of juvenile migraine plus a family history of migraine in 14 per cent allows one the conservative estimate that at least 10 to 20 per cent of these children had juvenile migraine. The commonest family association was a history of episodic abdominal pain in 46 per cent of parents, which suggests that episodic abdominal pain has a strong familial incidence. In part this could reflect a familial predilection to abdominal migraine as well as other etiologies such as psychogenic abdominal pain or undetermined metabolic factors: lactose intolerance, for example.

If the sample is restricted to children with presumptive migraine, then the incidence of an abdominal component is appreciable. Only nine patients (7 per cent) of Farquhar's study (1956) had recurrent abdominal pain alone, but 24 (21 per cent) had abdominal pain and vomiting, 21 (18.7 per cent) had abdominal pain and headaches while 30 (26.7 per cent) had abdominal pain, headache and vomiting. A series in which headache is the index criterion, such as that of Bille (1962), reveal that 20.5 per cent of his personally interviewed group had paroxysmal abdominal pain that alternated with attacks of migraine headache while only 4.1 per cent of the control group had episodic abdominal pain.

Estimates of the frequency of abdominal pain associated with the headache itself are also high as exemplified by the following reports: Holguin and Fenichel (1967) found 10.9 per cent; Prensky and Sommer (1979) found 19 per cent. Lanzi *et al.* (1983) found that 30 per cent of their migraine patients had abdominal pain, while only 5 per cent of their epileptic patients and 3 per cent of the controls experienced the complaint. The records of my own series are incomplete in this respect, but it is my impression that the Holguin and Fenichel estimate is close to my own experience.

Differential diagnosis
My own familiarity with the diagnosis of gastro-intestinal disorders is limited in that my personal experience for many years has consisted of patients who have been sent for neurologic consultation. Usually, the gastro-intestinal system has been thoroughly investigated and I seldom need to deal with a primary differential diagnosis of abdominal pain. For this reason my information on the extent of work-up necessary is not based on personal experience, nor do I have any personal views on the prevalence of recurring abdominal pain in children or the frequency of such issues as psychologic factors in the incidence of symptoms.

Abdominal pain is a symptom of a large number of clinical problems. Much of the differential diagnostic discussion of cyclic vomiting will apply here as well. Concern centers about anatomical disorders of the gastro-intestinal system and includes ulcer, the rare instances of Meckle's diverticulum, mesenteric adenitis and recurring appendicitis. At times distinction between migraine and appendicitis can be difficult, and it is not unusual for appendectomy to be done in this group of patients (Farquhar 1956, Cullen and MacDonald 1963). For example, the report of Blitzsten and Brams (1926) indicates that four of their 33 patients had undergone appendectomy. On the other hand, appendicitis can lead to recurring abdominal pain as exemplified by the following case presentation.

Recurrent abdominal pain due to appendicitis
This 11-year-old boy was referred for neurologic consultation because he **CASE** had had eight episodes of abdominal pain, vomiting and low-grade fever **14** over the previous year. On the last occasion he also complained of headache, and he was referred with the question of abdominal migraine. Each episode lasted two to four days and then spontaneously subsided. He had had a full GI work-up and was seen by his physician on several of these occasions. A paternal grandfather had migraine. The prolonged duration of the episode was atypical for abdominal migraine, and it was suggested that he return for examination at the time of the next recurrence. On this occasion, he was found to have abdominal tenderness, rebound pain that referred to the right lower quadrant and sensitivity in this area on rectal examination. Laparotomy showed an inflamed ruptured appendix in a bed of adhesions and pus. Removal resulted in complete relief and there was no recurrence.

Comment: The principal clinical clue in this patient who had had repeated episodes of appendicitis was the several-day duration of abdominal pain as contrasted with abdominal migraine where the duration is usually less than an hour to a few hours.

Lactose intolerance is probably the commonest metabolic basis of recurrent abdominal pain, and was found in 40 per cent of 80 children evaluated in a general pediatric clinic with this presenting complaint by Barr *et al.* (1979). This problem is discussed at greater length in Chapter 3. When abdominal pain is the primary manifestation, which is usually the case, one need not invoke the mechanism of triggering a migrainic reaction. Direct involvement of intestine by the products of intestinal bacterial action on the undigested lactose is a more likely answer. Other metabolic possibilities are less likely when abdominal pain dominates the clinical picture, but porphyria should be considered especially if the child is near puberty or in the adolescent age-group. Lead colic is possible especially in the younger child.

Psychologic factors form the basis of another large group of young people with recurring abdominal pain, and many believe they account for the majority of children with this complaint (Green 1967).

Finally we must address the issue of abdominal migraine *vs.* abdominal epilepsy in any paroxysmal abdominal pain syndrome without another explanation.

Abdominal migraine and abdominal epilepsy
A particularly troublesome problem has been the distinction between epilepsy and

migraine when the chief focus of the paroxysm is abdominal pain. It should be emphasized that the distinction should be based on clinical historical criteria and not on electroencephalographic observations. The emphasis on EEG findings in the differentiation of these entities is reponsible for much of the confusion over the years, confusion that persists to the present time. As is generally true of seizure disorder, it is the reported clinical phenomenology that is diagnostic, and the same may be said of migraine. The frequency of unusual EEGs in all varieties of juveniles with migraine, including focal spikes and paroxysmal discharges, was not fully appreciated when the concept of abdominal epilepsy became popular (see section on EEG in migraine, Chapter 4).

The enthusiasm for this diagnostic aid took precedence over clinical analysis in both abdominal pain (Livingston 1951) and cyclic vomiting, (Millichap *et al.* 1955) both of which became 'epilepsy' if the EEG was paroxysmally abnormal. The problem was compounded by the observation that phenobarbital and phenytoin were useful in the prophylaxis of episodic vomiting and abdominal pain. This observation is not a distinguishing feature in that both juvenile migraine and seizures may respond to these medications.

The distinction is of some importance. The diagnosis of epilepsy or seizure disorder has much more serious connotations in reality, as well as in the belief of most parents. Moreover, the commitment to prolonged drug treatment is quite different in seizures *vs.* migraine.

Abdominal sensations as a manifestation of the early phase of a generalized convulsion or of complex or simple partial epilepsies is a well known and common phenomenon. Moreover, the symptoms of any 'aura' may be isolated from the fully developed seizure. Hence there is no question as to whether abdominal epilepsy exists or not, as was the case made in the previous section where cyclic vomiting was the focus of discussion.

The characteristics of the abdominal aura of epilepsy is therefore a point of particular interest in the context of this discussion, and the study of van Buren (1963) is of particular value. The clinical findings of 100 seizure cases with abdominal aura were analyzed, as well as the results of depth stimulation of epileptic and non-epileptic patients. The nature of the abdominal sensation was described as painful in only eight instances, although nausea was more common (14 patients). In most cases the sensation was different from anything previously experienced and described as 'funny', 'peculiar' or 'odd', and sometimes unpleasant or uncomfortable. The sensation was midline and usually in the epigastrium. If it migrated, as about 50 per cent did, it moved upward to chest or neck. The various psychologic phenomena associated with temporal lobe seizures such as forced thinking, illusions and hallucinations were quite common. Facial pallor or flushing were noted occasionally. These findings could be reproduced by stimulation of the mesial temporal region and basal ganglia, which in effect probably means the insula.

The issue of careful distinction between abdominal epilepsy and migraine has been addressed in a helpful fashion by Prichard (1958) and by Douglas and White (1971).

TABLE IX

Comparison of Abdominal Migraine and Abdominal Epilepsy

	Migraine	*Epilepsy*
Family history of migraine	80–90%	10–20%
Duration	5–10 min. or longer	Less than 5 min, usually 1–2 min.
Altered consciousness	Rare	Expected in most episodes or associated with TL psychic phenomena.
Onset	Gradual	Abrupt
Quality of pain	Variable, usually severe	Discomfort less specific, may be sharp.
Appearance of illness	Usual (pallor, irritability, somnolence, *etc.*)	Rare
Vomiting	Common	Rare
Postictal drowsiness	Occasional	Frequent and sometimes sleep.
Associated symptoms	Other manifestations of juvenile migraine	Other varieties of seizures.
EEG	20% paroxysmal	80% or more have discharges.

Prichard (1958) reports 19 patients who had periodic abdominal pain without local cause that did not herald a generalized seizure. The patients fell into two clinical groups. In two cases the episode was abrupt, lasted from five to 10 minutes, was associated with confusion and followed by drowsiness. In one of these patients the episode was followed by a generalized seizure on occasion. Both patients had spike discharges in the temporal regions. The author believed these patients had abdominal epilepsy. In 17 cases the abdominal pain was of longer duration, usually between one and six hours; it was associated with pallor, often wih nausea and occasional vomiting. There was no alteration of consciousness, but the children often slept after the episode. In the larger group the EEG was normal in 11, three cases had minor slow-wave dysrhythmia and one had atypical spike-wave discharge. The abdominal pain in these 17 patients was attributed to migraine.

Douglas and White (1971) analyzed 28 consecutive hospitalized cases referred for neurologic consultation because of paroxysmal abdominal pain. On the basis of clinical criteria, which included pain lasting only a few minutes and associated disturbance of awareness or responsiveness in many but not necessarily all episodes, seven were identified as having abdominal epilepsy, five of whom had paroxysmal spike-wave or spike discharges. The three remaining patients and all 20 of the migrainic group had essentially normal or non-specific EEG findings. The authors make a particular point of recommending that positive clinical criteria be used in making the diagnosis of this variant of epilepsy and state 'the rigid criteria required for the diagnosis of other forms of epilepsy should also be applied to this syndrome'.

The same differential criteria as might be applied to seizures and migrainic phenomena in general are useful when the symptomatic focus is abdominal pain (Table IX). Abdominal epilepsy has a sharp onset in time, is brief, and usually lasts two to five minutes. It is accompanied by altered consciousness, and often amnesia for the event.

On the other hand, migrainic episodes last 10 minutes or more. The child remains alert and responsive, although usually crying and distracted by discomfort.

Nausea is more prominent and may occasionally be associated with vomiting. The EEG is more likely to be abnormal in abdominal epilepsy. Using these criteria, many more children with recurring abdominal pain will be found to have migraine than seizure disorder. Follow-up will often reveal the development of classic or common migraine in many of these patients, and seldom are seizures the outcome (Lanzi *et al.* 1983). For further relevant discussion of the issue of abdominal migraine and epilepsy see the sections on 'EEG and migraine' and 'seizures and migraine'.

The clinical presentation of abdominal migraine
Abdominal pain is the central feature of the disorder. The pain is variable in quality and severity. It is usually described as a diffuse aching sensation with a sense of fullness. At times it may become crampy or colicky, more or less continuous or developing in waves. In some patients a peri-umbilical location is indicated, but in many instances this is merely a reflection of the common tendency of the younger child to relate abdominal pain to this dramatic portion of their anatomy. In some, an epigastric location is indicated. The child will usually discontinue play and want to lie down. The abdominal discomfort may be mild, and in some it may be the consequence of repeated vomiting.

The duration of the episode is variable, but in most patients it lasts 30 to 60 minutes. It may be as brief as 10 minutes or as long as 12 hours. Between attacks the child is free of all symptoms. A pattern of recurring episodes over several days is also encountered, but this is unusual. In these instances there is continuous lower-grade abdominal discomfort, superimposed with more severe periods of pain.

Anorexia is the rule, associated nausea is common and vomiting occurs in a number of cases. Vomiting may be sufficiently prominent that the distinction between abdominal migraine and cyclic vomiting becomes arbitrary. Pallor is a common associated symptom as in most juvenile migraine syndromes, as is the tendency to seek quiet and rest. Food does not relieve the distress.

Abdominal pain is reasonably commonly associated with more characteristic migrainic concomitants such as headache, light-headedness or vertigo, and in rare instances it may be preceded by classic migrainic aura. Syncope and confusional states may also occur. Episodic abdominal pain may alternate with headache.

The frequency and severity of attacks can often be related to psychological tensions. The peak age-frequency of the patient is between seven and 10 years (Cullen and MacDonald 1963). A family history of migraine can often be elicited.

Pathogenesis
It is not known whether the episodic of abdominal pain is due to a central mechanism, to localized intestinal vasomotor factors, or to a local or systemic metabolic disorder.

Management
Diagnostic work-up should usually include x-ray study of the gastro-intestinal

system, especially an upper GI study. Stools should be examined for blood, perhaps for ova and parasites. Routine complete blood counts, urinalysis and an intravenous pyelogram on indication are also appropriate. Metabolic studies should include lactose tolerance test, and occasionally studies of urinary porphyrin excretion and measurement of blood lead. If episodes are brief and especially if associated with altered consciousness, an EEG should be done.

Symptomatic treatment of the abdominal pain is rarely indicated because of the relative brevity of the usual episode. If vomiting is severe and prolonged, measures indicated in the section on cyclic vomiting may be appropriate. The usual issue is the decision regarding continuous daily prophylactic medication. The range of drugs and the general principles of therapy are not different from headache, and the reader is referred to the section on the therapy of juvenile migraine (Chapter 8).

Abdominal migraine
When first seen, this boy was age six and had been having episodic **CASE** abdominal pain of increasing frequency for three years. The episodes **15** consisted of diffuse severe abdominal pain of about one hour in duration. He was noticeably pale and distracted. On one particularly memorable occasion, the abdominal pain began at the check-in counter of an airport and became very severe over the period of 10 to 20 minutes. He was cold and clammy and vomited during the flight. At one point he seemed to 'pass out' for about two minutes and subsequently was confused off and on for the remainder of the episode which was of several hours in duration.

The family history revealed that both mother and father had paroxysmal headaches with throbbing quality and nausea. His maternal grandmother had classic migraine.

Prior to his referral, he had various investigations including an upper GI and small bowel series, barium enema and an IVP, all of which were normal. His EEG done elsewhere was recorded as 'abnormal with intermittent paroxysmal high-voltage slow and sharp wave discharges'. EEG at Children's Hospital, Boston was normal both awake and during sleep. He was treated with phenytoin with good response.

Comment: This boy had clinically typical abdominal migraine, with a paroxysmally abnormal EEG on one occasion while a follow-up EEG was normal. On a single occasion he had a prolonged complex episode which was complicated by frequent vomiting ('cyclic vomiting') and periods of impaired consciousness and confusion.

Unusual associations with juvenile migraine
There are several symptoms or signs encountered in association with juvenile migraine syndromes that are perplexing because they are rare in migraine and usually suggest non-migrainic disorders. In this context one can mention fever, paroxysmal pain in legs or chest—symptoms that have been included in the concept of the 'periodic syndrome'. Migraine should not be the first thought when a patient

presents with any of these symptoms or signs, but it is useful to know that they may occur in association with paroxysms of migraine, or as separate episodes in some children.

Fever and migraine

The overwhelming majority of patients who present with fever and headache with or without vomiting, abdominal pain *etc.* will have the expected systemic infectious illness. The illness may involve the upper respiratory system, urinary tract, septicemia or meningitis. Possibilities range over the entire field of infectious and para-infectious diseases, and also includes certain intoxications such as atropine poisoning. It is only when the fever is 'unexplained' and occurs in a paroxysmal fashion associated with other more typical symptoms of migraine that it becomes acceptable to regard it as a part of this disorder.

In adults 'slight elevations of fever are common in migraine attacks' (Dalessio 1980). This is perhaps also true of children, but there is little documentation on this point. It is not common for body temperature to be measured in the relatively abbreviated episodes of migraine in this age-group. Fever is most often recorded in the history of patients with the 'periodic syndrome', especially those with the cyclic vomiting variant (Wyllie and Schlesinger 1933, Farquhar 1956). Perhaps this is in part accountable on the basis of the prolonged episodes and the accompanying dehydration in these children. Fever also may be prominent in those patients whose clinical presentation is abdominal pain.

Wyllie and Schlesinger (1933) also called attention to attacks in which fever dominates the clinical picture, without vomiting or abdominal pain but usually with some headache. They state that these episodes usually last two or three days, but may last as long as a fortnight. It is such episodes which test one's credibility, but after other causes of fever have been considered, such a patient may warrant a therapeutic trial of anti-migrainic therapy if episodes are of sufficient frequency.

The body temperature may be significantly elevated up to 102° to 105° F (39° to 40° c) (Wyllie and Schlesinger 1933, Cullen and MacDonald 1963). Most authors who refer to fever and migraine do not specify the degree of elevation (Burke and Peters 1956, Farquhar 1956, Kempton 1956). Fever is also mentioned by the authors who attribute the 'periodic disorder' to epilepsy (Millichap *et al.* 1955, Chao and Davis 1964).

The duration is brief and confined to the time period of the migrainic paroxysm in the usual circumstance. This feature may be of some diagnostic value inasmuch as fever due to infection may not correlate well with other symptoms. Treatment of the symptom, if necessary, may consist of any of the antipyretic preparations.

Paroxysmal leg pain

The prevalence of periodic limb pain in the Cullen and MacDonald (1963) survey of 3440 children was 4.5 per cent. It is a relatively common childhood complaint, most of the time quite non-specific and perhaps frequently a psychosomatic expression.

The benign nature of the complaint is responsible for the concept of 'growing pains', hardly a defensible medical concept, but useful in reporting failure of a better explanation to parents who are usually quite willing to accept this bit of medical sophistry.

In their description of the complex of symptoms in the 'periodic syndrome' Wyllie and Schlesinger (1933) state: 'Limb pains of considerable severity are common, and suggestive of rheumatism'. It is most apparent in the cyclic vomiting syndrome, unusual in abdominal migraine, and rare in association with headache. Paroxysmal leg pain as the major or only complaint as the manifestation of juvenile migraine is possible, but it is a difficult diagnosis to defend. I have occasionally seen patients who have isolated episodic leg pain who also have other migraine syndromes. An adult acquaintance with classic migraine has described episodic throbbing pain in one or both legs that occurs periodically, and bears qualitative resemblance to the throbbing hemicrania he also experiences.

Leg pain in a boy with migraine and confusional episodes
This seven-and-a-half-year-old boy had had episodes of periodic pounding **CASE** headache associated with nausea and stomach ache, usually lasting about **16** 20 to 30 minutes, since age two and a half years. Neurological consultation was prompted by two recent confusional episodes of several hours duration, characterized by screaming, agitation and fear. Of particular interest were episodes of severe pain in the legs, lasting three to four hours, and occasionally associated with headache. Further description of the quality of pain was not forthcoming.

Paroxysmal chest pain
Probably in the same general category as abdominal migraine are the very rare episodes of chest pain one encounters in the migrainic patient. It is a frightening development, because of the rarity of the symptom in children, and concern about myocardial ischemia at any age. The symptom is mentioned in the literature, for example in the Chao and Davis (1964) compilation of symptoms.

Juvenile migraine with an episode of chest pain
This 15-year-old girl was recognized to have physical exertion-related **CASE** abdominal migraine (pain, nausea and vomiting), and occasional **17** headaches. Her mother and grandmother had migraine. On one occasion she reported to the emergency room with severe left-sided chest pain that was accompanied by pallor, diaphoresis and nausea. She also mentioned milder epigastric pain. Physical examination was otherwise normal as was an electrocardiogram. She was treated with Fiorinal, which seemed to enhance recovery.

Comment: A girl with predominantly abdominal migraine presented with one episode of severe chest pain which was probably migrainic in origin.

91

Summary

This chapter has dealt with the major clinical phenomenology of what has been called 'the periodic syndrome'. It has been suggested that this syndrome is in fact another name for juvenile migraine. As such, it seems to me that the term 'migraine' is more specific and therefore preferable. Moreover, it allows for a meaningful separation of the various predominant symptoms, each of which has a somewhat different differential diagnosis and symptomatic therapy.

6
'COMPLEX' AND COMPLICATED MIGRAINE SYNDROMES

Introduction

The visual symptomatology of classic migraine reflects the first order of complexity in the hierarchy of vascular headaches. I have found it useful to designate the occurrence of other focal or multifocal neurologic symptoms or signs by the general term 'complex' whether they occur in the aura or develop later in the paroxysm. By the convention of general usage, neurological signs that develop during the headache phase and/or persist for hours or days beyond the headache, the term 'complicated' migraine is used. This can apply to certain of the visual symptoms of classic migraine such as hemianopsia or a retinal scotoma, as well as to other neurological signs such as hemiparesis or aphasia. If focal signs persist beyond approximately 24 hours, infarction of tissue becomes a serious consideration. This issue is considered in Chapter 7.

Complex migraine is less common than the visual symptoms of classic migraine at any age, but is more frequently seen in younger patients. The paroxysmal event is symptomatic of a structural lesion more often than in common or classic migraine. Consequently these complex syndromes, and especially complicated migraine, dictate a higher index of suspicion of organic disease. They require more extensive investigation than headache alone or headache associated with prodromal visual symptoms.

The following sections deal with the various hemisyndromes, confusional states, symptoms related to brainstem (basilar artery), ophthalmoplegia, and sympathoparesis.

Migrainic hemisyndromes

Definition

The development of unilateral neurologic signs and symptoms such as hemiparesis, aphasia and unilateral numbness associated with migraine headaches has been recognized for many years (Clarke 1910). These symptoms usually occur as part of the prodrome. Less commonly they develop after the vascular headache is well established. The designation usually refers to phenomena of the carotid artery territory, although the most common hemisyndrome in migraine is hemianopsia and hemianopsic scintillating scotomata. These visual symptoms are related to the posterior cerebral circulation, and are of such frequency in migrainic patients as to form a recognized feature of the syndrome of 'classic' migraine.

The symptomatology may not be restricted to the territory of a single cerebral artery in individual episodes. It may begin with visual symptoms (posterior cerebral artery) and then extend to hemiparesis and other symptoms of the middle cerebral artery territory. The most frequent symptom is unilateral numbness of face, arm

93

TABLE X
Migrainic Hemisyndromes

Sex	Age of Onset	Family history	Features	Type*	Trigger	Studies
M	14	+	Sensory Motor	I	—	Angio
M	10	+	Sensory Motor	I	—	CT
M	15	0	Dysarthria Motor	I	Exercise	CT
F	11	0	Visual Sensory	I	Trauma	—
M	12	+	Visual Sensory Dysarthria	I	Exercise	—
M	12	0	Visual Sensory	I	Trauma	—
F	13	+	Visual Sensory Aphasia	I	—	—
F	8	+	Visual Sensory	I	—	—
M	6	+	Sensory (mother with same)	I	—	—
F	12	+	Sensory	I	—	—
F	4	+	Motor	I	Hypoglycemia	—
F	12	+	Visual Aphasia	I + II	Exercise	CT
M	14	+	Sensory Motor Aphasia	I + II	—	CT Angio
F	12	+	Sensory Motor	II	—	CT
M	14	0	Motor Early cyclic vomiting	II	—	Angio
M	12	+	Sensory Motor	II	Exercise	—

Total patients: 16 (male 9, female 7).
Family history of migraine: 12 (75%); Family history of hemisyndrome: 3, 2 in one family.
Triggers: exercise 4, trauma 2, hypoglycemia 1.
*Classification of Whitty (1953): Type I refers to hemisyndrome confined to the aura, Type II in which it either continues into the headache phase or develops during the period of headache.

and less commonly the leg. This distribution is to be distinguished from the more common pattern in migraine, which consists of numbness of peri-oral region and bilateral involvement of hands and lower arms. Unilateral weakness (*i.e.* hemiplegic migraine) is next in frequency, and is what is usually envisaged when one thinks of a migraine hemisyndrome. The occurrence of aphasia is least common, usually occurs together with hemiparesis, and is found when the hemisphere dominant for speech happens to be involved. It is curious that the left hemisphere was affected more frequently than the right in a large series of reported patients with hemiplegic migraine (Bradshaw and Parsons 1965).

Epidemiology

The frequency of hemisyndrome as an expression of migraine in children is not precisely known, although it is one of the commoner complex syndromes. The series where the incidence is mentioned are all biased by selective referral to large pediatric centers, and deal with relatively small numbers of patients. These include 84 patients reported by Prensky and Sommer (1979) where nine (10.7 per cent) patients were affected, the 54 patients of Jay and Tomasi (1981) where four (7 per cent) were affected, and my own series of 300 patients where 16 (5 per cent) were found (Table X). In my own series, the hemisyndrome was confined to the aura in 11 patients, and in the remainder it persisted beyond the aura or developed during the headache phase.

Although the family history of migraine in hemisyndromes is about the same as in juvenile migraine in general, the striking feature of this form of complex migraine is the occurrence of families with hemiplegic migraine (Clarke 1910, Whitty 1953, Bradshaw and Parsons 1965, Bruyn 1968, Glista *et al.* 1975, Jensen *et al.* 1981). Most of these reported families have a stereotyped syndrome of hemiplegia that occurs quite suddenly during the headache phase, and is often accompanied by impaired consciousness (Bruyn 1968). In some, the hemiplegia regularly occurred on the same side in various members of the family (Whitty 1953, Bradshaw and Parsons 1965).

Differential diagnosis

The chief diagnostic concern is usually with the patient who is seen during the first episode, particularly if the hemisyndrome persists for several hours. In almost 60 per cent of patients with hemiplegic migraine, symptoms are of less than one hour in duration and confined to the aura (Bradshaw and Parsons 1965). If prodromal episodes have occurred in the past, are associated with a family history of hemiplegic migraine, and particularly if they have alternated sides or have consisted only of numbness of face and hand, it is usually sufficient to watch and wait without utilizing any reassuring ancillary tests.

However, transient focal vascular symptomatology with associated headache can be symptomatic of tumor or arteriovenous malformation, as well as transient ischemia due to intrinsic disease of the blood-vessel wall, systemic disorder of the clotting mechanism, or inborn metabolic errors such as hyper-cholesterolemia and homocystinuria. More extensive discussion of these issues is undertaken in Chapters 7, 12 and 13.

Another possibility accounting for transient hemiparesis is the postictal state, *i.e.* Todd's paresis. Postictal vascular headache is not uncommon and may add to the diagnostic uncertainty. The history of an immediately preceding convulsion is almost never ambiguous unless it is nocturnal.

Clinical presentation

Hemiplegic migraine is a disorder of the young. Bradshaw and Parsons (1965), in their review of the literature to 1965, found that two-thirds of 36 patients were under the age of 30 when they had their first episode, and in the 75 patients of their

95

own series, the average age of onset was 23 years with a range from 10 to 50 years. The condition is relatively common in adolescent patients. The age range of the 16 patients in my own series is four to 15 years, and most were over age 10 (Table X).

It is most common for the symptoms of the hemisyndrome to occur as a manifestation of the aura, and they are most often confined to this phase of the sequence. They are replaced by contralateral hemicranial headache although the headache may be bilateral, diffuse, or ipsilateral. Other symptoms such as nausea, vomiting, and light-headedness are common.

It is relatively common for the ictus to begin with visual symptoms in the ipsilateral field of vision. Subsequent unilateral sensorimotor symptoms character-istically evolve over a period of a number of minutes and are quite deliberate in their march over the face, arm and leg. This is most dramatic in the case of numbness, but slow progression of weakness of the arm or leg is also characteristic. This is in sharp contrast with the much more rapid march of a seizure which usually takes place in less than a minute. Sensory and motor phenomena frequently occur together and dysarthria is frequent in association with hemiparesis. The hemisyn-drome of the aura rarely lasts more than one hour, and is usually five to 15 minutes in duration.

Aphasia assumes the characteristics of childhood aphasia in general, *i.e.* usually non-fluent in the younger children with an accompanying receptive component, while in older children paraphasic errors, inability to repeat simple phrases, and reading-writing abnormalities are common. Some confusion and disturbance of mental status is frequently found whether or not the patient is aphasic.

Although there is some tendency for the hemisyndrome to recur on the same side, random alternation is the rule. It is usual for the patient to have other varieties of migraine as well, either classic or common in expression. Moreover, although a family history of migraine is as frequent as in juvenile vascular headaches generally, the other affected members only occasionally may have hemisyndromes during the aura.

Beginning with the reports of Whitty (1953) and Blau and Whitty (1955) it has been customary to refer to the generally benign and relatively common group of patients who have hemisyndromes confined to the aura as 'Type I', and other authors have supported this categorization (Ross 1958, Isler 1971). It would seem to be true that mild hemiparetic or hemisensory symptoms of the aura have little more significance than that they involve the carotid territory as contrasted with the posterior cerebral or retinal artery territory of the more common 'classic' expression.

A second variety of presentation is the less common but more troublesome 'Type II' (Whitty 1953). In this variety, hemiparesis and/or aphasia continues into the headache phase or develops during the period of headache. In some patients the symptoms have a biphasic expression during a single episode (see case 18 below).

The duration of symptoms in the second phase is longer and measured in hours, not minutes. The hemisyndrome may persist for one to several days, and may continue well after the headache has subsided (Bradshaw and Parsons 1965). Persistent neurologic signs past 24 hours brings up the question of infarction, a question that is difficult to resolve in the older literature, or in patients in whom angiograms or appropriately timed CT scans have not been done. CT or angiography may be negative even if stroke has occurred. The hemiparesis may become quite dense and proceed to fully developed hemiplegia, a degree of weakness most unusual in the brief hemiparesis that is confined to the aura. Among the patients with the second variety (Type II) of hemiplegic migraine, there may be a striking familial incidence of relatives with hemiplegic migraine as well (see p. 95).

The usual age of onset is in children of approximately eight years and older, and onset is common during adolescence and young adult life. Episodes tend to be infrequent, although periodic common migraine may be interposed with greater frequency. In most patients, the hemisyndrome occurs once or more over the period of six to 12 months and is confined to a relatively brief period in the lifespan of migraine in a given patient.

My personal series (see Table X) of 16 juvenile (age four to 15) patients (which excludes three additional patients who had hemisyndrome and associated migraine in whom infarction occurred) tends to conform to the general expectation as emphasized in the literature and as indicated in the above general discussion. The patients have been separated into two groups, *i.e.* Type I (11 patients) in whom the hemisyndrome was brief and confined to the aura, and Type II (three patients) in whom the hemisyndrome developed during the headache phase and was more prolonged. In two patients there were both Type I and Type II features.

In one of the latter patients (case 18 reported in more detail below) there was a biphasic course in which the initial sensory symptoms occurred as an aura, were replaced by headache, and then recurred as aphasia and hemiparesis on the same side. In another patient there were features of Types I and II (see case 20 below). It is clear that patients do not necessarily separate sharply into the two groups, and that intermediate expressions occur.

There were three patients in the series in whom a family history of hemisyndrome occurred. One was a six-year-old boy with an aura of numbness whose mother had a similar history. The others are sisters, both of whom have visual and hemisensory symptoms during the aura. In neither instance does the clinical description conform to true 'familial hemiplegic migraine' as recorded in the literature. Sexes were about equally distributed in the group and a family history of migraine (75 per cent) was somewhat lower than in my total series of juvenile migraine patients.

My own experience with this group of children would certainly support the greater frequency of hemisyndrome as part of the aura and the generally benign nature of this expression. I would add that in this group of juvenile patients there would seem to be an unexpected frequency of exercise stress (four patients) and minor head trauma (two patients) as precipitating factors.

The three additional patients who had strokes fall into Type II. In two of the three, migraine represented an ancillary risk factor, *i.e.* specifically to mitral valve prolapse and Marfan disease with a redundant aorta. Both of these conditions have familial predilection. It makes one wonder if the observations of higher family incidence of hemisyndromes, and more prolonged and more severe hemisyndromes in some Type II patients, does not represent the clustering of patients in whom migraine is an additional risk factor superimposed upon a variety of other inherited anatomical or metabolic disorders.

Verret and Steele (1971) have called attention to an unusual group of patients in whom attacks of hemiplegia are relatively frequent and begin in infancy as early as three months. This expression has a malignant outcome in that four of their eight patients had residual neurologic signs including intellectual impairment, motor disorder and seizures. It is uncertain whether this syndrome represents a pathogenetically distinct group or whether it represents the extremely malignant expression of ordinary migraine. The relatively benign expression in other family members would favor the latter possibility. Perhaps the early age of onset is accountable for the frequency of enduring signs and presumptive cerebral infarction. These patients are described in more detail in Chapter 7.

The EEG is usually abnormal during the period of hemiplegia. The expected change consists of focal slowing in the theta or delta range of frequencies, usually with high voltage. The abnormality is usually continuous, sometimes periodic, and may be unilateral or asymmetrical with most marked change contralateral to the hemisyndrome (Isler 1971). There may be focal voltage suppression toward the end of the attack. None of these changes are specific to migraine. The EEG reverts to the more normal baseline subsequent to the episode.

CSF may reveal moderate increase in protein and low-grade pleocytosis of four to eight cells (Whitty 1953, Rosenbaum 1960) or more (Symonds 1931, Rossi *et al.* 1984).

Pathogenesis
The principal neurologic phenomenology of hemiplegic migraine relates to the territory of cerebral hemisphere supplied by the carotid artery, principally the middle cerebral branch. Jensen *et al.* (1981) attributed the hemisyndrome in their patients to the vertebro-basilar territory and demonstrated 'marked and prolonged' spasm of the basilar artery in one case. It is noteworthy, however, that the symptoms of a given episode frequently cannot be explained by a single vascular territory as exemplified by the hemianopsic visual symptoms that precede hemisensory symptoms and hemiparesis in some of these patients. This observation is most frequent in patients whose hemisyndrome is confined to the aura (Type I). It lends clinical support to the hypothesis that some factor other than large artery vasospasm may be responsible for the aura, such as Leão's spreading depression (see Chapter 2, p. 23).

It is probable that the biphasic expression, *i.e.* Type I and Type II, is indicative of different pathogenesis in each phase. The more outspoken and enduring symptoms that persist, or develop later in the course of the headache, may have a more complex pathogenesis (see Chapter 2).

Management

The chief issue in the diagnostic assessment of patients with a presumed migrainic hemisyndrome is the question of the need for neuroradiologic studies, with the particular question of tumor or AVM. CT scan is to be recommended for most, with increasing likelihood of positive results in those patients with a hemisyndrome that continues for more than 10 to 20 minutes, extends into or begins during the headache phase, or persists beyond the headache for several hours or more.

Angiography should generally be reserved for patients in whom CT is abnormal and suggests further study, or on the basis of a strongly positive indication such as duration of hemiplegia of 24 hours or longer. Pearce and Foster (1965) in their arteriographic study of 40 patients with complicated migraine included 13 patients with Type II hemisyndromes. In six the neurologic signs were persistent beyond three days. The angiogram was normal in all patients. This experience indicates that the return from angiography will be predictably low. The frequency of angiographic abnormality in symptoms confined to the aura will be even lower especially if the CT scan is normal. If cerebral angiography is done, the patient should be pre-treated with corticosteriods. The possibility of inducing stroke with angiography in migrainic patients is not fully documented, and certainly must be a rare occurrence, but steroid pre-treatment is relatively innocuous and seems a wise precaution (see section on laboratory diagnostic procedures).

If the hemisyndrome persists beyond 24 hours and the question of infarction becomes an issue, the investigative work-up should be extended to include those studies as indicated in the section on migraine and stroke (Chapter 7).

Therapeutic management is not significantly different from the usual approach to the child with vascular headaches, and primarily dependent upon frequency and severity of episodes of all varieties. It is probably wise to recommend daily aspirin therapy on a prophylactic basis for three to six months after prolonged episodes of hemiplegia because of the possibility of cerebro-vascular accident in these patients.

Hemiplegic migraine with aphasia and a bi-phasic course

This 14-year-old boy had had occasional periodic headaches associated **CASE** with nausea that would last about a day and were not particularly **18** troublesome. Three days prior to admission he had a 24-hour period of nausea and vomiting. In mid-morning on the day of admission he experienced the acute onset of numbness and tingling of the right hand that gradually spread up the right arm, then involved the face and the right side of the tongue. After about 30 minutes he developed a severe left-sided headache that centered behind his eye. After an hour the right-sided symptoms subsided but the headache persisted and was associated with vomiting. The tingling of the arm and face recurred after about one hour. Shortly thereafter speech became slurred, weakness developed on the right side and he became aphasic. He was admitted to the hospital for further study.

Family history revealed that his father had had hemianopsic scotomata consisting of flashes of light for a number of years, but it was rare for headache to develop.

The general physical examination was normal, although he was drowsy, inattentive, and aphasic with paraphasic errors and neologisms. Verbal commands were misinterpreted, and he was unable to read with assurance, but was able to write effectively. Cranial nerve function was normal with the exception of a right homonymous hemianopsia. He had a mild right hemiparesis and both plantar responses were extensor. There was no sensory abnormality. A number of studies were done, all of which were normal, including a CT scan, lumbar puncture and left carotid cerebral angiogram.

On the following morning he had improved, although there was some residual right hemiparesis and hemianopsia. Aphasia had entirely cleared although the headache persisted at lesser intensity. Prior to the angiogram he had been treated with methylprednisone, and prednisone 12.5 mg t.i.d. was continued. Propranolol 10 mg q.i.d. was begun. The hemiparesis gradually improved over the period of 24 hours, and the following day it was no longer present.

However later on that day he developed numbness and tingling in the left hand which slowly spread up his left arm and involved the left neck. It lasted about an hour and was followed by a right frontal headache. The headache gradually improved over the course of the day and by the next morning he was entirely asymptomatic with neither headache nor any other neurological complaints.

Propranolol was increased to 20 mg t.i.d., Prednisone was discontinued and he was begun on aspirin one tablet per day. In the following months he remained free of hemiplegia. He had occasional headaches, but only at times when he was irregular about taking propranolol.

Comment: This patient had a biphasic expression of hemiplegic migraine. He developed right-sided hemisensory symptoms in the aura (Type I) replaced by contralateral throbbing headache. During the headache the hemianopsia and hemisensory symptoms recurred, along with aphasia (dyslexia without agraphia) and hemiparesis of about 24 hours duration (Type II). On the day he recovered, he developed a hemisensory aura on the opposite side, *i.e.* the left, which was followed by headache on the right. The vascular territory involved in this major episode probably included both carotid and posterior cerebral arteries on the left, and perhaps some dysfunction on the right side (left extensor plantar) as well.

Hemiplegic migraine

CASE 19   This girl was age 14 when first seen. At age 12 she awakened in the middle of the night with a severe pounding headache. She was able to get back to sleep, but when she awoke in the morning she was numb and weak on the left side of her body. Weakness persisted with gradual improvement over a period of approximately five days. A second similar left-sided episode occurred approximately five months before her initial visit. In addition to the hemiparetic episodes, she had had monthly headaches consisting of a pounding sensation without associated nausea or other symptoms. They occurred about once a month, and were of about one hour in duration.

Her mother had severe migraine headaches occasionally throughout much of her adult life, and an eight-year-old brother also had periodic headaches that were less specific in quality.

Examination revealed no abnormalities, and she had had a normal EEG, a normal technetium brain scan and skull x-ray and a normal spinal fluid examination at the time of her most recent episode of hemiplegia. It was decided that no further studies would be initiated at this time, nor was treatment prescribed.

She did relatively well until seen approximately a year later with the complaint that she had been having much more severe, almost daily, incapacitating headaches for approximately one month. The headache onset was usually during the morning, throbbing in quality and associated with nausea and dizziness. It would last about an hour, and occur from one to two times per day. On the basis of her past history of hemiplegic episodes she was admitted to the hospital for further study which included a CT scan, EEG and skull x-ray all of which were normal. A lumbar puncture revealed a pressure of 130 and a protein of 40 mg per cent.

Treatment with propranolol 10 mg t.i.d. was initiated which resulted in definite improvement. Headaches were mild, and reduced in frequency to one to two times per week with a duration of around 20 minutes. Improvement was sustained throughout the remainder of the school year. Medication was discontinued in the summer and there has been no subsequent follow-up visit.

Comment: This patient with common migraine had two episodes of Type II hemiplegic migraine on the same side during a period of two years. The duration of five days of hemiparesis without residual is noteworthy.

Migraine hemisyndrome with aphasia
This 13-year-old girl had two episodes of difficulty. On the first occasion **CASE** approximately six months before her visit she had been jogging, then **20** bathed and shortly thereafter became dizzy and light-headed. This was accompanied by a disorder of vision in which objects she was viewing would seem to 'break apart' and there were also colored spots throughout her field of vision. She then became aphasic and 'her speech made no sense' although she understood what people were saying to her relatively better. She was nauseated but there was no vomiting or associated headache. After a two- or three-hour period she went to sleep for two hours and awakened with a bitemporal throbbing headache that was gone on the following day.

On a second occasion just prior to her visit she had a similar episode but in addition both hands became numb and she had a headache early in the course. She was nauseous and vomited several times. During this period her speech became abnormal and she was unable to dial the telephone. She was exquisitely sensitive to light and sound. She then went to sleep and was normal on the following day.

She was hospitalized elsewhere on this occasion. She had a normal CT scan, and an EEG which was abnormal with asymmetrical slowing bilaterally with more marked changes in the right temporal region. This had improved on repeat examination several days later. She was treated with amitriptyline 20 mg per day and in the months subsequent to this episode she had no further difficulties.

The family history revealed that her mother had headaches with nausea during childhood into early adult life.

Comment: This girl had complex migrainic episodes on two occasions during a six-month period without any other expression of migraine before, between or since. The first episode was precipitated by physical exercise and began with a bilateral visual aura. After the headache developed she became aphasic for about two hours. The second episode was spontaneous in occurrence but otherwise similar except for the development of bilateral numbness of the hands during the aura. The episodes had both Type I and Type II features.

Hemiplegic migraine

CASE 21 This 14-year-old boy was first seen in October 1972 with a complaint of four episodes of numbness and weakness of his left arm and leg since late June 1972. During the first episode his left arm and leg became numb and weak and this lasted for about an hour followed by spontaneous improvement. There was no headache or associated symptoms.

On 4th July the same year he had a similar episode of left-sided weakness. On this occasion the hemiparesis was followed by a severe right-sided headache centering about the eye, accompanied by blurred vision, nausea and vomiting. The duration of headache was five to eight hours. Hospitalization elsewhere led to studies which included lumbar puncture, electroencephalogram, electrocardiogram, skull x-ray and isotope brain scan. All were negative.

On 16th July 1972 he awakened in the morning with left hemiparesis again followed by headache and vomiting lasting approximately the same length of time. He was hospitalized and had a normal right carotid arteriogram. The diagnosis of hemiplegic migraine was made and treatment with propranolol 20 mg three times a day was begun. This treatment seemed to ameliorate the spells, although on 10th August he had a slight headache during which time his arm became numb, and again on 7th September he had a headache associated with very transient numbness of the hand.

His mother had frontal headaches associated with nausea and a 27-year-old brother also had headaches lasting about 12 hours during which time one eye became swollen. A nine-year-old sister also had occasional mild headaches.

The general physical and neurological examination were all entirely normal.

In July 1973 it was learned by telephone that in the intervening period he had had only one brief episode in late October 1972. However, the reason for the call was the fact that while at camp he fell and struck his head. After a five to 10 minute asymptomatic interval, he had a 24-hour period of amnesia, dizziness and vomiting. He subsequently recovered totally from this incident.

Comment: This boy had a number of Type I hemiparetic episodes with and without headache during a four-month period, all on the same side. The following summer, he had a post-traumatic amnesic confusional state.

Basilar artery migraine

Definition

Bickerstaff (1961) described this syndrome in the early 1960s. Basilar artery migraine has been an established, frequently confirmed 'complicated' manifestation of migraine since that time. The central core of the clinical problem consists of a complex of cranial nerve, cerebellar, and corticobulbospinal signs that vary greatly from patient to patient, together with visual symptomatology attributable to the territory of the posterior cerebral artery, the terminal bifurcation of the basilar.

Any combination of signs and symptoms related to the tissue supplied by the basilar-vertebral system is possible. The unequivocal examples include patients who have signs that could only result from dysfunction of a sizeable extent of brainstem. If this restriction is applied, the majority of patients tend to be adolescent or pre-adolescent females as Bickerstaff first reported. However, migraine headaches are frequently associated with symptoms attributable to functions within the basilar artery territory such as vertigo and other distortions of equilibrium, most instances of syncope, and the visual scotomata that are the hallmark of 'classic' migraine. Lapkin and Golden (1978) have recognized this issue and have accepted cases with a single brainstem symptom in their series of 30 childhood cases, 23 of whom were collected in the short space of 18 months. The patients were divided into three groups, based on one, two and three or more basilar symptoms.

The diagnosis then becomes a matter of definition, with group 3 (in which patients had three or more brainstem symptoms) conforming to the more commonly accepted concept of the disorder. The inclusive concept has merit and certainly calls attention to the special vulnerability of the basilar artery system in migraine. Nevertheless, the features of the fully-developed syndrome are sufficiently distinctive to warrant special categorization for purposes of diagnosis and management. It is the expression with three or more signs that will be considered in this section.

Epidemiology

Estimation of the incidence of basilar artery migraine is heavily dependent upon one's definition. If one accepts the Lapkin and Golden (1978) concept then the incidence is very high in juvenile migraine. For example Watson and Steele (1974) found an incidence of vertigo in 23 per cent of their patients, and in my own series the incidence of vertigo and the closely related symptom of giddiness was 19 per cent.

However, the more restricted definition that requires several symptoms or signs is probably more useful. With this definition my own series includes seven patients (2.3 per cent) while that of Jay and Tomasi (1981) indicates an incidence of 3.7 per cent.

Bickerstaff (1961) emphasized the unusual frequency in girls in late childhood and adolescence. Most subsequent reports have tended to confirm this point (Golden and French 1975). In a study that includes several adult patients, all of the adults were women and only two of 12 were pre-pubertal boys (Swanson and Vick 1978). Lapkin and Golden (1978), however, in a review of 30 childhood cases with their broader definition of the syndrome, found an almost equal incidence in either sex. As indicated above, this report included patients who had only one or two basilar territory symptoms such as vertigo or visual phenomena, and is therefore open to argument with those who would apply a more restrictive definition to the syndrome of basilar migraine.

Although more data is probably necessary, the following demographic points can be made with regard to patients with three or more basilar symptoms: (i) age of onset can range from infancy to middle adult years, (ii) strong female predominance from puberty onwards, and (iii) lesser female bias in the younger pre-pubertal patients, who also are less likely to have evidence of headache as an index clue to the migrainic nature of their disorder. Familial occurrence of fully developed basilar migraine must be most rare indeed and has not been formally reported, although a family with several affected members has come to my attention.

Differential diagnosis
Although transient (lasting minutes to hours), recurring brainstem signs associated with headache in a patient with a family history of vascular headaches are highly likely to represent migraine. The physician is faced with a clinical problem in which serious, life-threatening, and in some instances remediable alternate diagnoses must be considered. Possibilities include other causes of transient ischemic vascular events of childhood, congenital malformation at the base of the brain and calvarium, tumor, certain intoxications and inborn metabolic disorders. For discussion of childhood vascular disease, the reader is referred to the section on stroke in Chapter 12.

Congenital malformations, which early in their course may give rise to transient neurologic symptoms and signs referrable to the brainstem, include: bony abnormalities of odontoid, platybasia and basilar impression, and the Chiari malformation of caudal brainstem. This category is of special importance because of the possibility of remediation in many.

Most posterior fossa tumors present with a sub-acutely evolving, relentlessly progressive course. Except for infiltrating lesions of the brainstem, the clinical presentation is dominated by symptoms and signs of raised intracranial pressure. This typical presentation will not be confused with migraine. However, one particular tumor is biologically unusual in that it consists of both vascular and neural elements, with the characteristic of slow growth if it grows at all. These tumors (perhaps better designated as hamartomas), are frequently located in the brainstem (the other favored site is thalamus), and tend to occur in pubertal and adolescent patients. There is a tendency to relapsing/remitting symptoms that may occur at widely spaced intervals early in the course, possibly related to transient low-grade edema or episodes of minimal bleeding. The exacerbations are most often several weeks or longer in duration, in a course more reminiscent of multiple sclerosis than the brief episodes of migraine, but confusion could arise (Abroms *et al.* 1971).

Several metabolic disorders such as pyruvate decarboxylase deficiency, Hartnup disease and Leigh's disease, all may present as a syndrome of intermittent ataxia and are sufficiently reminiscent of basilar migraine to warrant consideration. One should also consider the organic acidemias and disorders of the urea cycle, particularly if the clinical presentation involves impaired awareness or seizures (see Chapter 13).

Clinical features
The clinical presentation of basilar artery migraine is variable among patients, but there is a tendency for each episode to be similar in a given patient. The hallmark of the disorder is the development of symptoms and signs of multiple cranial nerve dysfunction, together with truncal or appendicular ataxia, and weakness related to the bulbocorticospinal system. The weakness may be hemiplegic, diplegic, or quadriplegic. Dysarthria is common. The leading cranial nerves are vestibular, auditory (tinnitus), oculomotor, abducens, facial and less commonly glosso-pharyngeal and vagus. Visual symptoms are common and are usually first in the sequence of development. They consist of dimming of vision that may become almost total blindness. Bickerstaff (1962) has made the point that if there are positive phenomena, they consist of 'flashes or blobs of light', rather than the more formed fortification spectra. Hemianopsic scotomata are also recorded. Additional ocular signs include nystagmus, and less commonly inter-nuclear ophthalmoplegia.

In fact, all one needs is a concept of the physiological anatomy of the brainstem and occipital cortex to give one a perspective of the possibilities. Clinically, the most useful symptoms are the visual scotomata: if these are present, and the patient is old enough to describe the characteristic migrainic scotomata. they may be taken as a positive indication of migraine, and perhaps spare the patient some aspects of the extensive diagnostic studies that may otherwise be necessary.

Consciousness is impaired in some instances. Patients may become stuporous, sometimes proceeding to light coma. These developments usually occur late in the sequence (Lee and Lance 1977). Syncope is fairly common, and true seizures that are triggered by the migrainic paroxysm have been described (Bickerstaff 1962).

Basilar-vertebral signs and symptoms are usually phenomena of the prodrome, and characteristically precede the development of headache. They last for minutes to a portion of an hour, and are replaced by throbbing headache with associated nausea and vomiting. Headache is frequently occipital in location if it can be localized at all. Some patients, especially the very young, seem to have little or no headache. Such patients can be worrisome particularly if there is no family history of vascular headaches.

In a number of recorded patients, the brainstem signs develop after the headache is well established, perhaps after visual scotomata have occurred in their proper sequence in the aura. Such occurrence is reminiscent of similar late occurrence of complex phenomena in the carotid territory (*i.e.* Type II hemiplegic migraine). In these patient the signs tend to be more persistent, and last for hours or as long as several days.

The EEG recorded during or shortly after the episode will show delta or theta slowing in the posterior leads as the most typical expression (Lapkin *et al.* 1977), but may also show epileptiform activity (Swanson and Vick 1978). Some patients, who are more fully discussed in Chapter 7, have severe and almost continuous EEG abnormality while eyes are closed, together with susceptibility to occasional seizures during episodes of migraine involving the basilar territory (Camfield *et al.* 1978).

Despite the dramatic and frightening symptomatology and signs, residual impairment is very rare. There are a few recorded examples of mild persistent signs. They are more likely in the variety of attack that appears late after the development of headache.

The possibility of early onset is well made by Lapkin and Golden (1978) who include a patient of age seven months. These authors found a uniform age-distribution to 14 years with the mean at age seven. Fully 20 per cent of patients in this series had no headache.

The periodicity of basilar involvement in susceptible patients is highly variable. It is usual for complex episodes to occur in a setting of pre-existing vascular headaches. Certain of the younger patients have a complex episode on the first, or first few occasions of their migraine career. There is also a tendency for basilar episodes to occur in series over a period of a number of months to a year and then become a lesser problem after the adult pattern of headache for the individual evolves. In the usual susceptible patient, fully developed basilar migraine is an uncommon event.

Pathogenesis
Pathogenesis of this sub-category of migraine is not different from the usual complex or complicated phenomenology in migrainic patients. The symptoms and signs tend to fall within a vascular territory and the frequency of cortical-visual symptoms in addition to the involvement of brainstem is consistent with the vertebral-basilar artery basis of the event. Basilar-vertebral symptoms have the usual biphasic expression of complex migraine, *i.e.* the largest number are relatively brief and part of the prodrome, while some persist for many hours or days and/or tend to begin during the peak of the headache (see Chapter 2, p. 26).

Management

Proper management begins with a solid diagnosis. This is achieved by exclusion of certain other possibilities. CT scan with special attention to the posterior fossa is clearly necessary, as are x-rays of the cervical spine and odontoid process.

Vertebral arteriography with prophylactic corticosteroid therapy may be appropriate, depending upon the clinical circumstances. It should probably be done in most instances when the episodes are of hours or days in duration and accompanied by multiple cranial nerve and long tract signs. When they are brief, confined to the prodrome and followed by throbbing headache in a patient with a strong family history, arteriography can be deferred, perhaps indefinitely. This invasive procedure should not be proposed in those patients with limited basilar symptomatology such as vertigo, most visual symptoms and other symptoms that were categorized as group 1 and 2 of Lapkin and Golden (1978). It is this practical issue that argues most tellingly against expanding the concept of the syndrome beyond Bickerstaff's original definition, however sound the theoretical concept may be.

Metabolic studies, toxic screening, and work-up of circulatory vascular factors should be undertaken on appropriate indication, based upon possibilities as outlined in the discussion of differential diagnosis.

Pharmacotherapy is based on the usual principles, continuous if all manifestations of juvenile migraine are of sufficient frequency, and probably in those in whom multiple basilar symptomatology occurs more often than once in two to three months. Swanson and Vick (1978) were particularly successful with continuous phenytoin in this group of patients. Although a number were adults, this observation should be kept in mind when choosing pharmacotherapeutic agents. The use of caffeine-ergot preparations may be useful in those individuals where either the aura is prolonged or if the basilar signs occur late in the episode. Finally it is reasonable to consider continuous low-dose aspirin for those patients who may be at risk of stroke, *i.e.* those whose symptoms are prolonged and develop late in the sequence.

Basilar artery migraine

This young girl of Azorean background was nine years old when first seen **CASE** for two complaints of the previous six months. The first was an incident of **22** fainting during a hot day in church, and then on three subsequent occasions she had episodes of head and stomach pain during which she screamed and cried and seemed feverish. The spells lasted from 10 to 30 minutes. During this six-month period she had also had more frequent episodes, consisting of poorly localized throbbing headache of lesser severity and about the same duration, some of which awakened her at night.

Past history was uneventful except for an episode when she was about five, when she was struck by a falling light fixture and fainted. The injury was of no serious consequence. She had developed normally and was doing well in the fourth grade in school.

Family history was incomplete because of parental separation for a number of years. Mother denied headache and knew little of the father and his family. Subsequently her 12-year-old brother was seen for psychogenic tic. In the course of attention for the presenting problem, a history of occasional throbbing headache with nausea and two episodes of abdominal pain with nausea and vomiting was obtained. It was believed that these complaints represented juvenile migraine.

After office evaluation she was believed to have juvenile migraine and syncope. Phenobarbital 30 mg b.i.d. was begun which was increased to three times a day when she had an episode of abdominal pain about three weeks later. During this episode her speech was noticeably slow and difficult to understand but was entirely sensible. Five days later she had a two-hour episode during which she could not speak at all, seemed confused but was responsive. When seen locally a diagnosis of otitis media was made and treatment with penicillin was initiated. Two days later she complained of pain centered about the right eye, loss of vision, and she developed a noticeable strabismus and unsteadiness of gait.

Admission to CHMC Boston was arranged. During her first hours in the hospital her condition altered between neurologic normality and periods of gross neurologic abnormality consisting of bilateral abducens palsy, anarthria, and truncal plus appendicular ataxia with intention myoclonus. Vision was impaired especially in the right visual field. She was able to follow commands but seemed somewhat confused. The following morning she was initally well and then had another personally observed episode which included a right peripheral facial weakness along with the other signs. It lasted the better part of an hour.

During this episode an EEG was arranged which showed asymmetrical posterior quadrant delta slowing, more on the right. Other studies during the hospitalization included a normal Technetium-99 brain scan, and a normal CSF examination. Four vessel arteriography was normal.

It was concluded that she had had a cluster of basilar migraine attacks. She was discharged to continue phenobarbital to which methysergide 2 mg b.i.d was added. Subsequent to this admission she did well except for a few mild episodes of headache and stomach ache. Methysergide was discontinued after three months.

She had no subsequent episodes of basilar artery insufficiency. On two occasions in the following year she had episodes of severe throbbing headache with syncope. The first was two months after methysergide was discontinued and it was resumed for a three-month period. During the second follow-up year she had only rare mild headaches.

Phenobarbital was discontinued on a slow reduction schedule after two years without difficulty.

Follow-up information has extended to four years subsequent to the initial visit and during that period she did well.

Comment: This girl had classical episodes of basilar artery migraine, together with other manifestations of juvenile migraine, *i.e.* periodic throbbing headache and episodic abdominal pain. The several basilar episodes were clustered during a period of several months, probably interrupted by methisergide, and did not recur.

Confusional migraine
Definition
Some element of mental confusion has been recognized in certain patients during migraine attacks for many years, although it is not particularly common. Lance and Anthony (1966) report an incidence of 6.8 per cent of 500 patients who became disoriented and confused to some extent during some aspects of their migrainic experience. In 1970, Gascon and Barlow reported that in some young patients an acute confusional state with amnesia could be the major feature of the presentation of a juvenile migraine syndrome. This was confirmed in several publications (Emery 1977, Ehyai and Fenichel 1978). A recent case report entitled *Transient Global Amnesia in Childhood* by T. S. Jensen (1980) emphasizes that memory disturbance and amnesia for the event may occur in relative isolation.

Epidemiology
The first indication of the frequency of confusional state as a manifestation of juvenile migraine was in the report of Ehyai and Fenichel (1978) who described a 5 per cent incidence in a series of 100 patients. In my own 300 patients the incidence was also 5 per cent including three in whom amnesia was more prominent than confusion. 14 of the 15 patients were boys between eight and 16 years of age. In six of these episodes, the confusional or amnesic state was precipitated by minor head trauma as first reported by Emery (1977).

The greater frequency in boys is apparent in all reports. It is partially explained by their more violent sports and play activities in those episodes precipitated by trauma, but male predominance still pertains in the remaining patients.

Differential diagnosis
The range of diagnostic possibilities in a child presenting with an acute agitated confusional state is wide, and only rarely is migraine the answer. Much more commonly the cause is intoxication with various drugs that have been accidentally ingested or used for thrills, either of which may be the case in the five to 15 age-group where migrainic confusional states are most common. Occasionally physician-prescribed medication is at fault. The value of the usual 'toxic screen' of blood is limited and may be only about 50 per cent effective in identifying the offending substance. Careful history of available medication in the household and of street drug opportunities (usually after the confusion has cleared) is often necessary.

Metabolic encephalopathies must also be considered. Reye's syndrome in its early phase is characterized by disordered mental status, hyperventilation, nausea and vomiting. Elevated blood ammonia, prolonged prothrombin time and other abnormal liver function tests will lead to a correct diagnosis. Hypoglycemic encephalopathy is also a possibility as are other rare causes of episodic metabolic aberrations of urea, amino acids and organic acids.

Viral encephalitis can present with confusion and agitation without significant fever or nuchal rigidity. Examination of CSF is therefore important in assessing the problem, and any elevation of leucocytes or protein favors a process other than juvenile migraine, although CSF protein may be transiently elevated in complex migraine syndromes, and pleocytosis has been recorded. Fever has been described in migraine in children, but has not been noted in those with confusional state. The presence of fever is nevertheless a strong point against migraine and in favor of an infectious process. The longer duration of encephalitis will usually settle the issue after the first 24 hours.

An additional point of differential consideration is seizure disorder. Post-seizure confusion is common, agitation is less often encountered. The duration of the postictal state is not as long as in most instances of confusional migraine. Moreover, the history of the convulsion is only rarely ambiguous. The clinical manifestations of *petit mal* and temporal lobe status epilepticus and electrical stupor, however, may be altogether similar to confusional migraine. The strongest clue in these cases is the known presence of convulsive disorder. Only rarely is minor status epilepticus the first or only manifestation of convulsive disorder. An EEG showing continuous discharge during the episode is the key feature of the diagnosis. The EEG in confusional migraine is usually abnormal. The abnormality consists of theta or delta slowing, which may be relatively focal and lateralized with temporo-parietal and occipital distributions.

An acute psychogenic panic state, acute schizophrenic reaction or the manic state of polar mood disorder may figure in the differential diagnosis of some children. In my experience these disorders are not as common as most of the diagnostic concerns indentified above: nor do they usually pose a serious differential problem. With the exception of the acute anxiety state, the onset is more gradual and the behavioral change occurs over several days at least. Moreover, in all of these psychiatric entities, orientation and intellectual functions including memory are better preserved and attention is better sustained. They all share with confusional migraine the feature of agitation. In exceptional instances differentiation may be impossible until the migrainic confusional state subsides rather suddenly, which it will do in less than 12 to 24 hours as a rule. The patient will then be normal, unlike the children with the psychiatric disorders mentioned above, with the possible exception of those with a panic reaction. The EEG will be relatively normal in the psychiatric disorders, another helpful distinction.

Clinical presentation
A point to emphasize is the insignificance of headache in the clinical picture. In only about half of the patients is it present, sometimes quite mild, or only recalled or mentioned as the confusion subsides. When present, it is not different from the usual expression of vascular headaches in childhood. The headache may be unilateral, and may be preceded by aura and accompanied by more ordinary migrainic symptoms such as dizziness and nausea and vomiting.

The confusional state, consisting of inattention, distractibility and inability to maintain a reasonable and coherent stream of speech or action, is compounded by agitation and disturbance of memory. It is either the first evidence of abnormality, or develops after the headache is established. Typically the period of confusion lasts several hours, although it may be as brief as 10 minutes or as prolonged as two days. Six to eight hours is about average, beginning sometime during the day, interrupted by nocturnal sleep, and absent or minimally present the following morning. It may wax and wane throughout the time course.

Patients are often quite agitated and even combative and violent (Brott and Leviton 1976). Pharmacologic and occasionally physical constraint may be necessary. Tremulousness is common, and fear and perplexity are manifest. Disorientation may be either complete or partial. In some instances the disorder of mental status progresses to a stuporous state (Lee and Lance 1977), from which a confused and disoriented patient can be relatively easily aroused. If stupor is manifested in an attack it is often associated with brainstem signs, an indication of the potential for involvement of the basilar-vertebral system in this syndrome (Lee and Lance 1977).

The patient is typically fluent in language production and obscenity is fairly common. There may be dysnomia or more definitive evidences of aphasic disorders of language such as paraphasic errors, but true aphasic phenomenology is uncommon.

In a few patients amnesia and memory disorder dominate the clinical presentation, so much so that 'transient global amnesia' becomes an appropriate description. However, there is probably little advantage in identifying such patients separately from the more common predominately confused and agitated patients. It only serves to add a distracting element to a troublesome clinical problem of older adult patients that has a different pathogenesis in most instances, although migraine is a recognized possibility in some adult patients as well (Olivarius and Jensen 1979, Crowell et al. 1984).

Confusional episodes tend to be rare events in the long-term course of a susceptible child or adolescent. Single episodes are common, and may be the first clinically significant manifestation of migraine. Emery (1977) has called attention to minor head trauma as a precipitating event in two of his four recorded patients. He makes the point that trauma in these cases was relatively trivial, not associated with loss of consciousness, and that there was an asymptomatic period of 30 to 60 minutes before confusion developed. He correctly calls attention to the similarity of this issue to the trauma-precipitated complex migrainic symptoms that are dealt with elsewhere in this monograph.

It is likely that many episodes of post-traumatic confusion in childhood are really not 'mild concussion', but expressions of migraine. The history of periodic headache in the child, positive family history of migraine and the important clinical clue of a latent interval between injury and symptoms should help resolve this question in an individual patient. In the acute situation the latent interval also serves to raise the more serious question of the possibility of subdural or epidural bleeding, only to be resolved in most circumstances by CT scanning (see Chapter 10).

Pathogenesis
A confusional state is a complication of the developed pathophysiologic state, not the prodrome. Discussion of this issue is dealt with elsewhere with regard to the pathogenesis of migraine. In contrast with our earlier speculations about the reticular activating system as the site of disturbance, I now believe that both Emery (1977) and Ehyai and Fenichel (1978) are correct in their emphasis on the carotid territory, particularly in view of the relevant observations of Mesulam *et al.* (1976) relating acute confusional state to right middle cerebral artery infarction in adults. In fact the clinical and EEG indications suggest that there is potential for involvement of several arterial territories including the vertebral basilar (Lee and Lance 1977). Moreover, the process is not infrequently bilateral, although asymmetrical based on EEG evidence in particular. Memory disorder probably relates to bilateral temporal lobe and hippocampal dysfunction, areas in the territory of terminal posterior cerebral or the choroidal artery.

Management
The time of the first acute incident is dominated at the outset by consideration of the differential diagnostic possibilities and appropriate ancillary procedures. The only secure answer usually comes when the episode subsides, often rather abruptly or more commonly after sleep. At this point the proper diagnosis can be made.

Ancillary laboratory studies that are appropriate early in the incident include a toxic screen of blood and urine to detect possible exogenous ingestion. As mentioned earlier, the usual available testing in this regard may overlook as many as 50 per cent of the agents for various reasons, and negative results cannot be taken as a final answer. Certain street drugs such as phencyclidine ('angel dust') may not be detected. The history, which may not be obtainable until after recovery and then may be unreliable, is a key element in the evaluation of the possibility of toxic reaction.

Metabolic studies should include a full battery of electrolytes, blood ammonia, BUN, lactate-pyruvate and tests of liver function. T_3 and T_4 or other measurements of thyroid function are indicated in some patients.

CSF should be examined and CT scan is also appropriate. The EEG may be most helpful. Fast activity in the beta range of frequency usually indicates drug ingestion, while diffuse symmetrical slow waves are found in many organic pathologies and may reflect encephalitis, intoxication or metabolic disorder. EEG slowing is also consistent with confusional migraine, although in migraine during complicated episodes it is more often asymmetrical or relatively focal with episodic slow waves. Epileptic confusional state is indicated by almost continuous discharges of various morphologies. Any striking EEG abnormality is inconsistent with psychiatric disorders.

Decision regarding continuous therapy is based on the frequency and severity of common migrainic symptoms. The agitation may be sufficient during the acute phase to require IM phenothiazine or perhaps oral or rectal paraldehyde.

Confusional migraine

This 11-year-old boy had had occasional headaches over the previous three to four years. They were periodic, associated with nausea and vomiting and occurred every two to three months. On the morning of admission, he complained of a mild occipital headache that had been preceded by diplopia and vertigo. Later that morning his mother found him to be disoriented and not making sense. He vomited several times and was brought to the emergency room for evaluation. His general physical examination was entirely normal with a normal temperature. He was relatively unco-operative, tended toward drowsiness and indicated that he wanted to be left alone. He acknowledged that he had a headache and pointed to his chin. There was difficulty in word-finding and some misnaming. Memory was defective. Cranial nerve function was entirely normal including fundi, as were reflexes, strength, co-ordination, sensory system and gait.

The family history revealed that there were migraine headaches on both the paternal and maternal side of his family.

A number of laboratory examinations were done including normal SGOT, LDH and ammonia level. A Technetium-99 flow study was done which showed normal flow and a normal static study. An electroencephalogram on the day of admission showed paroxysmal generalized bursts and slow background especially on the left. Toxic screen revealed no indication of ingested medication or other substances.

After six to eight hours the confusional state lifted. He became totally lucid, fully oriented and had no complaint of headache. He had only fragmentary memory of the day.

A repeat EEG on the second day revealed considerable improvement with some residual bilateral posterior slowing with left hemisphere predominance.

He was discharged to take phenobarbital 30 mg b.i.d. with the presumptive diagnosis of confusional migraine.

On follow-up four months later, he had had no severe headaches and only a few mild headaches without associated nausea and vomiting. Phenobarbital was continued for the duration of the school year and discontinued in the summer.

He had no subsequent difficulties until approximately one and a half years later at age 12 and a half, when he fell in gym without striking his head and subsequently developed a period of similar confusion which lasted a number of hours. He had another episode at age 15 when he fell down several steps and struck his head. This was followed by bizarre and confused behavior, headache and vomiting. He was admitted to a local hospital and on the following day he was entirely normal.

Comment: This boy had three episodes of confusional state associated with other migrainic symptomatology: one was spontaneous and two were precipitated by mild head trauma.

Confusional migraine

CASE
24

This young man was 16 years when first seen, and had had headaches since age 12. They occurred about twice a week, were bitemporal in location, and if severe they had a throbbing quality and were associated with nausea. The more severe headaches occurred once or twice a month.

Two months prior to his visit he had an episode in the evening while out with friends during which he became incoherent, was apparently hallucinating and said he was confused and 'couldn't control his thoughts'. He had alternate feelings of heat and cold, was nauseous and vomited although he did not remember headache. He was admitted to the hospital and after about six hours he improved, slept through the night and felt very much better the following day. A toxic screen for drugs and other substances was negative but no other examinations were made at that time. This was believed to represent a 'psychotic episode', presumably schizophrenic, and he had been receiving psychotherapy since the hospitalization. He was being treated with chlorpromazine 100 mg per day. Subsequent to the episode his school work fell off. He felt under increased pressure and was tense and nervous.

The family history revealed that his mother and maternal grandmother had periodic throbbing headaches associated with nausea.

General physical and neurological examinations were entirely normal.

The headaches and the episode of confusion were interpreted to be migraine and he was treated with propranolol 20 mg three times a day. chlorpromazine was discontinued. With this regimen his headaches became less frequent and less severe. In the intervening three years of follow-up there have been periods of more active headaches usually responsive to propranolol administration. There has not been another episode of confusion, and there is no indication of personality disorder.

Laboratory examinations consisted of a normal EEG and subsequently a normal CT scan. The latter was done because his mother developed a seizure disorder, and was found to have an AV malformation, which raised the question of a structural basis for the boy's headache problem as well.

Comment: This young man with common migraine had a single confusional episode which was incorrectly interpreted as an acute schizophrenic 'break'.

Transient global amnesia

CASE
25

This 14-year-old boy was admitted to the hospital with the complaint of acute memory loss. On the day of admission, approximately 20 minutes after beginning a soccer game, he stopped in the middle of the field and said 'What am I doing here?' At this time he was unable to recall any of the events of the day and was transported to a local hospital. Later that day he was transferred to CH, Boston. In retrospect his coach and team-mates noted that two minutes before the onset of amnesia he had taken two head balls and may have also had some head contact with another player.

Family history revealed that a paternal grandfather had severe migraine and there was probable migraine in the patient's father and brother.

Review of past history revealed that between ages six and 12 he had had a number of mild head traumas which were complicated by transient amnesia of less than an hour in duration. Birth and development and other aspects of past history were normal. He was a good student in the ninth grade. There was no history of drug abuse.

On examination he was slightly irritable and perplexed. There were no general physical abnormalities except a tender sterno-cleido-mastoid muscle and a complaint of neck pain. Neurologic abnormalities were confined to mental status. He was oriented to year but not month or day. When told the date and questioned again a short time later he did not remember. He had no understanding of why he was in the hospital nor memory of the events of the entire day. Speech, language, writing, reading, praxis in construction were all good and he did serial sevens well. He was better when awakened in the middle of the night but unable to remember the period shortly after the beginning of the soccer game until 8.30 p.m. On the following day he felt well. He did not develop headache at any time but the history was obtained that for a number of years he had had occasional headaches, some sufficiently severe for him to lie down. There was no associated nausea or vomiting.

Work-up consisted of a normal CT scan, a normal EEG including nasopharyngeal leads, and a normal toxic screen.

No treatment was instituted.

Comment: This boy from a migrainic family had a number of episodes of global amnesia subsequent to minor head trauma.

Ophthalmoplegic migraine

Definition

One of the earliest recognized 'complicated' migraine syndromes was ophthalmoplegic migraine. The association of a third nerve palsy that develops during or after ipsilateral orbital, peri-orbital, or temporal headache was recorded by several 19th-century authors. It was not until the development of cerebral arteriography that the crucial distinction between migraine and congenital berry aneurysm of the circle of Willis could be made. Today, the diagnosis of ophthalmoplegic migraine requires negative arteriography.

Epidemiology

Ophthalmoplegic migraine is probably the least common of the well-known complex syndromes. Perhaps the best indication of its frequency is the study by Friedman *et al.* (1962*b*) in which eight cases were found in over 5000 patients with migraine. In the Pearce and Foster (1965) series of 40 patients with complicated migraine, only one had overt oculomotor nerve palsy, although an additional patient had abducens palsy and several others mentioned diplopia during attacks.

115

In my experience of 300 patients, there were two patients who had the disorder, one had a single episode at age 12, and the other (case 27 below) had early onset and multiple episodes.

Several authors have stated that a family history of migraine is less frequent in patients with ophthalmoplegic migraine (Walsh and Hoyt 1969). Both of my patients had a positive family history, but in the eight patients reported by Friedman *et al.* (1962*b*) only three had a family history of migraine.

Differential diagnosis

The differential diagnosis of third nerve palsy at the time of first presentation requires consideration of a wide range of possibilities. These include congenital berry aneurysm, tumor, trauma, sinusitis, basilar meningitis and non-specific orbital inflammation (the Tolosa Hunt syndrome of painful ophthalmoplegia). Clinical features are usually present that permit a relatively high degree of confidence in separating ophthalmoplegic migraine from most of the other entities.

Where in adult practice the issue of ischemic infarction of the third cranial nerve, usually associated with diabetes mellitus (Green *et al.* 1964), is the most common single reason for the development of an isolated third nerve palsy, this entity is almost unknown in children, and then only after recognized juvenile diabetes of long standing.

Myasthenia gravis, which may occur at any age with ptosis as the most prominent sign, has only a superficial resemblance to third nerve palsy. Features such as bilaterality, the common association with orbicularis weakness (a seventh nerve function) or weakness of anterior neck flexion, a pattern of diplopia or ocular movement palsy inconsistent with third nerve innervation, and especially the presence of a dilated and sluggish or fixed pupil in third nerve palsy, usually settle the issue. If there is any ambiguity, the ptosis usually recovers dramatically with intravenous edrophonium chloride (Tensilon) administration in myasthenia gravis.

Entities in which true third nerve palsy occurs may present more of a diagnostic problem, chiefly those in which there is associated headache or painful discomfort, although painless ophthalmoplegia can occur in most, including juvenile migraine. Certainly a clinically provocative finding that suggests a cause other than ophthalmoplegic migraine is any sign of dysfunction of adjacent cranial nerves, such as depressed corneal reflex, abnormal facial sensation and abducens palsy, althogh involvement of other cranial nerves (trochlear, abducens and trigeminal) is known to occur in ophthalmoplegic migraine (Walsh and O'Doherty 1960, Friedman *et al.* 1962*b*, Loewenfeld 1980).

Tumor, trauma and inflammation are responsible for the majority of the third nerve palsies of childhood. No statistics are available for the age of childhood alone but Green *et al.* (1964) have prepared an excellent review of 130 patients that covers the full age spectrum. Tumor represents only a small fraction (3.8 per cent) of this series. Experience indicates that it is relatively higher in children, where most are related to infiltrating gliomas of the brainstem. These tumors are accompanied by other cranial nerve findings as well as signs of dysfunction in the corticospinal and cerebellar systems. They are seldom associated with head pain.

They usually pose no diagnostic problem *vis-à-vis* ophthalmoplegic migraine because of their progressive course rather than periodic expression. Very occasionally a single cranial nerve is the first manifestation of a brainstem tumor and months may elapse before the next sign develops. Extra-axial tumors of the parasellar region, leukemic infiltration, and tumors infiltrating the basis of the occipital or the temporal bone are more likely to pose a diagnostic problem. These patients more often have associated ipsilateral pain and headache.

There are several reports in which mucocele of the sphenoid sinus has produced periodic headaches associated with recurrent third nerve palsy in a syndrome that closely imitates ophthalmoplegic migraine (Herman and Hall 1944, Norman and Yanagisawa 1964, Hayes and Creston 1974). Unilateral periodic headache behind or around the eye had occurred for a number of years before it was associated with intermittent then persistent third nerve palsy. Duration of headache was characteristically several days. Certain distinguishing clinical features were apparent. These included chronic post-nasal drip, recurrent episodes of acute sinusitis and provocative inverse relationship between nasal and post-nasal drainage and the development and relief of headache. The headache was sometimes relieved by nasal decongestants, and was often present upon awakening.

Blunt head trauma is a fairly frequent cause of isolated third nerve palsy in the young, 10.8 per cent in the Green *et al.* (1964) series. No age is exempt, and post-traumatic headache is a frequent concomitant symptom. However, significant head trauma is so prominent in the history that the question of migraine does not seriously enter into the differential consideration. Nor has there been any implication that trauma triggers post-traumatic migrainic vasomotor reaction leading to ophthalmoplegia as is the case in other complex migraine syndromes such as cortical blindness, hemiplegia and confusional states (see Chapter 10).

Another important category of childhood third nerve palsy is inflammation. Most often the process is granulomatous basilar meningitis, the prototype being tuberculous meningitis, although less virulent organisms are more likely to be diagnostically troublesome. Systemic illness and mild to moderate meningeal signs are the key clinical features of these illnesses. Sinusitis with or without mucocoel is also an occasional cause of associated oculomotor nerve palsy in the young. The association with headache and the possibility of remission and exacerbation brings sinusitis into serious consideration in the differential diagnosis. Appropriate treatment of the sinusitis leads to full restoration of nerve function.

The Tolosa Hunt syndrome of painful ophthalmoplegia should also be mentioned. It is different from the usual expression of ophthalmoplegic migraine in that pain and ophthalmoplegia occur simultaneously, and the time course is more prolonged although there may be some remission and exacerbation. There is often some indication of orbital involvement such as mild proptosis or swelling of the eyelid. The syndrome is a symptom complex, but the purest examples seem to represent non-specific inflammation in the orbit that is variably responsive to corticosteroids (Blodi and Gass 1968).

Lastly there is the question of congenital berry aneurysm, which can fully reproduce the clinical presentation of ophthalmoplegic migraine, so much so that prior to the introduction of angiography, 100 years of reported cases must remain in some doubt. In aneurysm, ipsilateral pain is followed by the development of ophthalmoplegia in over 90 per cent of cases. This is also the usual sequence of ophthalmoplegic migraine. There may be scintillating scotomata, nausea and vomiting, and remission with recovery of an ophthalmoplegia that characteristically involves pupillomotor fibres (Reinecke 1961, Green *et al.* 1964). Cogan and Mount's study of 60 patients with aneurysms causing ophthalmoplegia (1963) makes it clear that it is the supraclinoid aneurysm that duplicates migraine, while important clinical differences are apparent when infraclinoid aneurysm is involved. In the latter, ophthalmoplegia not infrequently precedes pain, there is a high incidence of trigeminal nerve signs and the pain has neuralgic qualities. It is usually described as burning, or knife-like with associated tingling. In none of these patients was a throbbing quality noted.

The basic point of distinction between ophthalmoplegic migraine and aneurysm is the simple factor of *age*. In the large series of 60 aneurysm patients reported by Cogan and Mount (1963) the age-range was 20 to 72 years, while in the series of 38 similar patients of Green *et al.* (1964) the range was 25 to 69 years. On the other hand with ophthalmoplegic migraine, as Bickerstaff (1964*a*) pointed out, the first attack is almost always below the age of 12 years. In his report of 11 patients, eight had their first episode between five and 11 years, three between 12 and 17 years. In the series of eight patients reported by Friedman *et al.* (1962*b*), the onset in six was under age 10. When onset is in the age-period above 15 or 20 years, the age distinction becomes first ambiguous, then meaningless, with a strong bias with increasing age toward aneurysm as the cause of ophthalmoplegia with headache.

Clinical features
The chief distinguishing features of migrainic oculomotor palsy in contrast with most causes of third nerve palsy is its periodic occurrence, the typical sequence of ophthalmoplegia developing as the headache pain subsides, the relatively shorter duration of oculomotor signs, and onset below age 10.

The central issue is the development of objective ophthalmoplegia. Diplopia and blurred vision are frequent among the complaints of the prodrome or during the headache phase in vascular headache in general, but these subjective symptoms are usually evanescent and are not sufficient to establish a diagnosis of ophthalmoplegic migraine. The oculomotor nerve is affected in almost all cases. Much less commonly the trochlear and/or abducens are involved either alone or in combination with the third cranial nerve. In some instances, authors have reported patients in whom sensory elements of trigeminal nerve dysfunction were found in association with ophthalmoplegia. Most authors point out that the most consistent feature of third nerve dysfunction is that the pupillimotor fibres are often affected, a point that has been challenged recently by Vijayan, who reviewed the literature and added a new case in which pupils were relatively spared (Vijayan 1980). Nevertheless, an ipsilateral dilated pupil with sluggish or no reaction to light is usual, a point in favor of compression neuropathy as a major element in pathogenesis. Ptosis is next in frequency and serves as the sign that usually provokes parental attention and concern. Finally there is the disorder of ocular motility, with eye deviated outward and complaints of diplopia when the eyelid is manually elevated.

An important and distinctive feature is that oculomotor palsy in migraine characteristically develops during the course of the headache, or as long as three to five days after the headache has subsided (Friedman *et al.* 1962*b*). It may then persist after the headache for hours, days, weeks, or months. A two- to four-week period of gradual recovery is not unusual. Complete restoration of function is expected, but after repeated episodes, some residual dysfunction may be irreversible. The point has been made that aberrant regeneration does not occur in ophthalmoplegic migraine in contrast with the frequent occurrence of this phenomenon in patients with aneurysm (Loewenfeld 1980).

The headache of ophthalmoplegic migraine is not distinctive except that it is invariably ipsilateral to the ophthalmoplegia. It runs the gamut of migraine headaches from common to classic, and is often associated with anorexia, nausea and vomiting. Headache may be preceded by typical migrainic scotomata. Usually the patient has had uncomplicated periodic headache as well, but the headache that leads to ophthalmoplegia is exceptionally severe.

The pain centers about the eye, peri-orbital and temporal region. The headache and ophthalmoplegia tend to recur on the same side and typically do not shift from side to side. However, there are reported instances in which a sequence of headaches with ophthalmoplegia remit and then recur in series on the opposite side. In some patients, usually infants or very young children, the headache may be absent or overlooked because of mildness, brevity or lack of communication, and the only obvious expression of the disorder is ophthalmoplegia (Durkan *et al.* 1981).

The pattern of periodicity of the ophthalmoplegia and headache in a given individual is almost infinitely variable and unpredictable. The usual pattern is for ophthalmoplegia to occur at widely spaced intervals, although in some patients several ophthalmoplegic episodes occur in a series. Most patients continue to have more frequent uncomplicated vascular headaches. It seems that ophthalmoplegia develops when a headache of unusual severity occurs on the 'vulnerable' side.

A striking clinical feature of ophthalmoplegic migraine is the early age of onset, frequently under 20 years. Van Pelt and Anderman (1964) described an infant whose first episode occurred at age eight months, and Robertson and Schnitzler (1978) observed a patient who was 12 months at the time of the first episode.

Pathogenesis
The pathogenesis of the ophthalmoplegia has been controversial over the years. The site of involvement of the oculomotor nerve is generally agreed to be distal to the brainstem because of the absence of associated neurological signs. If there are additional signs, except for the very rare involvement of ipsilateral abducens, trochlear and trigeminal, the more appropriate designation is 'basilar artery migraine'.

119

Arteriography in most patients has revealed no abnormality but there have been reported cases of narrowing, presumably transient, of the intracavernous portion of the carotid artery (Walsh and O'Doherty 1960, Bickerstaff 1964a) and a segment of the basilar (Friedman *et al.* 1962b). The observed narrowing could reflect either segmental spasm or edema of the vessel wall. Either process could be indicative of the pathophysiologic basis of the ophthalmoplegia. If spasm, it would be necessary to postulate involvement of arteries of the vasa nervorum of the third cranial nerve.

The intimate relationships of the oculomotor nerve to the carotid, posterior communicating, posterior cerebral arterial complex, and segmental swelling of the vessel walls and compression of the nerve or nerves probably provides a more satisfactory answer. Vessel wall edema can occasionally be observed in the temporal artery after a severe bout of headache, and the time course of ophthalmoplegia with late rather than early manifestation is consistent with this hypothesis.

The only unusual feature of the prognosis of ophthalmoplegic migraine is the danger of persistent, usually partial, oculomotor nerve palsy. Pupillomotor fibres are most vulnerable. Any permanent alteration of nerve function characteristically occurs after a number of ophthalmoplegic incidents.

Management
With regard to management, the chief issue is the requirement of more extensive diagnostic study in this form of migraine, which must include carotid and vertebral arteriography and computerized tomography with special attention to the orbit, sinuses and the base of the brain. In most patients CSF examination is also appropriate, and in some an edrophonium (Tensilon) test. Most oculomotor nerve palsies occurring in childhood and most palsies associated with ipsilateral headache will have an explanation other than migraine.

Once the diagnosis is established, the therapeutic approach must be individualized. The decision for continuous pharmacologic prophylaxis should be based principally on frequency and severity of all vascular headaches, complex and common. In addition, any severe headache that may occur in spite of continuous treatment, and especially if the frequency and severity of headache does not warrant daily prophylaxis, should be treated with an ergot-caffeine preparation such as Cafergot. This should be done, even if the pain of the headache is well established, as an effort to limit the subsequent development of ophthalmoplegia. Although not reported or part of my personal experience, the use of dexamethasone as a possible method of reducing edema of the vascular wall may also be worthy of serious consideration. The principal objective of vigorous therapy should be the prevention of irreversible damage to the oculomotor nerve.

Ophthalmoplegic migraine
CASE This girl was three years old when first seen in January 1969 with her
26   second episode of ophthalmoplegic migraine. She was born after a normal
      pregnancy and delivery. Neonatal period was uneventful and she had

120

developed normally from all points of view.

She was the only child of healthy parents. Her father recalled severe throbbing headaches during high school and college years, many of which were precipitated by the exertion of distance running in track. Her mother had had relatively mild periodic headaches without associated symptoms. Shortly before her second birthday she developed a right oculomotor palsy over a period of several hours with complete ptosis, dilated pupil and outward deviation of the eye. It developed late in an afebrile period of irritability, vomiting and indications of abdominal pain that had lasted about two days. Full recovery of ophthalmoplegia required several weeks.

Her second episode prompted admission to CH Boston. Five days prior to admission she complained of stomach pain, was anorexic, somnolent and vomited on several occasions. On the third day of this illness she developed ptosis that progressed over the next 24 hours to full oculomotor palsy. During this period the systemic symptoms subsided.

On admission she was alert, comfortable, intellectually above average, and had no general physical or neurological abnormalities except complete right ptosis, pupillary dilatation and inability to move the right eye in any direction except laterally.

Studies included a right arch arteriogram, pneumoencephalogram, and examination of CSF, all of which were normal. An edrophonium (Tensilon) test was also negative.

She was discharged with a presumptive diagnosis of ophthalmoplegic migraine and treated with daily phenobarbital 30 mg to be taken twice a day. All aspects of the third nerve dysfunction cleared over a two month period.

During the ensuing year she did well, continued to use phenobarbital regularly, although her parents mentioned that one to three times per week she would awaken at night with complaints of abdominal pain that lasted three to five minutes.

Then at age four years, after a period of headache and vomiting on and off for one week, she developed total third nerve palsy over a period of two days followed by recovery over a one-week period.

At this juncture, it was decided to use Cafergot (1 tab q 30 min × 3) with the next episode while continuing phenobarbital on a regular basis. Two months later she developed a headache with nausea and vomiting. Cafergot was used and on the following day she felt fine with no evidence of ophthalmoplegia. Over the next two years she had headaches every one or two months, with occasional development of mild, transient ptosis. All were treated with Cafergot. On one occasion, when she did not receive Cafergot, she developed total ophthalmoplegia requiring six weeks for recovery; and when seen six weeks later, the right pupil was still enlarged. During her sixth year, the last year of personal follow-up, she developed a tendency to vomit Cafergot and in a series of three episodes spaced at two- to three-month intervals she developed ophthalmoplegia of variable

121

severity on each occasion. Cafergot suppositories were recommended.

    Comment: This girl had typical recurrent ophthalmoplegic migraine beginning under age two years. The early episodes were preceded by migrainic cyclic vomiting, later by ipsilateral headache. Ophthalmoplegia was always on the right side. Treatment during the headache seemed to ameliorate the subsequent development of ophthalmoplegia.

Oculosympathetic paresis in vascular headache syndromes
Definition

Elements of the Horner's syndrome, particularly miosis and ptosis, are probably among the more common neurologic signs that develop during migraine in adults. They are less often recognized in children. There are probably several reasons for this. The subtlety of the changes in most instances may be easily overlooked by the parents or patient. More pertinent is the rarity of migrainous neuralgia (cluster headache) in this age-group, and it is in this variety of vascular headache where it is most likely to be encountered (Kunkle and Anderson 1961). It is also a prominent part of the expression of traumatic carotidynia (Vijayan 1977, see also Chapter 10). Sympathoparesis is not limited to cluster headache and traumatic carotidynia. It may appear in the course of common or classic migraine.

Epidemiology

There are no observations on the frequency of overt ocular sympathetic involvement in children, and the occurrence in common and classic migraine in adults has not been studied in any definitive manner. The incidence of sympathoparesis in cluster headache varies in different series (Herman 1983). Kunkle and Anderson (1961) found that of 98 adult patients with cluster headache, seven had miosis during episodes while one had ptosis. Persisting ptosis and/or miosis had developed in seven patients. Nieman and Hurwitz (1961) found sympthoparesis in 22 per cent of their 50 patients. They also made the point that anhidrosis was not seen.

    Herman (1983) studied 20 unselected adult patients with vascular headache by pupillography with and without cocaine instillation. Only four of these patients had cluster headache. Anisocoria was identified in 65 per cent of the total group and this increased to 90 per cent with cocaine instillation. The findings were interpreted to indicate that most patients with both migraine and cluster headaches had subtle chronic sympathetic deficiency, and that in many the findings became more overt during the headache.

Differential diagnosis

The development of miosis and ptosis calls attention to the sympathetic chain in the neck and especially to the sympathetic plexus as it ascends to the eye *via* the internal carotid artery. Diagnostic considerations include inflammatory or neoplastic involvement of adjacent tissues as well as the aftermath of trauma to the neck. Congenital abnormalities of the carotid artery and arteritis also require consideration. Intermittent sympathoparesis associated with headache is less threatening of an anatomical lesion than is the persistence of signs.

Any patient who has oculosympathetic paresis and evidence of trigeminal nerve dysfunction (Raeder's syndrome) should be carefully studied for an infectious or neoplastic lesion at the base of the skull, paranasal sinuses *etc.* (Raeder 1924). The concept of Raeder's syndrome has been contaminated over the years by the inclusion of patients with migrainous neuralgia (Mokri 1982). The key issue of distinction is the presence of true trigeminal pain (see p. 57), sensory or motor signs referable to the trigeminal nerve and occasionally the fourth and sixth cranial nerves as well. When trigeminal nerve signs such as an absent corneal reflex are present, a lesion of the middle cranial fossa is likely, usually either tumor or post-traumatic, less commonly inflammation. Very rarely, an absent corneal reflex is said to occur in true cluster headache (Nieman and Hurwitz 1961).

One of the more common issues that I have encountered is the problem of a congenital ptosis that is intensified and becomes more manifest during the course of the headache. It should also be remembered that pupillary asymmetry is 'normal' or unexplained in 17 per cent of the population (Herman 1983).

Clinical presentation
The Horner's syndrome becomes manifest during the headache phase, almost invariably on the side of the headache if the pain is hemicranial. It usually subsides concomitant with the headache, but may persist beyond for hours to several days. Repeated episodes not infrequently leave a permanent residual mild ptosis and miosis. Anhidrosis apparently does not occur in those patients who develop sympathoparesis with cluster headache (Nieman and Hurwitz 1961).

Pathogenesis
The most favored locus of involvement of the sympathetic system is those fibers associated with the carotid artery, probably at the base of the skull. The postulated mechanism consists of swelling of the arterial wall and compression of the nerves against the adjacent bone (Walsh and Hoyt 1969). The mechanism is comparable to that proposed for ophthalmoplegic migraine and the similarities to this entity extend to the clinical phenomenology as well, *i.e.* involvement of a single neural element outside of the CNS, the invariable manifestation during the headache, and tendency to permanent deficit after a number of episodes.

Management
The chief issues in management relate to the need for special diagnostic procedures that may include x-rays of the base of the skull, paranasal sinus and chest, CT scan of orbit, base of skull and in unusual circumstances the cervical region as well. Arteriography should rarely be necessary to clarify the diagnostic issues.

Treatment is based upon the principals of treatment of juvenile migraine in general or of cluster headache in particular. These issues are considered in the appropriate sections of this monograph and will not be repeated here.

Papilledema in migraine

There is a single case report in the literature in which edema of the optic disc is associated with a severe migraine episode (Victor and Welch 1977). A similar patient has been studied at Children's Hospital, Boston (see case report below). Significant concomitant visual symptoms did not occur in either patient which sets them apart from the rare, but well-established ischemic papillopathy that occurs in migraine of all ages (Walsh and Hoyt 1969, McDonald and Sanders 1971, also see Chapter 7). The full range of arterial and venous occlusive syndromes of optic disc and retina are possible as a complication of migraine, but these entities are accompanied by overt acute and occasionally persisting visual symptoms.

The objective changes in the optic nerve-head and retina are very similar in both papillitis and papilledema. They may consist of hyperemia and elevation of the optic nerve-head together with retinal hemorrhage in both conditions. However, significant visual impairment is the rule in ischemic papillitis, and it is minimal if present at all in papilledema.

The Victor and Welch (1977) case involved a man of 27 years who had had migraine episodically since age eight. In the context of headaches of increasing frequency and severity he had two complex episodes of 15 minutes duration in which he had feelings of depersonalization and body rigidity without loss of awareness. There were no visual symptoms in either. In the context of these complex events he was found to have retinal hemorrhages in the first, and in the second there were bilateral elevated disc margins of low grade, with full veins and hemorrhage. CSF pressure was 205 mm H_2O and protein was 16 mg/100 ml. Fluorescein angiography showed hyperfluorescence of the optic disc. CT scans were normal. The papilledema subsided during hospitalization for study and treatment.

It is likely that this rare complication is a visible expression in the optic nerve of the permeability changes that may occur in severe migraine in the CNS as evidenced by the CT scan demonstration of white matter lucency in some cases (Mathew *et al.* 1977). Obviously the finding requires full neurological study, including CT scan and CSF examination, before it can be concluded that the papilledema is related to migraine. However, the close correlation with a complex migrainic episode in time, and rapid resolution, is convincing evidence that migraine is indeed responsible.

Migraine with papilledema

CASE 27 This seven-year-old girl was under the care of Dr. David van Dyke of Grand Rapids, Michigan, and seen through the courtesy of Dr. Michael Bresnan on the occasion of her neurological evaluation at Children's Hospital, Boston.

In the 12 months prior to admission she had had episodes of throbbing hemicrania, nausea, vomiting, pallor, followed by sleepiness which responded to cyproheptadine. Her mother had headaches consistent with migraine. Then six months before admission, after a fall in which she struck the back of her head, she was admitted to the hospital locally with symptoms of generalized headache, nausea, vomiting, lethargy and mildly blurred vision. The symptoms were a cause of particular concern because at age four she was involved in a bicycle-auto accident that had resulted in multiple injuries including subluxation of C2 on C3. There had been persistent concern and conflicting opinion concerning the question of continuing C2-C3 instability and the need for operative treatment.

The examination in the context of her post-traumatic episode revealed papilledema with venous pulsation. The CSF was under 180 mm H$_2$O pressure. She recovered in about two days and the papilledema subsided. It was remarked that significant clinical improvement seemed to occur following the LP. Three additional episodes occurred in the following two months, during the last of which she was again observed to have papilledema with normal visual acuity. CT and angiography were normal, and an EEG showed left temporal spikes.

She was treated with phenytoin 50 mg b.i.d. and sent to Boston for an additional opinion one month later. Examination was entirely negative including retina and visual fields. Review of cervical spine x-rays revealed a stable fusion.

Comment: This seven-year-old girl had juvenile migraine and a post-traumatic C2-C3 stable fusion. Exacerbation of migraine occurred following minor occipital trauma. During the first and fourth migrainic episode following this trauma she developed transient low-grade papilledema, with only mild elevation of CSF pressure.

7
MIGRAINE WITH SEIZURES, STROKE AND SYNCOPE

Migraine and seizures

The interrelationship between migraine and convulsive disorder has intrigued physicians for many years. Interest has centered on the simultaneous occurrence of these two common disorders of childhood. One involves paroxysmal symptomatic expression of poorly inhibited or over-excitable vascular tissue, while the other involves the expression of poorly inhibited or over-excitable central neuronal tissue. Both paroxysmal disorders are common, and between them they account for the majority of the recurring periodic symptoms of childhood, with a much less frequent contribution by transient metabolic events such as hypocalcemia or hypoglycemia. Parenthetically, it is of interest that systemic metabolic incidents can be symptomatic in their own right, or act as 'triggers' of either vasomotor reaction or seizure discharge.

Both migraine and seizures may be expressed in anyone if there is sufficient provocation. This intrinsic property of excitable tissue is influenced by hereditary and other factors leading to the concept of a variable excitability threshold. Both migrainic and seizure phenomena can therefore become symptomatic expressions of CNS disorders such as arteriovenous malformations, cerebral tumors, or fixed lesions of the CNS.

Clinical differences between vascular and epileptic symptoms

The usual symptomatology of migraine (*i.e.* headache) and of seizure disorder leads to a clear separation of the two and there is no serious confusion. However, problems may be posed by vasomotor events associated with migraine such as syncope, complex cerebral symptomatology such as the various hemisyndromes or confusional states, and brief migrainic auras occurring without subsequent headache. Moreover, it is reasonably common for headache to follow a seizure. Another relevant and common ambiguity is the distinction between abdominal migraine and abdominal epilepsy, between migrainic and epileptic vertigo, and in the differentiation between seizures and syncope. These subjects are considered elsewhere. The problem of headaches as an epileptic manifestation (epileptic cephalia) will be discussed below.

The chief points of distinction in favor of seizure relate to alteration or loss of consciousness together with amnesia for the event. Furthermore, the full development of a seizure occurs in seconds, while development of vasomotor phenomena usually evolves slowly over minutes. The duration of the ictus is also important. Seizures are customarily brief and can be measured in seconds or minutes, while migrainic episodes are usually measured in portions of an hour or longer. Seizures tend to emphasize positive phenomena, for example tonic or clonic

TABLE XI
Epilepsy and Migraine

	Migraine	Epilepsy
Paroxysmal expression	Primarily vascular	Neuronal
Principal manifestation	Headache, nausea, vomiting, pallor	Seizures
State of consciousness	Typically preserved	Typically altered
Duration	Portion of an hour or more	Seconds or minutes
Aura	Typically visual, characteristic content	Wide range of neurologic phenomena
Duration of aura	Minutes	Seconds
Postictal sleep	Occasional	Common
EEG	Low incidence discharges	High incidence discharges
Family history	90% migraine	Low for seizures
Onset	Characteristically gradual	Sudden
Influenced by emotion	High frequency	Low
Recognizable triggers	Moderate frequency	Low

movements, whereas the emphasis of clinical phenomena in migraine is negative, or deficit symptomatology such as hemiparesis, or scotomata. None of these distinctions are absolute, however, and one may not be able to make a definitive differentiation in a given situation. This is particularly true when dealing with complex symptoms, especially those relating to visual, auditory or somatic sensory symptoms or distortion of complex cortical function (Table XI).

The EEG can be helpful in the distinction. The incidence, quality and quantity of discharges may be sufficient to bias the final decision in favor of seizure disorder. A notable exception can be found in the discussion of the 'basilar migraine, seizures and severe epileptic form abnormalities' syndrome as discussed later in this section. On the other hand, the EEG in seizure disorder may be normal in a significant number of patients, even with activation or prolonged monitoring. If a record can be made during the attack it is usually diagnostic.

A full discussion of the EEG in epilepsy is beyond the scope of this monograph, and the EEG in migraine has been discussed in Chapter 4 and will not be repeated here.

Migraine and seizures in the same individual
Clinicians have been interested in the apparent frequency of expression of vascular headaches and other migrainic symptomatology, and of seizure disorder in the same individual. The frequency of overlap is not so common as to be obvious, and the significant frequency of migraine in the population and the relative frequency of seizure disorder, especially in childhood, increase the possibility of chance overlap. This difficulty is compounded by the fact that the final diagnosis is based upon clinical criteria in both conditions. The EEG is the only laboratory test that might help to differentiate between the two. Both clinical and electrical criteria are stronger in convulsive disorder. The clinical criteria for migraine are subject to variable interpretation among clinicians, especially in children.

A full review of this literature is not useful here and citation of selected papers at either pole of the controversy is sufficient. Lance and Anthony (1966) found a 2 per cent incidence of epilepsy in patients with either tension or vascular headaches in a series of 500 patients. On the other hand, Basser (1969) found that 5.9 per cent of his 1830 patients with migraine had epilepsy as contrasted with 1.1 per cent of 548 patients with tension headache. The observations of Lennox and Lennox (1960) were similar to those of Basser. Lennox and Lennox also contributed a study of five monozygotic twin pairs, all of whom had migraine, and three individuals in this group had epilepsy.

There is no report of a large series of migrainic children in which the occurrence of seizure disorder is compared with a control group comparable to the Lance and Anthony (1966) and Basser (1969) studies. The largest reported series of migrainic children is that of Congdon and Forsythe (1979) in which nine out of 300 migrainics had seizures. In my own 300 patients presenting with migraine, five had afebrile seizures not associated with the migraine attack. If one tabulates the frquency of seizures in several reported series (Burke and Peters 1956, Bille 1962, Holguin and Fenichel 1967, Congdon and Forsythe 1979, Prensky and Sommer 1979) the incidence is 3 per cent in a total of 904 patients. Bille's series of 73 personally interviewed patients is the only report in which a control group was studied as well, and the numbers are too small to be meaningful. In Bille's migraine group, five had seizures (four with fever), while in the control group four patients had seizures (two with fever).

It is not clear whether most reports include febrile seizures, which of course would make a major difference in any effort to make a comparison with the incidence in the general population. There must also be a selection bias in that the reported series were collected at referral centers where more complex problems are studied.

It is probable that there is a slightly higher incidence of overlap than would be expected by chance. It certainly does not necessarily follow that there is a fundamental identity of the two disorders, or that the pathogenesis of the ictus is the same, as has been implied on occasion over the years.

What, then, is the importance of this occasional association? First of all, each problem requires consideration in any management plan, although in a number of patients standard anticonvulsants are effective in both. Only the duration and consistency of treatment is different, *i.e.* years for seizure disorder and usually months for migraine. Perhaps the necessary anticonvulsant blood-level is also less for migraine, although this has not been documented. Treatment of the seizure disorder takes precedence, but if headache persists after the seizures are controlled, one can then turn to a consideration of treatment of this aspect with propranolol, behavior modification, *etc.* There is some concern about the use of ergot or methysergide in children with low seizure threshold because of the possibility of triggering seizures. I generally use phenobarbital in small doses, usually 30 mg b.i.d. in the rare migraine patient under 10 or 12 years who is begun on continuous ergot or methysergide.

The other important issue is the possible diagnostic implication of the association of migraine and seizures in the same individual. Does the presence of the two symptoms in the same patient imply the greater likelihood of a tumor or arteriovenous malformation? There is no systematic study of this issue in either children or adults, but I regard the association as carrying a greater risk of cerebral tumor, AV malformation or other organic lesions than does either problem occurring alone. The risk is compounded if either migraine or seizures have a focal signature. It follows that special diagnostic study, especially CT scans, should be requested in children who have both.

Migraine and seizures
This seven-and-a-half-year-old boy had been having bilateral throbbing **CASE** headaches associated with blurred vision and vertigo for the preceding six **28** months. They were often precipitated by unusual physical exercise and were of five to 10 minutes in duration. This led to an EEG two months prior to admission which showed persistent left mid- and posterior-temporal spiking and sharp wave discharge. No treatment was initiated. On the day before admission to CH Boston, while asleep in his mother's lap, he developed clonic movements with onset in the right leg that then became generalized. The attack lasted intermittently for approximately 30 minutes. Examination revealed no general abnormalities, and his neurological examination was entirely normal. A spinal fluid examination showed a protein of 20 mg per cent. CT scan was also normal and he was discharged to take phenytoin 50 mg in the morning and 75 mg at night. On follow-up examination after three months he had had no seizures and only two headaches.

His mother had classic migraine since age seven, and on his father's side a grandmother, cousin and cousin's children all were subject to periodic headaches.

After two years of no seizures, an EEG still showed brief discharges and it was elected to continue medication. Follow-up was continued to age 11, at which time he was having occasional mild brief headaches, and he had had no seizures.

Comment: This boy had both migraine headaches and a single focal seizure which led to neurologic study and a normal CT scan. Phenytoin treatment was effective in controlling the seizures and ameliorating the vascular headaches.

Alternating migraine (complex) and seizure with arteriovenous mal-formation
Birth, development and early history were normal. Family history included **CASE** a paternal aunt with migraine. **29**

At age 13 he had an episode while ski-ing: he saw 'blue' to the right, associated with blurred vision that lasted a few seconds. Subsequently he vomited and became confused, and had no memory for the next 30 minutes. When found on the ski-slope he complained of a severe throbbing headache that lasted the rest of the day. Subsequently there were occasional

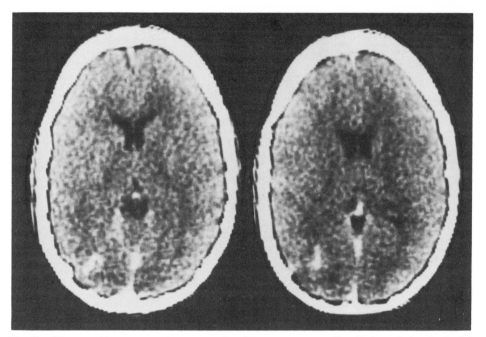

Fig. 7. CT scan with contrast enhancement that demonstrates a small radiodense lesion in the left occipital lobe that proved to be an AVM (case 29).

episodes of similar visual disturbance, followed by headache. An EEG showed theta slowing in the left posterior quadrant. A diagnosis of juvenile migraine was made and he was treated with phenytoin with good results.

At age 15, at a time when he was no longer on phenytoin, he had a full generalized major convulsion, and a month later he had repeated convulsions on and off for about three and a half hours which led to hospitalization. He had a postictal manic phase that lasted several days. This hospitalization was followed by a CT scan (Fig. 7) and an arteriogram that showed an arteriovenous malformation in the left occipital lobe. The malformation was totally removed by Dr. John Shillito.

In the postoperative period, he had right-sided visual scotomata accompanied by flashing lights. There was no alteration of consciousness, and only occasionally did headache follow the visual symptoms. These episodes were modified by anticonvulsants and further modified by propranolol, but they persist to the present.

Comment: This boy had classic migraine with one confusional episode and then two years later developed *grand mal* seizures. Neurologic study revealed a left occipital AVM.

Migraine and seizures in the same episode
This section deals with the uncommon but dramatic association of vascular and

130

epileptic clinical phenomenology in the same episode. The common postictal headache, a headache which may have vascular components clinically, is not under discussion. Rather, attention is drawn to episodes that *begin* with vascular headache or complex migrainic symptoms, which then seem to trigger a seizure. Just as seizure followed by headache is common and likely to be benign, the reverse sequence carries a high risk of organic cerebral lesions of surgical significance.

A definitive epidemiologic study of such patients that indicates the frequency of tumor or AVM has not been reported, but experience demands that one must take this association seriously. The risk of organic cause would seem to be at least as high as 20 per cent and may be higher. Review of my own series of patients has identified four patients who presented with this symptom complex who had tumor or AVM, as compared with only three who did not. These numbers cannot be considered more than suggestive because of the small total numbers of patients involved, selective referral, and the very likely possibility of overlooking patients in my chart review whose principal diagnosis was seizure disorder and whose migrainic symptoms were not included in the diagnostic formulation.

The importance of migraine and seizure in the same episode is emphasized in the report of Pearce and Foster (1965). These authors studied 40 patients with various types of complicated migraine. Three of their patients had migraine and seizures in the same episode, and two proved to have arteriovenous malformations. These two patients had the only surgically important disease in the entire series of patients which included those with ophthalmoplegia, transient and persisting hemisyndromes, and basilar artery syndrome.

I believe that intensive observation, certainly CT scan, and in some instances arteriography, are appropriate to the investigation. Perhaps even more important than initial studies is the continuing need for examination and re-appraisal, including repeat CT scan, if the early examinations have been negative. It should be recognized that it is quite possible to do a CT scan too early in the course of tumor, and before it becomes visible (see case 31 reported below).

Mixed seizures and migrainic phenomena associated with AVM
Pregnancy, delivery and early development were all normal. Family **CASE** history revealed a mother and maternal grandmother with classic migraine. **30**

At age 11 she began to have one-minute episodes during which her right hand became numb and she was unable to speak. The episode became more elaborate and was accompanied by what was described as partial blindness followed by a throbbing headache. She was diagnosed as having juvenile migraine and treated with phenytoin for several years.

At age 15 she came to Boston to attend boarding school. Shortly after arriving she had an episode during which her right hand became numb, she could not speak and she had headache and nausea. During this episode she had some clonic movements of the right arm. She was treated for two months with phenytoin. An EEG at that time was normal. Phenytoin was discontinued and shortly thereafter she had a similar episode leading to a full major convulsion which prompted admission to CH Boston where an

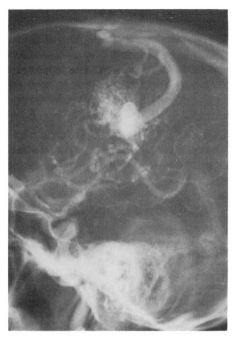 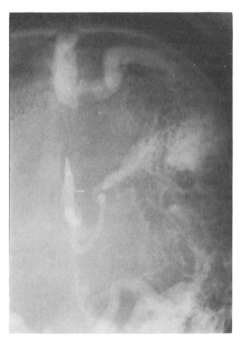

Fig. 8a. This lateral view of a carotid arteriogram demonstrates a 3 cm arteriovenous vascular malformation of the left anterior parietal region. Its arterial supply is principally the middle cerebral artery and its branches and the venous drainage is *via* a large superficial cortical vein into the sagittal sinus.

Fig. 8b. This AP view demonstrates the deep extension of the AVM into the left hemisphere and its additional venous drainage *via* the deep venous system into a dilated thalanostriate vein and the internal cerebral vein. There is no displacement of midline structures and no enlargement of the ventricular system (case 30).

arteriogram showed a large, deep, left-hemisphere arteriovenous malformation (Figs. 8a,b). This was inoperable.

Subsequent to the study she has had two varieties of episodes. The first was a periodic throbbing headache during which she had ptosis of the right eyelid, and the second consisted of focal sensory seizures with clonic twitching during which consciousness was preserved. Treatment consisted of phenytoin, at first on its own, and later with propranolol. The latter combination achieved total control.

Comment: This girl had migrainic attacks with persistent left hemisphere focal signature beginning at age 11. At age 15, convulsive activity during the attacks was manifest, leading to arteriographic demonstration of an inoperable AVM. Combined treatment with phenytoin and propranolol was successful in controlling both seizure and vascular phenomenology.

Mixed seizures, migrainic phenomenon with tumor

CASE 31 This boy was age six when first seen. He was well until March 1981, five months before admission to CH Boston. Subsequent to a streptococcal

132

infection, he awakened unable to speak and shortly afterwards it was noted that he had a right hemiparesis of several hours duration. He vomited, but there was no clonic movement and no headache. Hospitalization revealed a thoracic tumor and during myelography with metrizamide he had a right-sided clonic seizure. The thoracic tumor was removed, and proved to be a ganglioneuroma. Cranial CT scan and arteriogram at this time were both normal. The EEG showed left temporo-parietal slowing.

A month later he had another episode in which he could not speak. This was accompanied by severe headache and followed by intermittent twitching of his face accompanied by weakness of the right side of his body, all of which lasted about 30 minutes. Over the subsequent month he had several similar episodes that occurred despite anticonvulsant medication.

During his illness his parents noted a behavioral change and he became more temperamental and difficult. He also had four episodes during which his entire right face and body became red and sweaty and warm to the touch. There were also several independent episodes of micropsia lasting a few minutes.

The family history revealed that his mother and maternal grandfather had severe migraine.

The first general physical and neurologic examination at CH Boston in early June was normal in all respects as was the CT scan. He was admitted in mid-July 1981, when a repeat CT scan now showed a large enhancing tumor of the left posterior parietal region that was removed and proved to be a 'cerebral Schwanoma' (Fig. 9). Operative removal was followed by radiation therapy.

Radiation therapy went well, and he was continued on dexamethanone, carbamazepine and phenytoin. He had no significant postoperative neurological deficit except for slight awkwardness of his right leg.

Comment: The episodic phenomena in this boy consisted of complex migrainic phenomena and focal seizures. The CT scans were normal during the first four months of his illness, and a third study revealed a tumor.

Mixed headache and seizure with old infarcts
This boy was age 11 when first seen. For two months prior to his admission to the hospital he had weekly frontal throbbing headaches associated with nausea and vomiting lasting about one to two hours. The headaches were frequently preceded by flashing lights. On the day of admission he had an episode beginning with blurred vision, followed by nausea and vomiting, and after two hours he had a clonic seizure which spread from the right face to the arm and then generalized. **CASE 32**

On initial examination he was postictal, slightly ataxic with slurred speech but fundi and visual fields were normal.

Spinal fluid examination was entirely normal. CT scan showed the presence of bilateral occipital cystic lesions without mass effect probably related to an old perinatal infarction in the posterior cerebral artery

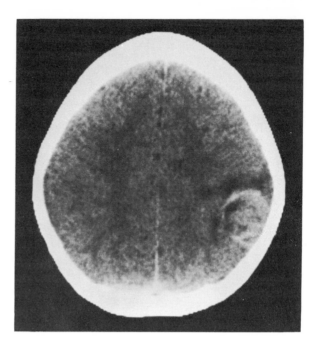

Fig. 9. This CT scan with contrast enhancement demonstrates an irregular density lesion with surrounding edema in the left posterior parietal region. Histologically it proved to be a 'cerebral Schwanoma'. A CT scan six weeks before this study was normal (case 31).

territory. The EEG showed bilateral slowing most marked on the left.

The history of the pregnancy was without an unusual event and he was delivered after a normal labor. However, he was cyanotic at birth and his deciduous teeth showed enamel dysplasia consistent with an event in the perinatal period. The family history was of interest in that a maternal grandmother had periodic headache.

He was treated with phenytoin and on follow-up had no subsequent seizures or headaches.

Comment: In this patient, migraine headaches complicated by a focal seizure were associated with a non-progressive lesion acquired in the perinatal period.

Basilar migraine, seizures and severe epileptiform EEG abnormalities

In contrast to the above-described patients is a most interesting group of patients reported by Camfield *et al.* (1978). Clinically these patients fall into the category of either 'migraine and seizures in the same individual', or 'migraine and seizure in the same episode'. They are distinguished by benign prognosis, particularly from the point of view of a structural etiologic basis. The migrainic aspect was frequently 'classic' in the initial presentation with visual scotomata, blindness or other complex symptomatology, and the seizures were either generalized clonic-tonic or had a focal motor signature.

The most dramatic feature of the clinical syndrome was almost continuous epileptiform discharges, predominantly posterior and of various morphologies. The other striking electroencephalographic finding was great sensitivity to eye closure. This latter point was emphasized in a second publication (Panayiotopoulos 1980) where this aspect was further examined. It was found that both darkness and eye closure precipitated the persistent discharge, but it did not occur in either an illuminated room or when central vision was retained in darkness. It might be said that this is one migraine-epilepsy syndrome in which the EEG is crucial to proper assessment, especially if time and a wider experience bears out the benign nature of the problem.

Summary of the relationship between migraine and seizures
The principal focus of this section is the practical diagnostic implication for a patient with migraine and seizures. It is almost impossible to be certain whether the vascular headache is a response to the tumor or AVM or whether it is a completely independent expression of migraine. It seems probable that when seizures *follow* vasomotor symptoms in the same episode, there is a strong indication that the total paroxysm is a symptomatic expression of the structural lesion. Here is a summary of the implications of the seizure-migraine relationship:
(1) Although migraine and seizures are separate and distinct phenomena, there is probably a higher incidence of overlap in the same patient than expected on the basis of chance.
(2) When migraine and seizures occur as separate events in the same individual there is probably a greater incidence of underlying structural disease, especially if either convulsions or migraine have a focal clinical expression. This clinical circumstance warrants CT investigation.
(3) When vasomotor (migrainic) phenomena and seizures follow as part of a single event, there is a highly significant likelihood of tumor, AVM or other structural lesions of brain (estimated 20 to 50 per cent). This clinical circumstance mandates CT scan, careful follow-up, and in many instances repeat CT scan at a later date.
(4) Both seizures and migraine may be treated with anticonvulsants, and combined phenomena may do well with combined therapy.

Headaches as an epileptic equivalent (epileptic cephalea)
As an addendum to the discussion of migraine and seizures, it is appropriate to include reference to seizure headaches or 'epileptic cephalea'. This designation refers to the concept of paroxysmal headache as an epileptic equivalent, as conceptualized by Weil (1952).
    Postictal headache is well known and quite common. Postictal headache not infrequently has a vascular quality although it is usually of a less specific nature. Moreover, a paroxysmal event may begin with vascular headache or complex migrainic symptomatology and then lead to a focal or *grand mal* seizure, a combination that has important diagnostic significance as indicated above. There are convincing examples reported in the literature where abnormal head sensations constitute the leading phenomenology of a seizure, which then may spread to focal expression or full generalization.

True epileptic headache must be quite rare, and I have no personal clinical experience to report. The cases reported by Laplante *et al.* (1983) are convincing and well documented by concomitant EEG during the abnormal head sensation. They point out that similar documentation is presented in only one other case in the literature. They report that the head sensations may or may not be 'painful' and are variously described as a sensation of 'swelling, fullness, pressure, heat, pounding or flush'. The episodes last one or two minutes and may not be accompanied by altered consciousness. The patients have other unequivocal epileptic phenomena, either occurring as separate events or following the head sensation.

Much of the literature that has developed around the theme of epileptic headache only makes a convincing case to those who accept paroxysmal discharges in the EEG, and favorable response to traditional anticonvulsants such as phenytoin, as acceptable criteria for the diagnosis of seizure disorder. These are the essential features upon which the usual concept of epileptic cephalea rests, and from my perspective these criteria represent insufficient grounds. The problem is similar to the issues previously discussed in relation to abdominal epilepsy.

As we have seen, paroxysmal discharges and Rolandic spikes are frequent in migraine, especially in children. It is debatable whether a group of otherwise clinically identical patients should be set aside on this basis as having a seizure disorder, with all of its implications (Halpern and Bental 1958, Chao and Davis 1964, Swaiman and Frank 1978). Moreover, the effect of phenytoin is not limited to the neuronal membrane, and is well known to be therapeutically effective in painful cranial (and less commonly peripheral) neuropathy, as well as in cardiac arrhythmias. Phenytoin and other anticonvulsants can have a favorable effect on the frequency and severity of all juvenile migrainic phenomena, quite unrelated to EEG findings.

My own reservations about the frequency of epileptic headaches seem to be shared by others. Several relatively recent authors of reviews on juvenile migraine avoid the issue by not mentioning the subject of epileptic headache (Prensky 1976, Brown 1977, Congdon and Forsythe 1979). Others seem to deal with the issue gingerly and without indication of a clear position other than to state that it is uncommon (Shinnar and D'Souza 1981) or that 'the diagnosis of the epilepsy equivalent syndrome is made far more frequently than the actual disorder occurs' (Rothner 1978). Rothner gives his own criteria for the diagnosis. The primary requirement is that consciousness be altered during the headache. Additional criteria include 'history of generalized seizures, an epileptiform EEG, a positive family history for seizures and a positive response to a trial of anticonvulsants'. It is also stated that nausea and vomiting are less often present than with migraine and that postictal drowsiness is common.

Jay and Tomasi (1981) were guarded in their comments, although they categorized 12 per cent of their 116 consecutive headache patients as having seizure equivalent headaches. These patients were described as having been 'given' (my emphasis) the diagnosis of 'seizure equivalent' headaches. Clinical criteria of the headache itself were not specified, but the 17 patients were distinguished by having a positive family history for headache in only 12 per cent: four patients had a prior history of seizures, four had mildly abnormal neurological examination, and 84 per cent had 'abnormal' EEGs in whom 35 per cent had 14 and six per second positive spikes.

When one reviews the clinical phenomenology of most reported seizure headache patients, the identity with juvenile migraine is obvious as may be pointed out by the authors themselves. For example: 'All subjects had unilateral cephalgia, teichopsia and vomiting' (Weil 1952); and 'The clinical picture of seizure headaches include the following features: they are usually diffuse or bifrontal; they begin abruptly at any time and last for minutes or several hours; in the majority of cases they are accompanied by nausea and vomiting and followed by postictal lethargy or sleep . . .' (Swaiman and Frank 1978). Review of the cases provided by Halpern and Bental (1958) reveals similar symptomatology.

Chao and Davis (1964) would go even further. The symptoms compiled as indicative of the 'convulsive equivalent syndrome of childhood' is a relatively complete listing of the various complaints in juvenile migraine. Each symptom was listed as belonging to group A, characterized by patients in whom the 14 and six per second positive spikes phenomena occurred (which is probably a normal configuration), and group B in which 40 per cent showed normal EEGs and the remainder had other EEG abnormalities. In the following compilation, group A is listed first and group B second. At the top of the list is headache in 84 and 85 per cent of patients, abdominal pain in 64 and 71 per cent, vomiting in 34 and 53 per cent, nausea in 19 and 24 per cent, dizziness or syncope 19 and 21 per cent, altered consciousness 16 and 19 per cent, and on through a list of symptoms such as fever, photophobia, pallor and pain in the extremities. Chao and Davis (1964) seem to propose that all juvenile migrainic phenomenology be incorporated into the concept of seizure disorder. The only surprise in the list is the frequency of altered consciousness. The basis of this contention is the frequency of EEG 'abnormality' (in quotes because of the inclusion of the 14 and six per second phenomena) and particularly the response to anticonvulsants.

Jonas (1966) takes a similar stand with regard to the definition of 'headache as seizure equivalents'. All of the patients in this small series responded to phenytoin or phenobarbital and the EEGs ranged from paroxysmal spike discharge to runs of four to six cycles per second. A clinical feature of Jonas's patients was the presence of symptomatology that the author attributes to temporal lobe dysfunction, although the headache itself had the quality of classic or common migraine. In one patient the character of the headache was that of migrainous neuralgia (cluster headache).

To summarize my own perspective on this issue, it can be said that migraine is a clinical concept and the diagnosis should rest on clinical grounds. The frequency of paroxysmal EEG changes is probably telling us something about the pathophysiology of this multisystem metabolic disorder, probably that the basic defect affects brain in some fashion together with blood vessels and other issues. It is probably not telling us that the disorder is the same as epilepsy. Finally, there are patients who have true epileptic cephalea, but they are very rare and usually identified by other clinical evidence of seizure disorder.

Migraine and stroke

Definition

Although juvenile migraine is generally benign from the point of view of morbidity and mortality, there are two circumstances in which this is not the case. The first refers to what may be called 'symptomatic' migraine where the vascular phenomenology is in some fashion triggered by a structural or metabolic lesion. This is the subject of Chapter 12 where the issue of headache as part of the acute symptomatology of a stroke is also considered. The second is the relationship of cerebral infarction to juvenile migraine, a problem that revolves about three questions:

1. DOES STROKE OCCUR IN THE COURSE OF A MIGRAINE ATTACK?

There are convincing reports in the literature, some with pathological verification, that cerebral infarcts can develop in the course of an attack of common, classic or complicated migraine (see review of the literature below). An infarct is more likely to occur in the territory of a vascular bed in which there have been transient neurological symptoms.

2. DOES JUVENILE MIGRAINE INCREASE THE RISK OF STROKE IN CHILDHOOD?

In a second, larger, group of young patients, it is less clear that their migrainic diathesis played a rôle in their stroke. They have migraine as expressed by typical periodic headache, but the headaches have not had complex features. The stroke may occur in the setting of headache, but the headache, although clinically consistent with a vascular headache, may be different in some respects from the headache of their usual juvenile migraine. An alternative cause of stroke is usually not ascertained, but this is frequently the case in juvenile stroke occurring in patients who do not have migraine.

It is the old problem of the possibility of the chance occurrence of a rare incident, such as stroke in childhood, in a patient who also has a common disorder, such as migraine. No systematic epidemiologic study has been done to address this issue.

3. DOES JUVENILE MIGRAINE INCREASE THE RISK OF STROKE IN PATIENTS WHO ALREADY HAVE ANOTHER KNOWN BASIC RISK FACTOR OF STROKE?

A more interesting and important question relates to the relevance of the metabolic and/or vascular defect of the migraine syndrome in children and young adults as a contributory factor to a lesion that has a recognized association with thrombotic or embolic stroke (Table XII). An excellent example is prolapse of the mitral valve, and perhaps other valvular and aortic anomalies, where the enhanced platelet aggregability of some patients with migraine could be an important contributory factor to intravascular coagulation, bland vegetation formation, and emboli. The availability of simple and safe measures to limit platelet aggregation, such as continuous aspirin therapy, may provide a therapeutic recourse in appropriate patients: an approach that should be considered when the association occurs.

TABLE XII
Conditions in which Migraine may Increase the Risk of Stroke

1. Oestrogen/Progesterone birth-control pills (Saper 1983), possibility of other medication.
2. Complicated migraine (Pearce and Foster 1965), especially when precipitated by trauma or physical effort (Lance 1976, Haas *et al.* 1975).
3. Prolapsed mitral valve (Litman and Friedman 1978, Conomy *et al.* 1982).
4. Fibromuscular dysplasia (Mettinger and Ericson 1982).

Epidemiology

Epidemiologic studies (Leviton *et al.* 1974) have indicated that there is an increased long-term risk of hypertension (1.7 times greater, $p = 0.05$) in migrainics, as well as a somewhat higher risk of heart attack. This epidemiologic study did not indicate an increased risk of stroke. The report dealt with people over age 40 years in whom the incidence of hypertension, heart disease and stroke is significant, and specifically excluded the young.

Therefore the problem considered in the Leviton *et al.* (1974) study and other epidemiologic studies of a similar nature is quite different from the issue of stroke in juvenile migrainics. Rather, they address the problem of the long-term consequences of migraine in the pathogenesis of hypertension. It would seem that a lifetime of symptomatic migraine does have a deleterious, albeit limited, contributory effect on the development of systemic hypertension, either in terms of: '1. common genetic features, 2. common psychological features, 3. shared aberrations of indoleamine or catecholamine metabolism, 4. adverse effects of therapy for migraine, and 5. common disturbances of vascular reactivity' (Leviton *et al.* 1974).

The study of Connor (1962) is the only indication of the frequency of the development of stroke in close association with the expression of migraine. He collected a total of 18 patients with ischemic stroke in a series of 500 migraine patients (3.6 per cent). Only one was a child, aged 12 years. Two additional patients had hemorrhage resulting from cerebral angiomas and are therefore examples of 'symptomatic migraine'. The basis of the diagnosis of stroke in this study was persistence of the focal defect. Only six patients had angiograms, most of which were normal. Selective referral perhaps accounts for what would seem to be a high incidence. In my own series there were five patients (1.7 per cent) with proved or presumptive stroke, one with a retinal infarct. In two of the five, an anatomical lesion of valve or great vessels was present (see cases 35 and 36 at the end of this section).

Patients with *complicated* migraine have a higher degree of vulnerability. In the series of 40 patients with various complicated migraine syndromes reported by Pearce and Foster (1965), 10 had permanent or persistent focal lesions, presumably stroke. All of these patients had angiograms, with the exception of one patient who had a retinal infarct, and none showed vascular occlusion.

The distribution of the infarct is illustrated by Connor's (1962) series. Five were retinal, 10 were in the cerebral hemisphere, predominantly in the posterior cerebral artery territory, and three were in the brainstem. In nine patients the infarct developed during an attack of migraine, and nine had had preceding transient symptoms in the area eventually affected by the stroke, with some overlap between the two groups. In the Pearce and Foster (1965) series, one was retinal, three were in the posterior cerebral territory and six were in the distribution of the middle cerebral artery.

Differential diagnosis
Issues relating to differential diagnosis are considered in Chapter 12 (especially in the sections on vascular disease).

Review of the literature
It is not consistent with the aims of this monograph to provide an extensive review of the literature on the subject of stroke in migraine. However, it is useful to have a degree of familiarity with it in order to place the problem in proper perspective. Most of the reported cases are well beyond the pediatric age-group, and some illustrate the issue of the relatively frequent ambiguity of migraine *vs.* another cause of the stroke in a patient who also happens to have migraine.

The most convincing situation is the development of persistent neurological signs for a minimum of a week beyond a clinically unequivocal migraine headache that is associated with complex symptomatology in the same vascular territory. Similar headaches, without complicating stroke, but with transient signs in the prodrome or during the headache, may have occurred in the past. The patient should be young, preferably under 20 years, and the family history should be positive for migraine. Finally, laboratory studies should be complete, including CT and angiography, and reveal no other cause.

Rarely in practice or in the literature is this hypothetical ideal case fulfilled. However, convincing cases in young adults have been recorded, and there is no question that infarction can occur in the course of migrainic episodes. Examples from the literature that give credibility to the close association, and sufficiently fulfil the above criteria, are the reports of Murphy (1955), cases 1 and 3 of Dorfman *et al.* (1979), and case 2 of Pearce and Foster (1965).

Reports in children are less common. Castaldo *et al.* (1982) reported a seven-year-old boy who developed an angiographically proved left middle cerebral-artery occlusion with CT evidence of infarction in the context of a severe and prolonged complex episode of migraine. He had been subject to abdominal migraine in his early years, then periodic headaches with anorexia and lethargy for two years before his stroke. His mother had common migraine and his father and paternal grandmother had complex migraine with hemiparesis and sensory disturbance.

When stroke occurs in migraine, it is usually a single event and the prognosis is good. The case of Ferguson and Robinson (1982) stands out as an exception to this general rule, and illustrates the malignant course in some patients. This 13-year-old girl had multiple complex episodes, several with persistent signs consistent with infarction over a period of months, the chief long-term residual of which was

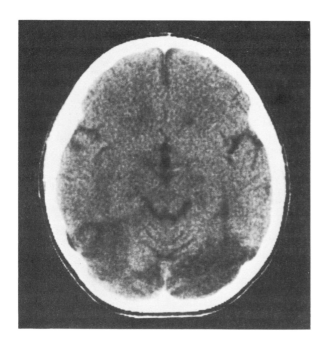

Fig. 10. This CT scan shows bilateral hypodense lesions of the occipital lobes secondary to infarction in a 15-year-old boy. The infarcts developed in the setting of severe migrainic episodes during a four-year period. The hypodense areas represent cumulative effect of both old and recent infarction.

amnesia for the period of frequent complex episodes. Control was eventually achieved subsequent to the discovery of a hypothyroid state and treatment with levothyroxine, amitriptyline, aspirin, relaxation therapy and continuation of the propranolol that she had been receiving throughout much of her illness.

Dr. Guiseppe Erba brought to my attention a 15-year-old boy who had had severe complex migraine, occasionally associated with seizures, since age nine. Four years previously he had had two CT-proved infarcts during severe attacks, one in each occipital lobe, which led to cortical blindness. He gradually recovered over a two-year period only to develop a third vascular accident in the same context at age 15 (Fig. 10).

A further indication of the malignant possibilities of stroke in some patients with migraine is reflected in the series of young children and infants reported by Verret and Steele (1971). The eight patients described had their first episode at three, four, seven and nine months, and at one and a half, two and three years. All patients had family members who gave reasonably convincing histories of migraine, including four with a parent or sibling who also had had transient hemiplegic migraine without complication. Two of the reported cases were siblings. In six patients the focal signs alternated; all occurred on multiple occasions, usually were of hours in duration, but were occasionally more persistent. Some had focal motor seizures as part of the ictal event and most had indication of significant pain with either verbal or non-verbal expression of contralateral headache. In some there was a brief vasomotor prodrome, and vomiting was usually prominent. The early onset of hemiplegic migraine in this group of patients led to significant mild to moderate

141

residual dysfunction (mental retardation, dyslexia, minor motor impairment) and the strong presumption that the culmination of multiple episodes was brain-damaging, probably related to small infarcts. Arteriography in five patients was negative. The report pre-dated the availability of CT scans, which might have been more revealing of findings suggesting infarction.

The principal issue that runs through any critical review of the literature on stroke and migraine is the question of the relationship of the two problems in a given patient. The majority of reported cases were in an older age-group where stroke is sufficiently common that embolic and thrombotic infarction of brain is not unusual, and in some the timing of the stroke bore no relationship to the headache. If headache was present, it may have been atypical of the usual vascular headaches of that particular patient. In those individuals in whom the stroke was hemorrhagic it is unlikely that migraine is more than incidental to the event, or alternatively, the vascular headache or other phenomena have been symptomatic of an underlying lesion right along.

The intriguing possibility has been suggested that migraine represents a significant increased risk factor added upon a lesion where there is already a basic risk of stroke (Table XII). For example, does the patient with prolapse of the mitral valve plus migraine have a higher incidence of stroke than the patient with a prolapsed valve alone (Litman and Friedman 1978, Conomy *et al.* 1982)? The same question might be posed in relation to other disorders of heart, anatomical abnormalities of various kinds of major and smaller cerebral blood-vessels, such as fibromuscular dysplasia (Mettinger and Ericson 1982), inherited disorders of clotting mechanism, or any risk factor of stroke in childhood (see Chapter 13 on causes of stroke in children as well as the section on pathogenesis in Chapter 2).

Clinical presentation
Among the most convincing examples of vascular occlusion in association with migraine are those which occur in the eye, where direct visual observation can be made with the ophthalmoscope. There are several reports of observed vasospasm of retinal arteries during the migraine aura (Walsh and Hoyt 1969). In some patients this leads to permanent occlusion of retinal arteries that can be documented by direct visualization and permanent segmental defects in the field of vision of one eye. Only one such patient has come to my attention.

When the infarction involves the optic nerve near the disc, pallid swelling of the optic disc results, along with a visual defect that may persist (Walsh and Hoyt 1969, McDonald and Sanders 1971). The retro-orbital ophthalmic artery may also be affected (Graveson 1949). When this occurs, the retina and disc become pale and vessels of the disc are attenuated. Optic atrophy is a later observation. Occlusion of the central retinal vein also occurs (Friedman 1951). This compli-cation results in gross swelling of the disc with hemorrhages.

The danger of cerebral infarction is greatest in those patients with focal neurological symptomatology. It usually occurs when symptoms that may have begun during the aura either persist into the headache phase or develop after the headache is well established. The clinical problem of whether a stroke may have occurred therefore blends into the issue of 'complicated' migraine. The problem for the clinician is similar to that of Todd's paralysis in seizure disorder. In both the acceptable time limit may be set at 24 hours beyond the paroxysm, but in both the duration of focal signs is usually less and is of several hours duration.

The infarct may occur in a territory distinct from that implicated in the aura. In some instances there is a biphasic course, *i.e.* brief symptoms and signs during the aura, which recur later with more persistence. Any vascular territory may be affected, and in some instances the process is quite clearly multifocal. It is probably significant that the vascular territories of retina and posterior cerebral artery, which correspond to the aura of 'classic' migraine, are those most frequently involved.

Migraine triggered by trauma or physical exertion may increase the risk of stroke: a statement based upon the unexpected number of persistent neurologic defects in reported series involving these factors (Haas *et al.* 1975, Lance 1976). The same may be said of the increased risk of stroke in migrainic women using birth-control pills (Saper 1983).

Otherwise there is nothing unusual about the focal symptoms or signs that develop. The principal feature of diagnostic significance is persistence of the deficit beyond the headache phase for at least 24 hours. Even at this point there may be some ambiguity as to whether infarction has occurred. However, persistent focal signs beyond several days must be regarded as significant.

The persistence of focal signs may not be the only diagnostic criteria. Mathew *et al.* (1977) have reported a series of 29 patients who had CT scan during the four to nine days after their last migraine attack. 10 scans were abnormal, and seven had areas of parenchymal lucency that could represent either focal edema or infarction. Clinically the patients ranged from normal at the time of the scan following an episode of severe 'common migraine' to those whose migraine was complex and associated with minimal residual signs. The low-density areas tended to disappear on subsequent scans. Five of these patients were 30 years or younger. On review of the limited clinical information given, one would not necessarily conclude that these patients had had an infarct on clinical grounds alone. Perhaps in some instances the CT scan will show the tissue change of infarction in migrainics when the clinical impression is ambiguous.

The same problem is addressed in the report of Dorfman *et al.* (1979) in which cerebral infarction was proved by arteriography and serial CT scans in four young adult migrainic patients. Two of these patients had neurologic defects that persisted for weeks or months. In the others the defect lasted less than three days, and the issue of an infarct might have been ambiguous had it not been for the CT scan findings. The authors concluded that 'cerebral infarction, as revealed by CT, may be more prevalent in "complicated" migraine than is generally appreciated'.

It is now clear that the CT scan is more likely than angiography to show changes consistent with stroke. The angiogram has been quite unproductive in demonstrating occlusion or other vascular changes in migrainic patients, as noted in the reports described above. This is not very surprising, in view of the frequency of negative angiography in strokes in general. This is especially the case when the stroke is mild as is usual in migraine-related incidents.

A young patient may also present with definite clinical indication of stroke, but the past migrainic symptomatology has consisted of common migraine without complex or classic phenomenology. The stroke may occur in the setting of a particularly severe common migraine attack, and in these circumstances the etiologic relationship to migraine is reasonably convincing, but in other circumstances the headache may be vascular in quality but significantly different from the patient's usual headache, or there may be no headache at all. All of these clinical circumstances have been reported as 'stroke with migraine'.

They may indeed reflect a direct or indirect pathogenetic relationship to migraine, especially if the patient is young, has a convincing history of prior vascular headache and a positive family history, and proves to have no other cause for stroke on full investigation. As alluded to above, even if certain putative causative factors are identified, the question remains open as to whether the basic inherited biochemical systemic-vascular disorder of migraine has played a contributory rôle in the catastrophe.

Pathogenesis
The pathologic physiology of the presumptive vascular occlusion, whether it be thrombosis or embolization from a distant site, centers about the issues of vasospasm and platelet hypercoagulability. These factors were considered in greater detail in Chapter 2.

Management
Supportive treatment in the acute phase usually poses no unique problems. Primary attention to diagnostic considerations is appropriate. This should include CT scan at an early point to resolve the question of parenchymal hemorrhage, the presence of AVM, or a mass lesion. The finding of edema is non-specific, but may be present especially if compromised tissue is extensive. A repeat CT scan seven to 10 days later is appropriate to define the extent of the infarct.

With the initial information of CT at hand, one may proceed to an examination of the CSF. Arteriography should usually wait for at least 24 hours to ascertain whether the focal signs are persistent. Because of the possibility of inducing further trouble by the injection of radiocontrast material, pre-treatment with dexamethasone is appropriate. Results of the nitroprusside urinary test for homocystinura should be available prior to angiography, and if positive would indicate deferring and perhaps cancelling the procedure.

During the early phase of investigation it is important to initiate other studies relevant to etiology of stroke in the young, such as sedimentation rate and other indicators of systemic vasculitis, *i.e.* wbc lupus preparation, ANA antibodies, and plasma globulin. When appropriate, a sickle cell preparation should be done. Cholesterol levels, clotting factors such as anti-thrombin III, as well as repeated blood cultures upon indication should all be considered. Echocardiogram is important in assessing the possibility of prolapse of the mitral valve, valvular vegetations, or myxoma, and should be part of the routine investigation of strokes in the pediatric and young adult age-group.

Cerebral arteriography of appropriate cerebral vessels is a necessary step in the investigation of most young people with stroke. If the patient has a previous history of migraine, in addition to pre-treatment with dexamethasone, the initiation of propranolol and aspirin therapy may be indicated. None of these measures are of proven benefit in preventing further emboli, thrombosis or spasm in the acute phase, but all are relatively innocuous and reasonable at this stage of our information.

Once the diagnostic phase is well under way, if no specific cause of the vascular accident is revealed and migraine remains a reasonable possibility as the only likely cause or as a factor in the pathogenesis, the most appropriate recommendation would be continuation of prophylactic anti-migrainic therapy (propranolol) and aspirin or aspirin-persantin or other anticoagulants for a period of several months. The chance of recurrence of stroke in these patients would seem to be very low although the reports of Ferguson and Robinson (1982) and Verret and Steele (1971) are indications of the potentially devastating consequences in some patients.

Migraine with basilar-vertebral stroke

This girl was nine and a half when first seen. She had been entirely well **CASE** until age seven when she fell and struck her head. Shortly thereafter she **33** vomited, became stuporous, then comatose, and had a seizure during which her head and eyes turned to the left and the left arm extended. The seizure lasted two minutes, after which she recovered relatively rapidly. She was admitted to a local hospital where bilateral angiograms were normal. An EEG five weeks later was normal. During the next one and a half years she had several attacks that were characterized by pain centering about the left eye, associated with numbness and tingling of the peri-oral region and the right upper extremity, accompanied by slurred speech.

Her father had severe, throbbing, hemicranial headaches preceded by visual disturbance and numbness of the arm and mouth. They usually involved the right arm although they occasionally occurred on the left.

The patient was treated with Cafergot at the first indication of numbness, which usually prevented any significant headache.

Two weeks prior to her admission to CH Boston, she developed an episode beginning with numbness of the right foot and hand, followed by dysarthria and then throbbing headache. She vomited two Cafergot tablets and was given intramuscular promazine, following which she became comatose and remained in coma for 10 days, requiring tracheostomy and initial respiratory support. Arteriograms were negative.

As she awakened, she had diplopia, ataxia, and weakness on the right side of her body. Two weeks after the original incident she was transferred to CH Boston where physical examination revealed her to be alert and co-operative with no general physical abnormalities. There was bilateral horizontal nystagmus and very mild right hemiparesis, and her most prominent sign was truncal ataxia with mild bilateral intention tremor in the upper extremities.

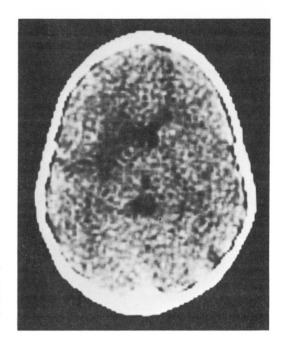

Fig. 11. This CT scan demonstrates a low-density lesion involving the basal ganglia and internal capsule of the left cerebral hemisphere, indicative of infarction in the territory of the middle cerebral artery (case 34).

The EEG showed asymmetrical slowing posteriorly and a pneumo-encephalogram was entirely normal.

Over the subsequent months she made full recovery. She was treated with phenytoin 100 mg b.i.d. and intermittent methysergide 1 mg b.i.d. In a two-year period while on this regimen she had no subsequent difficulties, with the exception of one mild episode approximately three months subsequent to her hospitalization. No additional follow-up information is available.

Comment: This child's first episode of migraine followed head trauma and was complicated by a seizure. Subsequently she had periodic complex migraine that was similar in expression to that of her father. During an otherwise relatively typical episode she became comatose and recovered with residual signs indicating infarction in the vertebral-basilar territory.

Migraine with stroke

CASE 34 This boy was six years old when first seen.* For the preceding two years he had had such severe headaches that he cried. They occurred every two to three months. Family history revealed that his father had had hemicranial throbbing headaches, occasionally preceded by flashing lights, for much of his lifetime. A paternal grandfather also suffered from classic migraine and the boy's mother had occasional bilateral frontal headaches attributed to

*Patient reported courtesy of Dr. Karl Kuban.

'sinusitis'.

Two days prior to admission he complained of a headache that was aggravated by jumping up and down. The quality of headache could not be ascertained but it continued throughout the day and he spent a restless night. On the following day he slept late but then seemed well until around 5.00 p.m., at which time he again complained of severe headache. He was nauseated but there was no vomiting. At 10.00 p.m. that night he awakened crying and by midnight his speech was thickened. When he went to the bathroom he used his left hand exclusively. At 3.00 a.m. it was noted that he had a right hemiparesis and was unable to walk. When seen a few hours later at the local hospital, he was found to have a right hemiparesis with lower facial weakness, and aphasia. Cerebrospinal fluid examination was normal.

On arrival at CH Boston, he seemed in no acute distress but vomited on one occasion. Temperature was 99.8 and blood pressure 106/60. General physical examination was unrevealing. Neurological evaluation found him to be anxious, frightened and somnolent. His understanding of spoken words was incomplete and he had a right hemianopsia. There was lower facial paresis and weakness of the right arm and leg with diminished tone, increased reflexes and an extensor plantar response on that side.

A CT scan (Fig. 11) demonstrated loosening of tissue in the left middle cerebral distribution, and EEG showed slowing over the left hemisphere. CSF revealed three mononuclear cells and a protein of 24 mg per cent. Nitroprusside urine test was negative as were a number of other examinations, including sedimentation rate and latex fixation. Arteriography showed multiple irregularities in the vessel wall which were interpreted as consistent with a restricted vasculitis (Fig. 12).

Prednisone therapy was initiated, and in the two months subsequent to admission he had seven episodes of headache, one of which was a severe pounding headache accompanied by nausea but no scotomata or vomiting. Fiorinal was given for the severe headaches and prednisone was tapered and discontinued. There was gradual improvement in the hemiparesis. Over the subsequent four years of observation he had occasional headaches usually managed by Fiorinal and aspirin. The headaches had a throbbing quality, were associated with nausea, but no vomiting. When most recently seen, approximately four years after the initial incident, he continued to have mild to moderate hemiparesis and at that point had had very little trouble from headaches during the previous year.

Comment: This boy was subject to vascular headaches as were several members of his family. During a particularly persistent headache he developed a hemiparesis, with CT-demonstrated infarction. Arteriograms revealed findings consistent with 'arteritis'. There was no indication of systemic disorder and it is possible that the arteriographic abnormality was a reflection of abnormal flow in the system. It is difficult to be certain whether the stroke was exclusively a migraine complication, or whether he

147

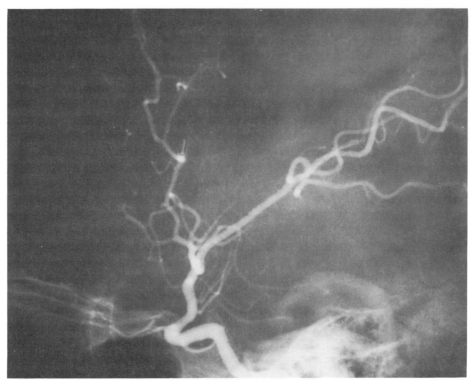

Fig. 12. This left cerebral arteriogram shows multiple vascular occlusions of smaller branches of the middle cerebral artery together with a long straight middle cerebral with multiple irregularities in the wall (case 34). This patient raises the question of interpretation of the vascular changes. Are they due to 'arteritis' or are the abnormalities due to changes related to migraine? (Serdaru *et al.* 1984.)

did indeed have a restricted cerebral arteritis and the migraine was a contributor in some fashion, or was incidental and irrelevant (Serdaru *et al.* 1984).

Migraine and stroke in a patient with Marfan's syndrome

CASE 35 This young man was age 13 when first seen. For the previous year he had had bilateral frontal pounding headaches that occurred about once a week. During the early phase of the headache he noted yellow or green colored spots in his entire visual field. The headaches usually occurred in the afternoon, lasted about three hours, and were not accompanied by other symptoms such as nausea or vomiting. His father, mother, paternal grandfather and paternal uncle all suffered from vascular headaches.

One day prior to admission he experienced the onset of severe pain behind his left eye that was worse than his usual headaches. It was not preceded by visual scotomata. He was released from school, the headache

148

remained severe and he vomited three times, and then lay down for a nap. After approximately two hours he was awakened by his parents and found to be confused with an unsteady gait, slurred speech and weakness on the right side of his body. He was admitted to a local hospital and on the following morning had a dense right hemiparesis with facial weakness. A CT scan was normal with and without contrast media. He was then transferred to CH Boston.

On admission he no longer had headache (actually none since the first day). Blood pressure was 112/78. There were no carotid or cranial bruits. He had an asymmetrical and atrophic right hemithorax with protrusion of the left anterior hemithorax. Cardiac examination revealed a systolic ejection click followed by a systolic ejection murmur, loudest at the apex, which radiated to the left and right lower sternal borders. There was a 2/6 blowing decrescendo diastolic murmur, heard loudest at the apex. He was tall for age (97th percentile). He had elongated fingers and toes and an arm span of 176 cm equal to his body length, and consistent with Marfan syndrome. There was no dislocation of lenses.

Neurological examination revealed him to be oriented and alert. Calculations were poor and in reading and speaking there were occasional paraphasic errors. He was dysarthric with right lower facial weakness and right hemiparesis.

Various laboratory tests were normal including a normal platelet count, prothrombin time, and sedimentation rate. Nitroprusside urine test for homocystinuria was negative. Arteriogram of the left carotid and vertebral-basilar circulation showed moderate tortuosity of the vessels including the aortic arch, internal carotid, and left vertebral circulations. There was no evidence of vasculitis and no vascular occlusion. 2D cardiac echo revealed an abnormal aortic valve with partial fusion of the right and left coronary leaflets. There was mild dilatation of the aortic root, and some thickening of the cusps of the aortic valves, but no thrombus.

Repeat CT scan after about a week remained normal. He was treated with daily aspirin and propranolol 20 mg t.i.d. On the sixth day of illness in the early morning he developed an episode of transient aphasia that lasted several hours. It was decided that anticoagulant therapy should be more vigorous. He was begun on Coumadin, and aspirin was discontinued. Throughout the remainder of his hospital stay he made continuous improvement in the hemiparesis and was discharged after a hospitalization of nine days.

In the period subsequent to discharge he continued to improve, making an excellent recovery, and was free of headache while taking propranolol and anticoagulants, first Coumadin, then aspirin and dipyridamole.

Comment: This boy developed a stroke in the setting of migraine and Marfan's syndrome with an abnormal aortic arch and its major branches. The circumstances raise the question of the possible contribution of both conditions acting together to enhance the risk of embolic stroke.

Migraine and stroke in a patient with prolapsed mitral valve

This 15-year-old girl had had periodic headaches for approximately one year. They occurred one to two times per month, were of low-grade severity and usually lasted 30 to 60 minutes. Aspirin gave relief. They were not associated with nausea, vomiting or photophobia and were not pulsatile. The quality of the sensation was more an aching pressure.

There was a strong family history of migraine. The mother had classic migraine with episodes of right hemiparesis and a 24-year-old sister also had hemiplegic migraine. Both grandmothers had migraine headaches. Her father had chocolate-precipitated severe abdominal pain and vomiting of several hours duration, and a sister also had periodic abdominal pain with no precipitant and no explanation during her high school years.

Pertinent past history included the recognition of mitral valve prolapse that was discovered in the context of exertional chest pain and proved on cardiac echo study.

She was athletically inclined and accustomed to running six miles per day. At the end of one of her running episodes she complained of stomach ache and her coach noted her to be pale. This occurred the evening prior to admission. On the day of admission, after running four miles (less than usual) she developed a stomach ache and felt ill. She went home, lay on the couch, then suddenly felt very faint and fell from the couch onto the floor. She was alert but it was noted by her parents that she had left facial weakness, slurred speech and weakness of the left arm. She was brought to the emergency room of CH Boston and at that time had a severe right frontal headache associated with nausea and mild photophobia.

On examination, her mental status was clear. She was dysarthric and had left lower facial weakness and a left hemiparesis affecting arm more than leg. Reflexes were equal and there was an extensor plantar response on the left. Cardiac consultation reported an apical ejection click followed by a soft blowing grade 1 systolic murmur that radiated to the left axilla, consistent with mitral valve prolapse. She had a normal CT scan on the day of admission. An EEG done on the same day showed slowing in the right posterior quadrant which was irregular and at about three to four HZ, indicative of right hemisphere dysfunction. No epileptiform discharges were seen. The sedimentation rate was 18, and latex fixation was negative as was nitroprusside test for homocystinuria.

Over the next several hospital days she improved gradually. On the day following admission she had a brief headache lasting about 30 minute associated with photophobia and slight exacerbation of weakness in the left arm. Treatment with propranolol 20 mg t.i.d. and aspirin 325 mg was initiated in the hospital.

When seen on follow-up two weeks later she had had no subsequent headache, and reported that her left side had returned to normal shortly after discharge. The total duration of noticeable weakness from the onset was approximately six days. However, examination on the two-week follow-up visit still indicated very minimal dysfunction consisting of slight inturning of the left foot as she walked.

Comment: This girl, with known mitral valve prolapse, was also subject to mild periodic headaches in a setting of a strong family history of migraine. She developed a stroke subsequent to distance running which seemed to provoke abdominal migraine symptoms. As in case 35 (above), this patient also brings up the question of enhanced risk of stroke in migrainic patients with anatomical abnormality of cardiac valves, in this instance the much more common mitral valve prolapse.

Migraine and syncope
Definition
The basis of loss of consciousness due to syncope is circulatory insufficiency, primarily, whether induced by brief cardiac asystole, profound bradycardia or cerebral hypotension related to other mechanisms including orthostatic hypotension. Less commonly, direct neural brainstem mechanisms may be responsible. It may occur as part of the phenomenology of the migraine attack, or as an independent episode in both migrainics and others. Because loss of consciousness is the central feature of the disorder it must be distinguished from seizures. Syncope is a relatively common phenomenon, and in most people who are subject to it, it occurs occasionally as the result of an identifiable inciting event.

Epidemiology
The population incidence is not known, nor has it been systematically studied. It probably reaches a peak expression during adolescence and early adult years. Orthostatic hypotension with occasional syncope is particularly common in boys during their adolescent growth spurt. If one includes the 'breath-holding spells' of young children as an expression of syncope, which is probably appropriate, then it becomes a very common phenomenon and affects 4 to 5 per cent of children between 18 months and five years (Lombroso and Lerman 1967). Certainly the less common 'pallid' variety of breath-holding spell, that is based upon cardiac asystole in response to injury, as well as frustration and crying, is a frequent predictor of the adult or older child who faints at the sight of blood or as a response to personal injury.

Syncope also occurs as an expression of the vasomotor instability of migraine, both as an independent event or as part of the migraine paroxysm. Syncope is most convincingly attributed to the migrainic process when it occurs during an attack as it did in 4.6 per cent of the Lance and Anthony (1966) adult series, as contrasted with a lower incidence in childhood. Prensky and Sommer (1979) recorded only 1.2 per cent in their series of children. The incidence is distinctly higher when one looks at individuals with associated symptoms and signs in the basilar artery territory. In a study of 29 patients of all ages that focused on loss of consciousness in migraine, seven had other symptoms attributable to the basilar-vertebral arterial territory, while 13 of the total group had syncope during 'ordinary migraine' (Lees and Watkins 1963). The remainder of the patients described in this report had epilepsy

151

either as a separate phenomenon (six patients) or during migraine (three patients). Lapkin and Golden (1978) identified three patients with loss of consciousness, and three with transient confusion or disorientation, out of 17 patients who had two or more symptoms of vertebral-basilar artery insufficiency during their migraine attacks. None had convulsive activity.

Bille's (1962) personally interviewed patient group gives some insight into the problem of independent episodes of syncope in juvenile migrainic patients. In this series 28.8 per cent of the index group had symptoms related to orthostatic events, as compared with 8.2 per cent of controls. 12.3 per cent of the migraine patients with orthostatic symptomatology fainted occasionally, as compared with 5.5 per cent of the control group. In my own series, 10 of 300 juvenile migrainics had independent episodes of syncope.

In summary one can say that syncope occurs with reasonable frequency during the migrainic episode, especially those with basilar-vertebral artery symptoms. Orthostatic symptoms short of syncope are common amongst juvenile migrainics, and syncope occurs on occasion. However, syncope occurring as an isolated event is not a common concomitant of the migraine syndrome, nor does it herald the appearance of classic or common migraine as does paroxysmal abdominal pain or cyclic vomiting. Infantile syncope (breath-holding spells) does not seem to be a precursor of migraine, although follow-up studies on a large series of patients have not been done. In Bille's (1962) 73 personally interviewed migrainic patients there were two who had had breath-holding spells as compared with one in the controls. The numbers are much too low to detect a small difference, but a major difference should have been apparent.

Differential diagnosis
Syncope must be differentiated from seizures. At times this may be difficult or even impossible, at least in part because an adequate description may not be available. It is not necessary to reiterate the various criteria that identify seizures, but it is appropriate to review the positive features upon which the diagnosis of syncope is made.

The clinical presentation of syncope
The event is sudden in onset, but almost invariably begins with a warning that consists of a feeling of light-headedness or giddiness. At this point, the attack may be aborted if the head is lowered. Much of the time, loss of postural tone precedes loss of consciousness and the patient is thereby able to recall falling. Facial pallor and cold sweatiness is a common observation. The patient becomes limp and unconscious for a time-period measured in seconds and seldom longer than a minute. Then the patient begins to rouse and consciousness is restored rather quickly. There may be residual symptoms of giddiness and unease for several minutes. Continence is maintained throughout and there is no post-event sleepiness.

Syncope is usually triggered by an identifiable provocation. In orthostatic syncope the event is either sudden postural changes which results in elevation of the head from its previous position, or the maintenance of the upright posture for an unusual length of time. The sight of blood, injury to self or others, a hot stuffy room, sudden and unexpected fright or emotional events are all recounted as precipitating factors.

Breath-holding spells (Lombroso and Lerman 1967, Laxdal *et al.* 1969), although perhaps out of context in this discussion, may be briefly mentioned. They are a common problem of infants and children aged six to 18 months and occasionally in younger infants (Laxdal *et al.* 1969). They are rarely encountered after age four or five years. Familial incidence is apparent in about 25 per cent of patients. In the commonest expression the child is frustrated, frightened or injured, begins to cry for a few seconds at which point the breath is held in inspiration and the child becomes cyanotic. Shortly thereafter consciousness is lost, and the child becomes limp and flaccid. On occasion the child may stiffen in an opisthotonic posture. If the episode is prolonged, convulsive twitching may occur.

In another scenario, the stimulus that leads to the event is usually pain, often a minor blow to the head. Reactive crying is usually less obvious and may not occur at all. Pallor occurs rather than cyanosis. This has been identified as the principal distinguishing feature of this variety of attack, *i.e.* the pallid breath-holding spell (Lombroso and Lerman 1967). Consciousness is lost and episthotonus and convulsive activity with occasional incontinence are all more frequent than in the cyanotic type. There is a high incidence of sustained cardiac asystole induced by ocular compression in this group of patients, which probably is a direct expression of the pathophysiologic basis of the disorder. In a number of instances the clinical distinction based on skin change is ambiguous, as is the result of ocular compression. Individuals with classic pallid breath-holding spells are likely to be subject to syncope as adults.

Pathogenesis
The most easily understood pathogenetic mechanisms are based upon cerebral circulatory insufficiency, either as a result of cardiac asystole or profound bradycardia, or of sudden hypotension attributable to other mechanisms.

In the context of migrainic episodes, the central nervous system and especially the brainstem must be entered into the pathogenetic equation. This may be operative *via* influence on circulatory events, but is more likely to be a direct effect *via* neural mechanisms involving the brainstem reticular systems.

Management
The diagnostic issues raised by syncope can usually be settled clinically, but an EEG is appropriate and reassuring if normal, as is usually the case. In breath-holding spells, the EEG should include an electrocardiographic lead and be accompanied by ocular compression to ascertain whether this maneuver produces cardiac asystole and concomitant EEG changes (Lombroso and Lerman 1967). Measurement of blood pressure before and after rising to full standing from the supine can be helpful, especially if the clinical story suggests an orthostatic component. This is particularly convincing if symptoms are reproduced. One should give particular

attention to cardiac examination and an electrocardiogram may be indicated.

Prevention of the syncope that may occur in the context of a migrainic episode is handled by prophylaxis of migraine. Syncope that occurs in isolation is usually managed by avoidance of precipitating events if this is possible. This may be impractical except when episodes have an orthostatic component. Advice to change position slowly can be helpful.

In those individuals who demonstrate cardiac asystole with ocular compression, including young children with the 'pallid' variety of breath-holding spell, one may consider continuous treatment with atropine or preparations with similar properties (Lombroso and Lerman 1967, Laxdal *et al.* 1969). This is only appropriate when the frequency of episodes is sufficient to warrant this measure.

Basilar migraine with syncope

CASE 37 This 13-year-old girl had had spells of increasing frequency over a period of two years. The spells began with double vision and a feeling that the ground was moving. She became unsteady, and would usually sit down. On two occasions she fainted during a particularly severe episode. These episodes would last five to 10 minutes and were followed by a retro-orbital and frontal throbbing headache. Nausea was present throughout the episode and on occasion she vomited. Her mother recalled periodic throbbing headaches that occurred when she was a teenager.

Examination was normal and she was treated with propranolol 10 mg t.i.d. with almost complete control.

Comment: Syncope occurred in this girl during an episode of migraine on two occasions. The migrainic episodes had symptoms indicative of vertebral-basilar artery insufficiency.

8
TREATMENT OF JUVENILE MIGRAINE

Introduction

There are limitations in any program of treatment for juvenile migraine. Without an understanding of the basic cause or causes of the inherited abnormality, a rational approach to the fundamental problem cannot be designed. Nor is genetic counseling a consideration. The disorder is much too common, and on the scale of serious morbidity it must fall near the bottom of the list.

It is, nevertheless, a significant cause of repeated incapacity and therefore an important annoyance in life. Moreover, until the diagnostic uncertainty of the relatively benign nature of the recurrent symptoms is settled, the existence of repeated headache, or other symptoms of the migraine syndrome, is a source of uncertainty and anxiety that serves to aggravate the problem. Differential diagnostic considerations comprise most of this monograph. A solid diagnosis is the first step in therapy.

The current goal of therapy is to interrupt a step or steps in the pathogenesis of the paroxysm in order to afford symptomatic relief. The measures used consist of a combination of pharmacotherapy and formal or informal behavioral modification. It is my estimate that the rate of success is at least 80 per cent.

Any treatment program should be planned in the context of what is known of the natural course of the disorder. It is worth reconsidering several fundamental points about juvenile migraine in the context of therapy. Adult migraine as it presents to the physician tends to be a persistent problem that may wax and wane in relation to biological and psychological factors (Graham 1956). The biological factors include the hormonal influence of pregnancy, menopause, and menstruation in women and intercurrent illness of many varieties. The environmental factors that can be responsible for remission or exacerbation include those related to school, marriage, work, vacations, deaths and all of the individual events of life which produce stress (exacerbation) or equanimity (remission). The adult pattern is probably established at about 18 years.

The childhood pattern is somewhat different, although the basic theme of stress-induced exacerbation is quite apparent. As Prensky and Sommer (1979) pointed out, most children had exacerbation of six months duration 'regardless of the type of therapy'. I accept the statement that six to eight months is the usual duration of an exacerbation in childhood, but am not as pessimistic about the effectiveness of therapy. As stated before, exacerbation in childhood is often correlated with the school year; this is so regularly so, that duration of continuous pharmacologic treatment can be based on this association. It is my contention that significant amelioration or suppression of migraine expression can be achieved in most children during this period of school-related exacerbation.

It is less clear whether pharmacologic suppression for a period of time will result in a sustained remission of months or longer. This may be true of adults, or adolescents who have assumed the adult pattern, but it is not yet clear in children.

A two- to four-year period of school-related exacerbations is a frequent experience in children, followed by an indefinite period of remission. The remission tends to occur between nine and 16 years as the Congdon and Forsythe (1979) data show. These authors also pointed out that between 3 and 14 per cent of the young patients in their series had a remission each year; and that of the 228 children followed for eight years, 29 per cent had had an eight-year remission. Boys are more likely to undergo prolonged remission than girls.

The above epidemiologic points provide the background for decision regarding the therapeutic plan in the individual patient. Several options are available.
(1) Reassurance of the benign nature of the recurring symptoms based upon careful history, examination and any ancillary examinations that may be indicated may be all that is necessary. This should be combined with general advice about lifestyle, including avoidance of trigger factors. The approach of total reassurance should not be adopted unless or until the problem has lasted longer than six months, because of the possibility of symptomatic migraine, especially tumor.
(2) Treatment may be focused on the individual attack, either to ameliorate the headache, vomiting or other symptoms, or to abort it at the first evidence of trouble. The approach may emphasize pharmacotherapy, or biofeedback and other behavioral measures.
(3) If headaches are of sufficient frequency and/or severity, daily prophylactic pharmacotherapy may be the treatment mode of choice.
(4) Behavioural modification therapy is preferred by some patients and parents who are reluctant to use drugs or where the simpler drugs have failed. Once learned, it has the advantage of lasting a lifetime. Intensive psychotherapy is seldom necessary in the treatment of juvenile migraine.

The choice of therapeutic approach is principally contingent upon the judgement of need based on the frequency and severity of the paroxysms in each individual. Infrequent episodes (less than one per month) seldom warrant aggressive treatment unless the episodes are devastating and/or prolonged. Frequent episodes (several per week), even if relatively mild, can lead to sufficient disability to warrant active therapeutic intervention. The inevitable gray area lies between.

General approach to migrainic children and their families
This section applies to the management of all patients. The approach is probably sufficient for many. The chief point to be communicated is the importance of psychological factors that may be identified as the responsible circumstance in any given attack, or as the basic substrate for a more sustained exacerbation. These issues account for the placebo effect in migraine that is probably more prominent in adults but is also operative in children. In double blind studies in adults 20 to 30 per cent and occasionally more will respond to administered placebo. Children may not be as responsive, but the reassurance of a careful, confident and caring manner is important and helpful to both the child and parents.

In discussions with the patient and their family, it is important to emphasize that migraine is not the equivalent of psychogenic headache, however important psychologic factors may be in the problem. The basic problem can be described as an inherited predisposition to overresponsive vascular reaction. It is useful to cite the other members in the family with similar problems. It is also useful to indicate that the psychologic stresses may be no greater than others are subjected to, but that it is the body's built-in reaction that is different. It nevertheless follows that the young person with migraine must accommodate certain aspects of their lifestyle or suffer some consequences. Regular bedtime and arising, reasonable meals and avoidance of overload in curricular and extra-curricular school activities are important and worth assessing (see Chapter 3 for discussion of the many factors that may trigger migraine in certain individuals).

In some, the regular school curriculum amounts to stress because of concomitant dyslexia and other learning disabilities. The numbers of boys in whom this is a factor in migraine headache seems disproportionate, but there are no hard data on this point. Certainly information regarding learning problems is worth specific inquiry in any migrainic patient, especially in boys.

Other psychologic forces can be important in individual patients. The issues in migraine are no different than those of psychogenic headache, and the reader is referred to that section for further discussion.

Another major area of general advice is to suggest that patient and parents make an effort to identify other factors which precipitate the attack, and then avoid them to the extent that this is possible. A headache diary can be useful in this regard. In general, easily identifiable triggers only account for a minority of headaches in a given individual. Food factors are among the more obvious. For practical purposes in children this amounts to chocolate and hot dogs, sometimes cheddar cheese or milk. Adolescents may have a wider range of possibilities, including over-indulgence in wine and cigarettes, skimpy breakfasts, and delayed or no lunch. Prolonged physical exertion is also a reasonably frequent precipitating cause in young people, and bright light and sun exposure may also be identified. In some instances hypoglycemia or lactose intolerance can be proved, and appropriate dietary action recommended.

The treatment of the episode
Even with the best regulated life or the most successful prophylactic regimen, the patient with juvenile migraine will have an occasional episode. Early treatment is the first principle in the symptomatic management of the paroxysm. The earlier the effort is made, the more likely it will be successful. It is this very issue, however, that tends to defeat this approach to management in children. The headache is not usually reported or recognized until it is well established, and by then it may be too late. The alternative of having the child carry medication is usually impractical, and in most instances inappropriate as well. These statements apply to pharmaco-therapy, and are much less relevant to the behavioral therapies. It is one of the distinct advantages of the behavioral approach.

The child will often spontaneously interrupt activity and want to lie down. This should be encouraged and he or she be given a quiet place and an opportunity to go to sleep. Sleep is the most dependable method of interrupting a paroxysm.

A simultaneous effort should be made to obtain symptomatic relief with medication. Aspirin in a dosage of 60 to 120 mg may be useful, and it is the first thing to try. Usually this already has been done as a home remedy in the past and the value of this approach ascertained before consultation. It will often be reported that milder headaches have responded to some extent, while the more severe have not.

There are several preparations consisting of a mixture of drugs that have been marketed by pharmaceutical houses for headache relief, usually containing sedative, analgesic and various other drugs. The combination that has the greatest value is a mixture of butalbital 50 mg, aspirin 200 mg, phenacetin 130 mg and caffeine 40 mg (Fiorinal). It can be effective in children as well as adults. Adolescents may be given the recommended adult dose of one or two capsules every four hours with a maximum of six on a headache day, while children should have half this amount. Because of the shorter duration of headache in childhood, usually one or two capsules are sufficient, but it should be given early. This preparation is also available with codeine in various amounts. Although codeine enhances analgesic properties, it should not be used in migraine because of the chronicity of the problem and the possibility of abuse and habituation. Fiorinal has been a useful preparation in my own experience, and although drug mixtures in a single tablet or capsule limit flexibility, this seems to be a generally useful combination for migraine therapy.

Another approach to intermittent therapy is somewhat more elegant in that the effort has greater theoretical specificity. The essential feature is the use of ergot derivatives, preferably at the stage of the aura in order to interrupt the presumed pathophysiologic sequence of 'vasospasm followed by vasodilatation.' Theoretically, ergot and related materials are valuable because of their vasoconstrictor action. There is good reason to doubt that this is the actual basis of the therapeutic effect of these preparations in the dosage used. For example, continuous use of ergot and related vasoconstrictor medications can effectively prevent the aura of migraine in those individuals who experience the aura alone. Also the dosage as used in many successful therapeutic regimens is insufficient to promote vasoconstriction. What may be a more accurate working hypothesis is that the effect in some way relates to modification of vascular tone and a reduction of responsiveness in either direction.

Whatever the basis of their effectiveness, derivatives of ergot have a long history of successful use in the treatment of migraine. There are a number of preparations available that can be used to abort an attack, many of which are compounded in tablet or suppository form in combination with other medications that may also have an additive favorable effect. They are of greater value in adolescents and adults than in younger children for the reasons cited above, *i.e.* the problem of the child carrying medication and the related problem of early administration. In addition the relative infrequency and brevity of well-developed auras in children tends to reduce the number of patients who are good candidates. The greatest value of these preparations results when they are administered during the aura.

The study of Congdon and Forsythe (1979) illustrates the general limitation of intermittent therapy at the onset of the headache in children. In an effort to assess the effectiveness of ergotamine tartrate *vs.* placebo, a double blind crossover study was planned. The drop-out rate of 66 per cent precluded any statistical treatment of results, a point which illustrates the problem very well. The lifestyle of childhood does not lend itself to this mode of therapy. Parenthetically, neither the inhaler nor sublingual ergotamine tablets in a dose of 1 mg every half hour to a total of 3 mg seemed to have any advantage, insofar as the data could be analyzed.

The ideal indication for the use of preparations to abort the attack is in adolescent patients who have classic and relatively severe migraine at intervals of one month or more in frequency, an incidence that tends to preclude the use of the continuous prophylactic mode of pharmacotherapy. Obviously the ideal patient is not common in pediatric practice. Exceptions may be made to any of the above descriptors when the individual circumstances warrant a therapeutic trial. This applies to age (younger patients may be responsible enough to carry medication or to report at the earliest phase of aura or headache), frequency (for whatever reason continuous treatment may not be warranted and other features such as a prolonged aura may be present), or aura (a discernible prodrome without classic aura may provide sufficient time for effective treatment or a slow build-up of the headache may encourage this approach). As a result of the limitations of intermittent therapy, I seldom use it. In my group of patients there are very few where a regimen based on interrupting the individual headache sequence has become the principal feature of the management.

Combination tablets of ergotamine tartrate and other active principals
The most widely-used preparation of this type is a combination of 2 mg ergotamine tartrate, and 100 mg caffeine (Cafergot) that is supplied in tablet form. The recommended schedule of administration for adults consists of two tablets at the outset followed by one tablet every half hour to a maximum of six tablets, and a recommended maximum of 10 tablets per week. This dosage is appropriate for most adolescents but should be scaled down for children. Usually four tablets are adequate, but best effect results from use of two at the outset at any age. Side-effects are minimal, but can include increased nausea, and rarely evidence of systemic vascoconstriction.

Preparations are also available that include barbiturate, analgesics and belladonna derivatives (the latter included for their anti-emetic properties). These include Cafergot p-b (see above plus belladonna alkaloids 0.125 mg and pento-barbital 30 mg), Wigraine (ergotamine tartrate 1 mg, caffeine 100 mg, belladonna alkaloids 0.1 mg, phenacetin 130 mg), and Bellergal (ergotamine tartrate 0.3 mg, phenobarbital 20 mg, belladonna alkaloids 0.1 mg). Note that Bellergal contains much less ergotamine tartrate. This accounts for its very limited value in aborting attacks, but for the same reason it can be used as daily prophylactic therapy. Several of the above preparations are also available as suppositories. Adminis-tration per rectum has the obvious advantage over the oral route when vomiting is a significant aspect of the clinical presentation. Absorption is more rapid and reliable. Suppositories have the disadvantage that they must be kept at home under refrigeration and often must be administered by others. They are available as Cafergot and Cafergot P-B in the same dosage as the tablet. One half suppository may be effective and is appropriate as the first step in children. Wigraine (same dosage as tablets) is also available in suppository form.

Ergotamine tartrate is also available for parenteral use. It is given by subcutaneous or intramuscular injection in a usual dosage of 0.25 mg (0.5 ml). It is the most immediate and effective method of delivering ergotamine but has the great limitation of requiring syringe, needles and a certain expertise, and should usually be administered by a physician or nurse. Its value in childhood is limited to those patients who have the most severe and prolonged paroxysm, especially if sustained vomiting occurs.

Dihydroergotamine is a hydrogenated ergotamine, available for intramuscular use in 1 ml ampules containing 1 mg of the drug. It has tended to replace ergotamine tartrate for parenteral use in migraine. Indications and contra-indications are generally similar, and the dose for adolescent patients is 0.5 to 1.0 mg which may be repeated three times in the course of a headache. Weekly dosage should be limited to 6 ml.

Anti-emetics
Symptomatic anti-emetic therapy also plays a rôle in the management of the acute attack in those patients in whom repeated vomiting is either a significant aspect of the attack or in the cyclic vomiting variant. Commonly used anti-emetics include trimethobenzamide HCL (Tigan) that is available as tablets (100 mg or 250 mg), suppositories (200 mg) or 2 ml ampules (100 mg/ml). Extrapyramidal reactions have been known to occur. Dosage in children is 100 to 200 mg t.i.d. by mouth and 100 mg t.i.d. by suppository, while parenteral administration has not been recommended in this age-group.

Hydroxyzine pamoate (Vistaril) is available in 25, 50 and 100 mg/5 ml. It has an anti-emetic effect but also has sedative and anti-anxiety properties. Adverse effects consist of over-sedation and occasional tremors. Dosage in children is 25 mg, b.i.d. to t.i.d. and in adults 25 mg t.i.d. to q.i.d.

Chlorpromazine has a well-deserved reputation as an effective anti-emetic and acts to control apprehension as well. Both properties are useful in migraine with vomiting. It is available as 10, 25 and 50 mg tablets, suppositories of 25 and 100 mg and in ampules of 1 and 2 ml (25 mg/ml). Adverse effects include drowsiness and acute dystonic reactions, postural hypotension, and very rarely more serious reactions such as agranulocytosis or jaundice. Oral dosage for children is 10 to 25 mg t.i.d., by suppository 12.5 to 25 mg b.i.d. or t.i.d., and the maximum IM dosage is 75 mg per day.

Metoclopramide HCL (Reglan) is a newer anti-emetic that has potential value in migrainic vomiting. It is a dopamine antagonist that stimulates motility of the upper gastro-intestinal tract. It is available as 10 mg tablets and two ml ampules containing 5 mg/ml. Adverse effects include drowsiness and extrapyramidal reactions in children. Oral dosage in children is 5 to 10 mg b.i.d. or t.i.d.

Intravenous administration should be reserved for hospitalized individuals with sustained vomiting over several days.

Continuous prophylactic treatment
The cornerstone of the treatment of juvenile migraine is the use of a rather long list of potentially beneficial medications on a continuous daily basis. The objective is the reduction in frequency and/or severity of attacks of migraine. The ideal result is complete suppression of attacks during a significant period of vulnerability. This usually means treatment for the duration of the school year in most patients. Medication may be discontinued during the period of the prolonged summer holiday. This is possible largely because of the strong correlation of migraine expression with the stress of the school year. There also may be an element of sustained beneficial effect based on interruption of the cycle of frequent expression over a period of time.

One might ask whether continuous prophylaxis is worthwhile in a benign episodic disorder in which most of the hours of most days are asymptomatic, particularly if the problem will spontaneously improve in six to eight months. One could also make the point that the principal aggravating factor is psychologic tension and this should be approached directly. However it is not necessarily undue individual reactions to psychologic stress or personality disorder that lie behind the aggravation of symptoms in migraine. Migraine consists of an unusual physiologic response to stresses that are handled without overt symptoms by the non-migrainic child in most instances. Psychotherapy would need to achieve a superhuman degree of equanimity in order to be totally successful. This is not meant to disparage the behavioral modification techniques that have great and enduring value in migraine. These are not methods of personality adjustment. They are based upon conscious interruption of the pathophysiologic sequence in migraine by achieving control of these processes.

Finally, why should a child experience repeated unpleasant and painful disruptions in the normal flow of life, if relatively simple measures can succeed in reducing the number or severity of attacks? The final answer in each case comes down to the combined judgement of physician, parents and child, of which the most important is the doctor who must make the initial recommendation.

The principal factor in the decision to recommend prophylactic treatment is the frequency and severity of the attacks. One or more episodes per week, particularly if they are of sufficient severity to interrupt activity, is ordinarily sufficient indication. It is more difficult to decide about episode frequency of one or two per month. If they are severe and prolonged or complex in expression, the bias is in favor of continuous treatment. Episodes less frequent than monthly seldom warrant treatment on a continuous daily basis.

An additional element that requires judicious decision relates to the potential adverse effects of medication. When the simpler measures with propranolol, phenytoin, cyproheptadine or phenobarbital have not proved effective, a serious reconsideration of the posture is necessary before proceeding to the more toxic methysergide, ergot preparations or less well-established therapies whose

161

effectiveness and toxicity are less well known.

Before embarking on a discussion of individual drugs that have value on a continuous-use basis, it should be pointed out that there have been very few studies in which the effectiveness of any of them has been validated by proper clinical pharmacologic study. Most such studies deal with drugs that have come into use in the modern era. Even fewer studies have dealt with children as the principal subject. Based upon my own experience, I believe that there may be a significant age difference, particularly with respect to the more favorable response to some drugs such as the anticonvulsants phenobarbital and phenytoin. This issue of compliance in the daily use of medication in the treatment of migraine has not been addressed, nor are medication levels customarily employed to ascertain compliance or determine therapeutic level.

Moreover, the studies that have been done are plagued by a high incidence of placebo effect. Although this may confound the clinical investigator, it should serve as a reminder to the clinician whose chief aim is relief for an individual patient. The conviction and confidence with which the treatment plan is offered may carry him 20 per cent along the route to success, at least temporarily. No apology need be made for this. The art of medicine demands results, while the science of medicine demands unbiased facts. The goals therefore differ.

Propranolol

Propranolol has come to occupy the key position in the therapy of migraine in my own practice and I suspect in that of many others who deal with juvenile migraine on a regular basis. It is a beta-adrenergic blocker and is active on both beta-1 (cardiac) and beta-2 receptors (smooth muscle of blood vessels and bronchi). In addition it has been shown to increase the threshold for aggregability of platelets, and affects the release of serotonin from platelets (Weksler *et al.* 1977). This may provide an additional pharmacologic advantage in its use in migraine, particularly in those patients in whom stroke may be threatened. Metabolism takes place in the liver. It is lipid soluble and therefore has access to the CNS. Propranolol is available in 10, 20, 40 and 80 mg tablets, the first two sizes of which are useful in children. The drug is contra-indicated in patients with cardiac decompensation, certain arrhythmias, asthma and depression. The low doses needed in children allow for careful use in some patients whose asthma is mild and occurs at widely spaced intervals. The same can be said of its use in children with mild depressive reactions. In both conditions, parents should be warned of possible adverse effects and advised to discontinue the drug at the first indication of trouble. There is relative contra-indication of propranolol in children with diabetes because it may block the adrenergic symptoms of a hypoglycemic reaction and make detection of this serious complication more difficult.

Propranolol therapy is initiated in a dosage of 10 mg t.i.d. in children of eight to 12 years for a trial period of two to four weeks and then increased to 20 mg t.i.d. Most young people of 13 or 14 years and above may be treated as adults. The adult starting dose is 20 mg t.i.d. with gradual increase to as much as 80 mg t.i.d. in those adolescent patients who have attained adult proportions. A two- to three-month period of gradually increasing dosage is required to give the drug an adequate trial, usually encouraged by some reduction of severity or frequency at lower doses.

In a study involving adults primarily, Rosen (1983) has pointed out that the efficacy of propranolol increased between three and 12 months of continuous usage in maximal dosage. 30 per cent of the patients who responded did so after three months. The total eventual response rate was 84 per cent, a highly significant result as compared with controls. This author found that only 3 per cent of patients had a relapse in the one- to eight-year period of follow-up if they had responded to propranolol and maintained the regimen for 12 months, as compared with an 85 per cent recurrence rate in those who discontinued medication at an earlier time.

The implications of the study are very significant in the management of migraine because they suggest that the lessons learned from the management of seizure disorder may apply to migraine as well. That is, a prolonged period of effective suppression may interrupt the cycle of periodicity and lead to sustained remission in many patients. This will be somewhat easier to establish in the adult patient with a more standardized and prolonged headache pattern than in children where summer remissions are commonplace, and prolonged remissions after several years of difficulty are also frequent (Congdon and Forsythe 1979).

At present trying a summer drug 'holiday' is probably the most appropriate course of action in children, but a course of sustained therapy for one year should be considered in patients who approach age 18 without remission. This suggestion is based on the Congdon and Forsythe (1979) data that the adult pattern is established at that age, and that the frequent sustained remission of childhood does not occur thereafter.

Lechin and van der Dijs (1977) have called attention to the highly favorable synergistic effect of dextroamphetamine and propranolol when used together in small doses in the prophylaxis of migraine. The age-range of patients was 12 to 75 years and presumably mostly adults. The dosage was propranolol 10 mg and dexedrene 2.5 mg one to three times per day. Response was rapid and sustained. A double blind study indicated dramatic relief in 94.3 per cent of patients as compared to 45.6 per cent response to other methods of therapy. Other 'depressive' symptoms were improved as well. I have no personal experience with this therapeutic approach, but it may warrant careful trial in children. To my knowledge there have not been confirmatory reports regarding combined propranolol-dexedrene therapy in either adults or children.

Primarily for the reason that propranolol became available in the modern era of clinical pharmacology, there have been several reports dealing with its effectiveness in children and many more in adults. The report of Diamond *et al.* (1982) can be taken as an example to illustrate the experience with adults who had classic and common migraine. Of 245 patients, 72 per cent were propranolol-responders at a dose of 160 mg/day as measured by a scale of headache frequency and severity. Only 5.7 per cent of patients had bothersome side-effects. Of patients who remained on propranolol six months or longer, 46 per cent maintained their improvement and only 11 per cent of patients had a rebound reaction. The suggestion of sustained effect supports the Rosen (1983) data cited above.

163

Ludvigsson (1974) reported the results of a double blind crossover study in 28 children age seven to 16 years. Dosage was 20 mg t.i.d. in children of less than 35 kg, and 40 mg t.i.d. for those weighing more. Results were excellent in 20 (71 per cent), good in three, and moderate in three, while two patients failed to respond. The attack-frequency was 10.2/month on placebo and 2.5 while on propranolol. Similar results were reported in the second three-month period of the study. In addition to the reduction in frequency, headaches were also less severe; only one patient complained of a side-effect which was trouble getting to sleep at night.

Side-effects of propranolol have been minimal in my own experience as well. There have been a few complaints of nausea, easily managed by post-prandial administration. There have been a few patients where CNS side-effects have necessitated discontinuation. These have consisted of light-headedness and a 'spacey' feeling and occasionally insomnia. There have been no serious adverse effects. Relative bradycardia is sometimes observed, but it has not been symptomatic nor has hypotension been an observation. Postural symptoms have neither developed, nor have they been aggravated if they were part of the history prior to the use of propranolol.

Other beta-adrenergic blockers have become available. An example of such a drug is nadolal which has shown promise of results comparable but probably not superior to propranolol (Ryan *et al.* 1983). As more selective preparations become available, there will probably be other effective drugs in this class found. The group of 'beta-blockers' must be watched for the appearance of preparations that may be superior to propranolol.

Phenytoin

Prior to the introduction of propranolol, my own first choice in the treatment of juvenile migraine was phenytoin. It is probably slightly less useful than propranolol. It is utilized as the drug of first choice when propranolol is contra-indicated, most commonly in patients who have asthma and less commonly in those with significant childhood endogenous depression. It can also be useful in those patients who do not respond to propranolol.

The dosage is usually 50 mg b.i.d. or 50 a.m. and 100 noc. in children up to 10 or 12 years. It is my impression that levels less than those required for anticonvulsant action are needed, usually ranging from 5 to 10 micrograms/ml. Adolescent patients may also respond, but are more likely to require larger dosage, *i.e.* 200 to 300 mg/day. Phenytoin has not been particularly useful with adult patients. The duration of therapy, if it proves to be successful, is in accordance with the usual program of treatment, that is until the end of the school year, followed by summer respite, and resumption in the autumn if indicated by recurrence.

Adverse effects of phenytoin are generally well known and will not be reviewed in detail. The occasional morbilliform rash is usually transient, gingival hypertrophy and hirsutism are not usually a problem in the lower doses and with only periodic use, and the symptoms of direct toxicity such as truncal ataxia and diplopia are unusual for the same reason. The more serious lymphoid hyperplasia syndrome or bone marrow depression (fortunately very rare with phenytoin) are always a risk, and constitute a good reason to place propranolol before phenytoin as the therapy of first choice.

The efficacy of phenytoin has not been put to the test of formal study. I have used it extensively over the years and can only say that based on my clinical impression it is almost as effective as propranolol in reducing frequency and/or severity of juvenile migraine. Perhaps as good an indication as any is the reported results of the treatment of the 'convulsive equivalent syndrome' (Chao and Davis 1964) that was discussed in a previous section of this monograph, where the case was made that the authors were describing juvenile migraine. In this series of almost 350 patients, approximately 30 to 35 per cent achieved complete remission with anticonvulsants, primarily phenytoin, while as many as 40 per cent additional patients had marked improvement in frequency and severity. Aside from a preoccupation with the 14 and six second positive spike phenomenon as a putative EEG abnormality, the EEG incidence of spike and discharges was about the same as in any migrainic population. The symptomatology in the Chao and Davis (1964) series was most commonly headache, abdominal pain and other visceral symptoms. In my view this represents a reasonable cross-section of children with manifest migraine, and the results of 'anticonvulsant' treatment are close to my own experience with juvenile migraine.

Phenobarbital
This drug was my first choice in the treatment of juvenile migraine in the earlier years of my work as a neurologist. It is still preferred for the younger patients, especially those less than four or five years of age. Its use in older children was gradually replaced by phenytoin prior to the introduction of propranolol, although the effectiveness was probably about the same except in adolescent patients where its value is limited. The recommended dosage is 30 mg b.i.d., or 30 mg a.m. and 60 mg at night. Use may be limited by either overactivity or sedation. More serious side-effects are virtually unknown. The usual course of treatment is employed, *i.e.* during the school year, or for six to eight months in pre-school children.

Cyproheptadine
This drug has had widespread use in the prophylaxis of migraine in childhood and is the drug of choice of a number of physicians (Saper 1983). It is a histamine and serotonin antagonist with sedative and anti-cholinergic effect. It is supplied in 4 mg scored tablets as well as in liquid form containing 2 mg per 5 ml. It is well tolerated but may cause sedation, appetite stimulation and rare confusional states. The dosage recommended is 2 to 4 mg two to four times a day for the usual course of therapy during the school year. Bille *et al.* (1977) has reported an uncontrolled pilot study in 19 children in whom treatment was continued for three to six months. Four had no attacks for seven to 24 months, 13 improved significantly and there was no benefit in two. Side-effects consisted of persistent drowsiness in three and bothersome weight gain in three.

Amitriptyline

This tricyclic compound has had widespread use as an anti-depressant. It also has been successfully employed in the prophylaxis of migraine in adult patients where its effect is thought to be relatively independent of its anti-depressive effect. Couch *et al.* (1976) have found that migraine was improved by '50 per cent in 72 per cent of patients and more than 80 per cent in 57 per cent of patients'. Because of its double pharmacologic effect, it can be the first choice agent in the therapy of young people in whom depression as well as migraine is recognized. My own experience with it has not been extensive as a first choice medication. Ling *et al.* (1970) studied a small group of children with depression and undifferentiated headache and found that anti-depressants (amitriptyline and imipramine) had a definite advantage over phenytoin in their depressed patients, most of whom were under age 12 years. Prensky (1976) suggests that anti-depressants in combination with phenytoin or phenobarbital may have an advantage over either class of drugs used alone.

Amitriptyline is available in tablets of 10, 25, 50 mg and larger. Treatment should begin with 25 mg per day, increasing after one or two weeks to 25 mg b.i.d. and perhaps higher dependent upon tolerance and indication of beneficial effect. It is probably inappropriate to exceed 75 mg per day in children 12 years or below. Side-effects include the usual range of gastro-intestinal upset, rashes and CNS symptoms of problems with concentration, anxiety, *etc.* coupled with such anti-cholinergic symptoms as dry mouth and blurred vision. The usual program of summer drug 'holiday' is employed. Patients with overt depression usually require psychotherapy as well.

Imipramine

This tricyclic anti-depressant can be used in migraine with the same indication and in the same dosage as amitriptyline. It has the advantage of a wider experience in younger children where it has been used with success for many years in the treatment of nocturnal enuresis.

Methysergide

This drug was developed for migrainic therapy as a synthetic ergot-like preparation. It has a strong vasoconstrictor action and has been shown to block the effects of serotonin. Its use in juvenile migraine should be restricted to those patients in whom other preparations have failed and who are severely incapacitated by their migraine. This approach is necessary because of its significant adverse effects, principally fibrotic disorders of retroperitoneal and pulmonary regions. This serious side-effect is uncommon and has only been reported in patients who have used the drug continuously for over six months (Graham *et al.* 1966). It can be avoided if methysergide is used intermittently. It has been my own policy to use it continuously in young people for no more than three months, after which one month without methysergide is advisable. It may not be necessary to resume methysergide, apparently because the cycle of severe headache has been interrupted. At that point either no medication or a less potentially toxic drug such as propranolol, cyproheptadine or anticonvulsants can then be used. I have not hesitated to use it in adolescent patients, but have not employed it in children younger than age 10.

The effectiveness of methysergide in migraine in adults is well established (Friedman and Elkind 1963, Graham 1964, Saper 1983). Its use has declined considerably since the introduction of propranolol, although in both children and adults it remains valuable as a back-up drug if other methods fail and the problem is of sufficient severity. There is very little information in the literature on its use in children. Holguin and Fenichel (1967) report on six patients in whom intermittent therapy with methysergide was used, three of whom were completely free of headache with 2 mg t.i.d. Whitehouse *et al.* (1967) reported that seven of 13 children with migraine 'improved' with methysergide. Prensky (1976) commented on its value, but pointed out the limitation based on the danger of retroperitoneal fibrosis.

Methysergide is available in 2 mg scored tablets. The usual dose is one to 2 mg b.i.d. in older children, to 2 mg b.i.d. or t.i.d. in the adolescent patients. It is wise to advise that it be taken after meals. Side-effects are usually minimal, perhaps consisting of nausea, dizziness or drowsiness. The development of paresthesias, leg, abdominal or chest pain are more serious indicators of adverse reaction and require discontinuation of the drug. The problem of retroperitoneal fibrosis resulting from prolonged continuous use is mentioned above.

Ergot preparations
Various preparations and combinations of ergot alkaloids are also occasionally used for continuous prophylaxis, with indications similar to methysergide. Although they are not as clearly associated with fibrotic reaction, they probably have the same potential as methysergide in this respect and similar caution is appropriate. Bellergal (ergotamine tartrate 0.3 mg, phenobarbital 20 mg and belladonna alkaloids 0.1 mg) is favored by some for continuous usage because of the small amount of ergot. Children can be treated with a b.i.d. or t.i.d. schedule. The inclusion of phenobarbital can perhaps be useful, but the belladonna probably has little or no value in continuous prophylactic use. Ergonovine maleate in a dose of 0.2 mg b.i.d. or t.i.d. has not been widely discussed in textbooks or in the literature, but it can be very useful in migraine prophylaxis. In my own experience, it was a frequently used approach in the therapy of adults and occasionally in children in the period before propranolol and methysergide became available.

Calcium channel-blocking agents
It is too early to assess the value of these compounds in the therapy of migraine in childhood although work with adults has been encouraging (Diamond and Schenbaum 1983). If they are established as safe and effective with adult patients, it is highly likely that they will be useful in younger patients as well. Recent work has indicated that cyproheptadine has calcium channel-blocking properties which may play a rôle in its antimigrainic effectiveness (Peroutka and Allen 1984).

Indomethacin
This drug is in general use as an anti-inflammatory agent. A major pharmacologic

effect relates to its inhibition of prostaglandin synthesis. It has been reported to be effective in the treatment of several rather specific headache syndromes including chronic cluster headache, ice-pick headache and both brief and prolonged exertional headache (Mathew 1981). All of these forms of headache, with the possible exception of 'prolonged exertional headache' are uncommon in childhood, although more common in adolescents. It is uncertain in my own view as to whether the exertion-precipitated migraine of childhood (see Chapter 3) is the same entity as prolonged exertional headaches as described in the adult literature (Diamond 1982). Although I have had no personal experience, it is worth recording the excellent results of continuous use of indomethacin in doses averaging 25 mg t.i.d. in these patients.

Miscellaneous drugs
It is probably inappropriate to continue the list of drugs indefinitely. As long as continuous prophylactic therapy is used and as long as therapy with one or a few such drugs leave patients behind who are still having headaches, there will be new candidates to replace the old.

Clonidine, a drug used extensively in the treatment of hypertension, has been studied in children by Sillanpää (1977). The effect on vascular headache was marginal at best and does not encourage additional study. Pizotifen, a tricyclic preparation with structure similar to cyproheptadine, is not generally available. However, reports indicate that it significantly improves patients with migraine with few side-effects, and that a single dose per day is as effective as spaced medication (Capildeo and Rose 1982). Sillanpää and Koponen (1978) have reported on the value of papaverine in a small number of children with migraine. 11 of 19 children had a 75 to 100 per cent reduction of headache frequency on a dose of 5 to 10 mg/kg, while only five of 18 responded similarly to placebo. There were no side-effects, and classic migraine seemed to respond better than common.

Cluster headache (migrainous neuralgia)
The treatment of this variant of vascular headache is described in Chapter 4.

Anti-platelet drugs
Platelet aggregation may be an aspect of the pathophysiology in some patients with migraine. It becomes a significant issue in those individuals who have neurological-ly complex migraine that develops during the headache phase, particularly if the duration of neurologic signs extends beyond 12 to 24 hours. There is also reason for concern about possible stroke in those patients with migraine who also have anatomical abnormality of the heart or great vessels, particularly prolapsed mitral valve. At the present state of our information, it is prudent to treat such patients with 'anti-platelet' drugs such as aspirin, and dipyridamole as well as propranolol, which also has an effect on platelet aggregability (Weksler *et al.* 1977).

Summary
To summarize my personal approach to the pharmacotherapy of juvenile migraine:

(1) The first decision that must be made is whether to treat with drugs at all. This judgement is made on the basis of the frequency and severity of the headache or other migrainic phenomena and the presence of aura.

(2) If an aura occurs regularly, trial with an ergot, caffeine mixture (usually Cafergot) is worthwhile if the patient is old enough or sufficiently responsible to carry medication. If the patient is not, it may be worthwhile to have it on hand for those episodes which develop at a time when the child can report to a parent.

(3) Pain relief with aspirin or a preparation such as Fiorinal may be all that is necessary or reasonable for headaches that occur sporadically once every two weeks, or less frequently. It is also useful for headaches that occur despite a program of continuous prophylactic pharmacotherapy or a program of behavioral modification.

(4) For headaches with a frequency of one per week or more, continuous daily medication is usually the treatment of choice. Propranolol is the first choice followed by phenytoin, cyprohepatidine or phenobarbital in younger patients. If depression is apparent, amitriptyline or imipramine is used early. The duration of treatment usually coincides with the school year.

(5) For patients whose headaches are resistant to several of the drugs mentioned under (4), serious consideration is usually given to referral for behavioral therapy.

(6) Simultaneously with or perhaps before referral I may use methysergide, especially if the episodes are frequent, neurologically complex or severe and prolonged.

(7) For those patients who have developed complex symptomatology during the headache phase and have had neurologic signs that persist for 12 to 24 hours, continuous low-dose aspirin therapy is recommended for a period of six to 12 months. If the patient has a prolapsed mitral valve or another potential source of emboli, aspirin, dipyridamole and propranolol should probably be continued indefinitely if episodes of complicated migraine or stroke have occurred.

Dietary treatment
For a discussion of dietary treatment see Chapter 3.

Behavioral treatment
Behavioral modification techniques have become increasingly popular and useful for the management of migraine as well as psychogenic headache. Most of the published results deal with adult patients, but it is now clear that many children are highly responsive, intrigued and challenged by these techniques. Certainly the methods are adaptable in children aged seven and above (Diamond 1979, Masek *et al.* 1984, Mehegan *et al.* 1984). There is general agreement that the specific techniques employed are more successful if combined with situational adjustment and psychotherapy (Adler and Adler 1976).

The behavior modification techniques employed can be considered from two aspects, 'meditative relaxation training' and 'biofeedback'. Relaxation training is to be regarded as the basic issue, and is the goal of the treatment however it is achieved. As an isolated procedure it consists of a systematic effort to instruct the patient to bring pathophysiologic processes under conscious control as the yogi have done for centuries. At a higher level of achievement, control becomes an almost unconscious reaction.

This may be accomplished by progressive systematic relation of body musculature in the 'relaxation training' ritual. It is perhaps less meaningful for children than the use of 'biofeedback', in which the visual or auditory trace of an electromyogram of fronto-temporal musculature is displayed as a challenge to relax. The immediate visible evidence of successful accomplishment is positive reinforcement, particularly in a society where video games are a familiar feature. The method is taught in a series of sessions, usually weekly, with additional sessions at home. For migraine, temperature feedback control has had a somewhat higher rate of success in adults. This technique employs a finger thermistor that senses heat, and is therefore directly related to skin and subcutaneous blood-flow. The patient learns to elevate finger temperature. This is believed to be an index of generalized activation of neurogenic and perhaps humoral factors of the sympathetic nervous system.

The potential importance of behavioral treatment of migraine is well illustrated by the preliminary report of a group of investigators from the Departments of Psychiatry and Neurology at Children's Hospital, Boston (Masek et al. 1984, Mehegan et al. 1984). These include Doctors Dennis Russo, Bruce Masek, James Mehegan (graduate student), Robert Harrison (thesis supervisor, Boston University) and Alan Leviton from the Department of Neurology. It has been possible for me to observe the progress of their work at close hand, and the success of the behavioral treatment approach has led to a steady and increasing number of referrals from my office practice. It is useful to consider their findings in some detail in order to give the reader an indication of the methodologic issues and time involved in the therapeutic program as well as the results.

These investigators have studied 20 children, age seven to 12 years, with periodic migraine headache, four of whom had classic expression of the migraine syndrome. None were using continuous pharmacotherapy at the time of the study. The patients were having three or more headaches per month. Documentation was accomplished by a headache 'chronicle' which included data on headache frequency and duration, severity, headache-free days, medication requirement for headache relief and behavioral antecedents. The baseline collection period varied from three to 12 weeks.

Treatment was carried out in nine sessions, the first seven at weekly intervals, and the final two sessions were spaced two weeks apart. Each session required approximately 50 to 60 minutes. The components of treatment involved training in meditative relaxation procedures (resting in a reclining chair, deep rhythmic breathing, and concentration on a single thought), EMG biofeedback (frontalis EMG electrode with TV display and thermistor recording of finger temperature), and behavior therapy (assessment of headache occurrence, individualization of relaxation procedures and working with parents in techniques of pain-control management).

The first session was given to orientation, followed by six weekly sessions consisting of four-minute periods of '1. resting baseline, 2. relaxation with feedback, 3. relaxation without feedback, 4. resting baseline, 5. relaxation without feedback, 6. relaxation with feedback, and 7. resting baseline'. During the final two sessions biofeedback was eliminated. Children were instructed to practise relaxation for five to seven minutes twice daily at home.

Improvement occurred in all parameters examined and usually began in the first few weeks of treatment. Headache frequency was reduced from a mean of 2.6 per week to 0.5 per week after 22 weeks, and total hours of headache went from 14.6 per week to 1.1 per week in the same period of time. Intensity and duration of individual headaches were also reduced. Moreover follow-up at six months and one year indicated that the degree of improvement was well sustained. Half of the children continued to use relaxation on a regular basis and five used the technique sporadically and in association with headache onset.

It was the authors' impression that improvement occurred in relation to the child's development of relaxation skills and in the recognition of environmental influences. It had less to do with the more dramatic biofeedback instrumentation, and this was confirmed by the reports of the children themselves. It is my own impression that children are intrigued by the prospect of EMG and TV display and that this facilitates referral and commitment to the program. Certainly the basic issue is for them to become skilful in the techniques of relaxation, whatever the method.

Although this study dealt with juvenile migraine, the method is equally adaptable to psychogenic headaches (Masek 1984). Systematic study of this group of children has not been done, but the indication of results in my own referrals is that improvement is comparable. It is the preferred method of management for psychogenic headache.

These techniques are all quite specialized and not adaptable to the time available or the personality and background of the general physician, pediatrician and most neurologists. They have the great advantage of providing a strategy that may last for the duration of the life of the patient. This advantage may be more applicable to migraine than to childhood psychogenic headaches. Migraine is often a disorder which remits and exacerbates in the long term. Psychogenic headaches in children are usually restricted to a period of months or at most several years. In those individuals who have expressed nervous tension by this somatic symptom, the basic issue may be the danger of developing an enduring personality disorder. If the personality is at sufficient risk, the real hope for these patients is psychotherapy.

9
PSYCHOGENIC HEADACHE

Introduction

Psychological factors are a central feature in the consideration of all types of headache in childhood as well as in adults. However, the psychogenic headache syndrome as the principal expression of emotional disorder is comparatively uncommon in children. It is also undoubtedly true that many psychogenic headaches are short-lived, and minor in expression; parents seldom think they warrant general medical attention, let alone neurologic assessment. In my own referral practice, psychogenic headaches are uncommon under 12 or 13 years (about 5 per cent of all headaches), but increase significantly in adolescent patients (about 10 per cent of all headaches). The diagnosis is based on both the clinical characteristics of the headache pattern, together with some positive indication of significant emotional disorder in the child.

In some patients, the clinical expression consists of a mixture of both vascular and psychogenic headaches. This relatively common experience in adult medicine is not frequently encountered in children (Rothner 1978). On the other hand, it is common for juvenile migraine to be aggravated by psychologic factors. These factors may be quite minor in degree and not greatly different from the tensions to which many of their fellows are subjected. These issues are treated at greater length in Chapter 3.

Apart from headache, what are the usual somatic expressions of psychologic tensions in children in whom the principal symptoms consist of abnormalities of behavior? It is not the purpose of this monograph to attempt to recapitulate the content of a textbook of child psychiatry. For a discussion of behavioral symptoms, psychodynamics and related issues, the reader is referred to appropriate sources. Somatic expression of emotional distress is much more commonly centered on the abdomen and gastro-intestinal system. This may eventuate in abdominal pain, vomiting, diarrhea or constipation (Green 1967).

Despite the frequency of psychologic illness in childhood, expression in terms of headache is not usual. When headache does become part of the symptomatology, it is not usually monosymptomatic, and occurs in a setting where other psychogenic behavioral or somatic symptomatology is manifested as well. Even then, the headache more often has the quality of migraine than of psychogenic or muscle tension headaches. Another illustration of the lack of predilection of the child to headache of the psychogenic type is the infrequency of muscle contraction headache in the post-traumatic syndrome in children as compared with adults. The incidence of behavioral disorder is high after childhood head trauma, but the common 'tension type' headache of adults is not. These points are further discussed in Chapter 10.

The concept of the relative infrequency of psychogenic headache in childhood and adolescence as presented above is not generally accepted by some authors who have written on the subject. For example, Rothner (1978) states: 'Psychogenic headaches are the most common type of headache in children and adolescents'. No estimate of the relative percentages is given, nor is literature cited. On the other hand, Prensky (1976) states: 'Tension headaches are unusual prior to puberty'. As pointed out in the previous discussion of epidemiology, there are no population surveys in the literature that deal directly with the issue of the frequency of psychogenic headaches in childhood, except to say that headache is not a common presenting complaint in the usual child psychiatry clinic. In a small series of 116 consecutive patients with headache seen in a child neurology clinic, that were reported recently by Jay and Tomasi (1981), 28 per cent had tension headache.

These varying indications of frequency can only be indicative of quite different referral patterns or of a significant difference in definition and interpretation among neurologists who deal with children. It is probable that the latter is the case and there is an area of overlap and clinical ambiguity between migraine and psychogenic headaches in children. There is general agreement that psychologic issues are important in the etiology and expression of both, including juvenile migraine where psychologic factors play a critical rôle in influencing frequency and severity.

The problem of an ambiguous group of patients where qualified physicians might not agree about the diagnostic category is not restricted to childhood headache. For example, Butler and Thomas (1947) believed that adult 'tension headaches' were basically vascular but could be distinguished from migraine. This point of view brings us to the concept of 'cephalia vasomotoria' of European authors. It seems to occupy a middle ground between psychogenic headache and common migraine. This issue is neatly summarized in Bille's monograph (1962). Cephalia vasomotoria is not widely used as a diagnostic category and is practically unknown in English and American literature on headache. Nor does it appear in the 'Classification of Headache' by the NIH Ad Hoc Committee (Friedman *et al.* 1962*a*). Cephalia vasomotoria serves to illustrate the fact that there is a significant middle ground of diagnostic uncertainty in the classification of headaches in adults as well as in children.

The problem of both vascular and psychogenic headache in the same individual adds complexity to the diagnostic issues, but is even more serious as a complicating factor in treatment and management. Once one accepts the proposition that both may occur in the same patient, the ambiguity of an overlap in terminology tends to disappear. A mixture of migraine and psychogenic headaches in the same patient is common in adults, but much less so in children. In this, my own experience agrees with Rothner (1978). There are only 15 such patients in my series. They have all presented management problems, and unlike the simpler and common problem of migraine aggravated by emotional factors, many have required formal psychotherapy.

To summarize these general comments, the principal issues are:
(1) Headache that has the characteristics of either psychogenic or tension headache may reflect organic intracranial disease.
(2) The successful management of all remaining 'benign' headaches requires

attention to the whole patient, including the environment and the mental health of the patient.

(3) Nevertheless, the separation of migraine and psychogenic headaches on clinical grounds may lead to more expeditious management of the symptom. This is what most patients desire. Pharmacotherapy for migraine will be a waste of time in psychogenic headaches of childhood, and should be avoided. Behavioral treatment is useful in both.

Characteristics of psychogenic headache

The objective of the clinical history is to extract sufficient key information to allow a specific diagnosis to be made. This in turn depends on relatively few key points that differentiate psychogenic headache from vascular headache. These clinical features consist of historical information relating to (i) occurrence, (ii) quality of pain, and (iii) associated symptoms.

Occurrence

Headaches due to nervous tension tend to be relatively continuous in occurrence. They are 'always' present, or occur daily. This key historical point must be qualified to stipulate that it is those psychogenic headaches which are *brought to medical attention* that are continuous or daily in occurrence. It is certainly true that children as well as adults will have an occasional headache of short duration that is clearly related to a stressful situation such as over-stimulation and excitement, fatigue, oppressive workload or the debility of systemic illness. The headache itself has the quality of psychogenic headaches to which a minor throbbing component may occasionally be added. This latter brings up the issue of vascular reactivity in any painful process. It is probably indicative of a universality of vascular contribution to pain which is based upon a variable individual threshold. A different interpretation is that many people who cannot be labelled migrainic nevertheless have occasional common migraine headaches closely correlated with occasional stressful circumstances.

In any event, a history of a continuum of headache points towards psychologic factors as the key issue in pathogenesis. The duration of the complaint varies widely from weeks and months, to years. Typically the headache waxes and wanes and usually builds in intensity during the day. Only a vestige is apparent in the morning on awakening, or it may not appear until the day wears on. Perhaps a better occurrence descriptor of the psychogenic headache syndrome is 'daily' rather than 'continuous', and certainly this is a more accurate description of occurrence in some patients.

Quality of pain

Another principal distinguishing feature of psychogenic headache is the quality of the pain. The limitations of childhood and even adolescent vocabulary pose a restriction here. The commonest description used is probably 'ache' or 'it hurts'. More articulate children will refer to the discomfort as pressing or tightness. Although a band of discomfort encircling the head may be frequently described by

174

adults, this is seldom if ever heard from children and only occasionally from adolescent patients. A further goal in the description of the quality of pain is to learn that a predominantly throbbing quality is not present, a point that is usually settled by direct questioning.

The commonest location is frontal, sometimes vertex or occiput. The frequent occipital muscle contraction headache of adults is less common among the psychogenic headaches of children. The severity of the described discomfort is difficult to determine. It is always a surprise, after hearing a rather dramatic story of persistent and troublesome headache, to learn that the child sitting comfortably in the office is having a 'severe' headache at that moment. It is also wise to inquire if the parents can tell if the child is having a headache without asking. The usual answer is no. This is in contrast with migraine, where pallor and desire for quiet and rest, provide the parent with certain knowledge that their child is ill.

The family turmoil caused by psychogenic headache is usually out of proportion to the objective evidence of discomfort. The consequences of the headache in terms of poor school attendance is also excessive. The child with migraine may miss school or be sent home from school with headache, but weeks and months of continuous school absence is almost pathognomonic of a psychogenic headache syndrome (Rothner 1978).

Associated symptoms
A third clinincal feature relates to *associated symptoms*. In psychogenic headaches this involves the symptoms of the basic personality or emotional disorder that forms the substrate of the chronic headache problem. In practical terms this usually centers on anxiety, phobias (especially those relating to school), and childhood depression. Headaches due to hysterical elaboration must be quite uncommon, as are the elaborate and bizarre delusional head symptoms of the schizophrenic. A brief review of these personality disorders will be discussed below.

Family history
There is no systematic information on the frequency of psychogenic headache in family members of children who have headaches of this variety. Nor does chart review of my own small number of patients give any insight, other than to say that the incidence does not seem to be disproportionate. In individual instances there may be some indication of child imitating parent, but this is not common.

On the other hand, family history of major affective illness is an important clue to the possibility of depression in childhood. As discussed below, depressive reaction, both situational and especially the endogenous variety, are important considerations in some childhood headache problems.

Childhood behavior disturbance
As mentioned above, it is inappropriate to attempt an in-depth discussion of child psychiatry, but a brief, somewhat superficial treatment is in order. The manifestations of childhood anxiety and fears take many forms, and are basic to many of the psychiatric disorders of this age-group. They reflect the reaction of a

175

child who is usually sensitized by past experience, and this is compounded by current environmental stress. The situational factors that recur frequently are family stresses due to parental interpersonal tensions, such as separation and divorce, parental alcoholism and financial reverses.

In other circumstances, parental expectations may be unrealistic and excessive: characteristically an expression of a parent's own frustrated personal goals which the child is expected to fulfil. The child-object of those expectations may be entirely normal, and only lack the interest or talent to fulfil the parent's desires, or have some biological limitation that places him in double jeopardy and open to frustration. The possibility of developmental or neuropsychological handicap is suggested by a history of poor or borderline school performance. If there is any question on this score, the child should be referred for formal psychological appraisal by a psychologist sensitive to both organic and experiential factors. At times projective testing can be helpful.

Peer pressures can also provoke anxiety, especially in immediately pre-teen and teenage patients. Exclusion by peers may be based on what seems to be minor issues of appearance or personality. Acne can be a great social burden both in real terms and in terms of self-image. Acne is a specific problem that can be addressed medically with some hope of success.

At times the basic problem is less complex and has to do with authority figures other than parents such as teachers or athletic coaches. If true, and not a displaced focus of reaction to parental authority, or a reaction to unappreciated neuropsychological disability in the child, the solution may simply be a matter of time and readjustment to a new school year and a new teacher.

Identification of a source of conflict and tension does not imply etiology. In fact, it is often impressive how a child can manage to carry on emotionally in the face of what would seem to be devastating environmental circumstances. Moreover, when symptomatology results it is seldom monosymptomatic, and perhaps this is especially the case with headache. Juvenile migraine is a notable exception, but in this circumstance emotional factors trigger an inborn pathophysiologic response. In the case of psychogenic headache, it is expected that other associated psychogenic symptoms will be part of the syndrome.

As indicated above, headache is among these associated symptoms, and when present, tends to have the characteristics already outlined. The most common additional symptoms are abnormalities of behavior. Children and many adolescents are sufficiently naive that reaction to situational stresses leads to a response in kind. Temper tantrums are probably the most common in the young child, accompanied by less overtly challenging behaviors such as negative verbal response ('talking back'). Resistance may be either active or passive. To some degree these behaviors are a normal developmental expectation as the younger child tests his or her environment. The child expects that limits will be set by the parents, and when this is not forthcoming, an anxiety-provoking sequence may be established. This leads to more tantrums and greater parental frustration. The anxiety of the child is compounded, and becomes truly pathological. The older the child, the more abnormal tantrums become.

Childhood aggression directed at peers is another relatively common behavioral manifestation, together with disruptive behavior in group activities such as school. This is also a phenomenon where age and degree are important criteria of abnormality. Overtly antisocial acts and delinquency such as stealing, lighting fires, destroying household and neighborhood property, or habitual truancy, occur less commonly and are more unequivocally abnormal. On the other hand, the child may become painfully shy. He or she may withdraw from family and school activities, a development which may be even more indicative of psychopathology. Any of these behaviors often have a deleterious effect on school performance.

A number of behavioral and somatic symptoms are centered about what has been termed school phobia, a form of separation anxiety that is more common in younger children. It is probably best considered a variation on the general theme of anxiety. The somatic symptoms are most frequently focused upon the abdomen, although headache may also be a part of the symptomatology.

Abdominal pain, sometimes with nausea and vomiting, is a common somatic expression of school phobia, but it also occurs in other anxiety states of childhood (Green 1967). In school phobia it tends to occur in the morning before setting off, in other circumstances it can occur at any time. The differential diagnosis includes organic gastro-intestinal disorders such as peptic ulcer as well as abdominal migraine. These differential diagnostic considerations are discussed at greater length in the section on abdominal migraine (Chapter 5).

Other somatic expressions of psychologic tensions include constipation, refusal of food and overeating, psychogenic tics and sleep disorders, as well as classic anxiety attacks.

Childhood depression
In recent years there has been a major awakening of interest in childhood depression, as well as an appreciation of its frequency in the psychopathology of the young. The manifestations are somewhat modified in children, but the essential features are comparable to the symptoms of adults. Often there is a suggestive history of depressive or manic-depressive illness in the family. This information may provide the first clue to what may turn out to be the fundamental issue in a child presenting with a headache problem, whether migraine or psychogenic in its characteristics (Ling *et al.* 1970). Headache does not appear to be a common symptom of depression in childhood.

The criteria for the diagnosis of childhood depression have been concisely stated in the Diagnostic and Statistical Manual of Mental Disorders (DSM-III) of the American Psychiatric Association. They consist of (i) dysphoric mood, which must be present, and at least four of the following: (ii) poor appetite or weight loss, or increased appetite and weight gain; (iii) sleeping difficulty or sleeping too much; (iv) loss of energy; (v) psychomotor agitation or retardation; (vi) loss of interest or pleasure in usual activities; (vii) diminished ability to concentrate; (viii) feeling of self-reproach or excessive guilt; and (ix) recurrent thoughts of death or suicide. These symptoms must be present for at least one week.

Using DSM criteria, the incidence of significant depressive reaction in children between seven and 12 years has been estimated at 1.9 per cent (Kashani and Simonds 1979). This is much lower than in adults, but appreciable nevertheless. An incidence of almost 30 per cent has been identified in a relatively unselected pediatric psychiatric clinic, which indicates the highly significant frequency among emotionally disturbed children (Carlson and Cantwell 1980). A further elaboration of these criteria, and a presentation in developmental age-related sequence, has been set forth by Herzog and Rathbun (1982). They include 'vague complaints, abdominal pain, eczema, seizure-like episodes, asthma, eneuresis and encopresis' in the six to eight and nine to 12 year-groups; and 'anorexia nervosa, ulcerative colitis, abdominal pain and conversion reactions' in the post-pubertal group. Headache does not appear in this listing. It unquestionably occurs, but this compilation gives an indication of its relative infrequency.

Brumback *et al.* (1980) called attention to impaired cognitive function in depressed children, and its reversibility with effective anti-depressant pharmaco-therapy. In a later report, these same authors extended their observations to additional children, identified the right hemisphere and frontal lobes as the principal focus of the neuropsychological dysfunction and reported the highly interesting finding of mild left hemiparesis in two patients in the study. Of particular interest is the observation that the hemiparesis also improved with drug therapy (Stalon *et al.* 1981).

In summary, depression is a significant aspect of the psychopathology of childhood and may be an occasional cause of psychogenic headache. It may also be a significant aspect of the psychopathology of migraine. Recognition is important in pointing the way to appropriate therapy.

Conversion reaction and hysteria
The 'conversion headache' is well established in adult psychiatric formulation (Saper 1983). It has no identifying clinical characteristics, although it is usually described in dramatic terms and there is a predilection for face as well as head localization. Typically it is relatively monosymptomatic, and accompanied by the detached indifference characteristic of hysterical symptoms in general. There is no doubt that hysterical sensorimotor phenomena occur in childhood and during adolescence, the basis of which may be either neurosis or less commonly schizophrenic or depressive illness. A hysterical basis of headache has been cited in children (Rothner 1978), but it must be very rare. It may be more common in adolescence. My own reaction is to include the headaches which some may prefer to categorize as hysterical in the relatively less specific, more general, category of undifferentiated psychogenic headache.

Management of psychogenic headache
Therapy of psychogenic headache is based upon the fundamental psychiatric diagnosis (*i.e.* whether depression or anxiety), and an assessment of the complexity of the problem. Either may be of sufficient ambiguity at the outset to require specialized psychiatric referral for advice. Usually, however, although the headache itself may be clinically characteristic of psychogenic headaches, the basic

psychopathology and its degree is less obvious. Several visits may be necessary to sort this out. It is important to inform the parents and usually the patient of the psychiatric aspects of the problem, to set the stage for exploration of relevant emotional issues. It is unusual to encounter resistance to this suggestion, perhaps because headache is so commonly linked to emotional factors in the mind of the public.

The first step in therapy is the reassurance provided by a thorough clinical assessment, including a careful neurological examination. Further studies are not necessary in most instances, although some parents are not fully reassured without additional studies such as CT scan or EEG. The lack of purely medical indication is seldom worth a confrontation on this point.

If continuing situational factors can be identified, they can sometimes be addressed directly. An effort should be made to correlate exacerbation or onset of the headache with such factors as time of day, what may have happened during the day or the night before, and school examination schedules. The anxieties relating to learning disabilities are more complex and require long-term attention and special arrangements.

Pharmacotherapy is much more useful in depressive reaction than when the psychiatric basis of the problem is anxiety. Both amitriptyline and imipramine have proved useful (Ling *et al.* 1970, Brumback *et al.* 1980, Stalon *et al.* 1981) in childhood cyclic depression. The treatment schedule should begin with a 25 mg tablet of either amitriptyline or imipramine given at bedtime. Then increases are made every one or two weeks until a remission is established. Stalon *et al.* (1981) found that therapeutic effect was obtained at approximately 2.5 mg/kg on average, with a range of 1.1 to 3.5 mg/kg. Ideally, drug treatment should be combined with psychotherapy. Under most circumstances, the total treatment of the more serious depressive reactions is best managed by someone who has specialized in these problems.

Pharmacotherapy of anxiety syndromes is less effective in general, but can have some value on occasion. It may be sufficient to tide the child over difficult situations, or as an initial effort before other interventions can be initiated. Meprobamate in a dosage of 200 mg t.i.d. for younger patients, to 400 t.i.d for adolescents, may be worth a period of trial. Phenobarbital in small amounts (for example 30 mg b.i.d. or t.i.d.) may also be useful. These medications should be presented to the patient and family as nothing more than an effort to reduce the level of nervous tension in order to obtain some relief while more significant plans are being made in terms of situational adjustment, behavioral modification, or psychotherapy.

Referral for psychotherapy should usually be made only after the ground is well prepared and the plan is found to be acceptable to the parents in particular, and hopefully the child as well. In younger children, it will usually consist of a program which involves parents as well as child, and this should be fully understood. In the adolescent, the patient will often be the focus of attention. Details of psychotherapeutic techniques are well beyond the scope of this monograph, and they will not be considered further. The methods of 'meditative

179

relaxation' and 'biofeedback' are equally applicable and effective in both psychogenic headaches and juvenile migraine syndromes. It probably represents the most useful management technique available for many psychogenic headache problems (Masek 1984), and should be employed if the problem is resistant to simple situational adjustment, discussion, and perhaps a brief period of pharmaco-therapy.

The exceptions to this approach are those children whose basic psychiatric disorder is depression, where attention directed to the depressive reaction is usually more appropriate. Depressed children may also respond to behavioral treatment, and it can be useful for symptomatic management while the depression is being attended. For a more extended discussion of behavioral treatment, see Chapter 8, p. 169.

10
TRAUMATIC HEADACHE SYNDROMES

Introduction

The basic reaction of the child or adolescent to head trauma is similar to the adult, but the details of the resulting clinical problems may be quite different. The incidence of certain post-traumatic headache syndromes and complications is very different.

Minor head trauma is very common in children because of their lifestyle. The effects are evanescent as a rule, and their chaotic life proceeds as usual. However the lifestyle of adults also plays a rôle in head injury in children, only in this instance the consequences are much more serious and can be fatal. Automobile accidents, either with children in the vehicle or struck on the street, are the leading cause of death in children of the western world. Drunken drivers play a significant rôle in the problem. In children who survive, neurologic disability is a significant and frequent long-term consequence of major head trauma. The fact that many of these catastrophes could be prevented by careful driving and seat-belts and moderation of alcohol intake is a sad commentary on the recalcitrance of human nature.

Of lesser frequency, but not of lesser importance, are accidents in the home such as falling down steps or from windows. Sporting injuries become prominent in older children and adolescents, and the motorcycle is an additional invitation to disaster. Protective headgear is mandatory in some parts of the world and should be used everywhere.

The curtailment of accidental childhood trauma is one of the greatest challenges of preventive medicine.

Knowledge of acute and sub-acute head trauma is consequently an important body of information for the physician or surgeon who deals with children. On the other hand, the chronic post-traumatic headache syndromes are distinctly less common in children than in adults. In my office practice, trauma has figured significantly in the history or pathogenesis of approximately 5 per cent of headache patients.

Acute post-traumatic syndromes

Almost any degree of head trauma must have some effect on intracranial contents, and especially some effect on the larger tethered arteries where they traverse the space between skull and brain. This is usually well compensated by the buffering effect of the cerebrospinal fluid. When mild, or moderate and well compensated, symptoms amount to little more than non-specific headache, mild confusion, light-headedness, and perhaps nausea and vomiting. These symptoms begin immediately after the injury and last for a few minutes to a few hours. The other benign group of reactions to head trauma can be encompassed by a discussion of migraine and trauma.

Migraine and head trauma

There are three aspects of the relationship of migraine and head trauma that require consideration. The simplest relationship is the vascular component of the pain resulting from head trauma in the acute phase following injury. This pain frequently has a throbbing quality and may be associated with nausea and vomiting. It probably illustrates the innate potential of blood vessels to react in almost anyone, and possibly reflects a threshold of reactivity that is individually variable. Those individuals who have inherited the migrainic diathesis have the greatest degree of susceptibility to vascular headache following head trauma, just as they tend to stand out as the patients with more prolonged and severe post-lumbar puncture headaches.

There are two additional phenomena that will be considered at greater length: (i) a single common, classic or complex migrainic reaction to trauma that usually develops after a brief post-traumatic latent period; and (ii) trauma-precipitated periodic vascular headache syndrome that may persist for weeks or months. It accounts for the majority of chronic post-traumatic headaches in childhood. This will be discussed later (p. 193).

Post-traumatic migrainic episodes

In a large number of patients with juvenile migraine, even relatively mild head trauma will precipitate a vascular headache or cyclic vomiting, usually after a latent interval of two to 10 minutes and sometimes several hours later. It is characteristically more severe than the patient's usual headache, and the circumstances often lead to medical consultation, particularly if it is the first migraine episode of the patient's life. The history of prior headaches in the patient, reinforced by a history of vascular headache in the family, is important and reassuring.

In small children, usually boys, this may be the only circumstance in which vascular headaches occur, but the relative frequency of minor buffeting at this age can lead to headaches several times a year. Once the relationship is established, the resulting headache, vomiting, *etc.* is expected, and can usually be viewed with relative equanimity (Matthews 1972). It is probable that many 'mild concussions' in childhood can be best explained on this basis.

Migraine precipitated by trauma

CASE 38 This 15-year-old girl gave the history that at age 11 she was running down cellar steps and struck her head on the top of the doorway. After a few minutes she found that she was unable to see from the left field of vision and subsequently developed a severe headache which had a throbbing quality and was associated with nausea. The headache continued for two days.

Subsequently, with a frequency of about every three months, she was subject to periodic headaches with complex symptomatology. The aura consisted of numbness of the left hand and arm during which time she saw black spots throughout her entire visual field. About 30 minutes later she developed a right lateralized throbbing headache associated with nausea.

Vomiting then occurred which led to some relief although the usual headache lasted about 12 hours. In addition, with a frequency of about once per week, she had throbbing headaches that lasted about two hours and were usually responsive to aspirin.

General physical and neurological examination was entirely normal.

It was suggested that she be treated with Cafergot for the headaches with prodrome. No follow-up was obtained and she was returned to the care of her referring physician.

Comment: This girl had classic and common migraine, the first paroxysm of which was precipitated by head trauma.

Cyclic vomiting precipitated by trauma

This girl was seven years of age when first seen with a chief complaint of four episodes of repeated vomiting. They were all precipitated by an accident, usually a fall in which she struck her head. The parents were certain that she did not lose consciousness either before, during or after the fall. She then began to cry and after about 15 minutes became drowsy and nauseous and she vomited repeatedly. She was pale and her speech was somewhat thick although she was entirely conscious. On each occasion she was hospitalized and was well within 24 hours. The first episode occurred when she was three, the second when she was four and the third one month before she was seen in neurologic consultation. Previous studies included normal skull x-rays on each occasion and an EEG which showed no abnormalities on two occasions. **CASE 39**

The family history revealed that the father was subject to migraine headaches throughout his lifetime.

Examination was entirely normal.

It was believed that the basis of her trauma-precipitated episodes was migrainic cyclic vomiting. Because of their infrequency, continuous treatment was not prescribed.

Comment: This child had several episodes of cyclic vomiting triggered by mild head injury.

Much more provocative, but probably similar in its essential pathogenesis, is the development of complex vasomotor phenomenology after trauma. The most comprehensive review of the subject is that of Haas *et al.* (1975). They report 50 incidents in 25 patients. The greatest susceptibility was between age four and 14 years, during which period 40 of the episodes occurred. Head trauma was usually sufficient to 'daze the patient momentarily', although two incidents followed a brief period of unconsciousness.

The neurologic phenomenology developed after a latency of several seconds to four hours, but the majority of episodes occurred between one to 10 minutes after the trauma. Expression varied from (i) hemisyndrome (hemiparesis and/or hemianopsia), (ii) somnolence, irritability and vomiting, (iii) cortical blindness (fundi and pupillary light response normal, but no useful vision), and (iv) brainstem

TABLE XIII

Complex Migraine Syndromes Triggered by Trauma

Sex	Age	Trauma	Unconscious	Latent interval	Event	Duration
a. Female	14	Struck head playing basketball	? brief	1 hour	Blindness	3–4 hours
b. Male (case 21)	14	Fell and struck head	0	5–10 minutes	Global amnesia, dizziness and vomiting	24 hours
c. Male (case 23)	12½	Fell in gym and struck head	0	?	Confusional state, headache and vomiting	4–5 hours
		Fell down steps	0	5 minutes	Confusional state, headache and vomiting	8 hours
d. Male (case 25)	14	Headed ball in soccer	0	2 minutes	Global amnesia	12 hours
e. Male	5	Fell from bike	0	?	Confusion and headache	6 hours
	10	Fell from bunkbed	0	?	Confusion and nausea	4 hours
	12	Fell while playing	0	5 minutes	Lost vision, headache	2 hours
	15	Basketball	0	2 minutes	Aphasia	6 hours
f. Male (case 40)	12	Fell while playing	0	30 minutes	Scotomata, numbness and weakness on left	5 min.
					Headache	4 hours
g. Male	5	Fell from bike	?	5 minutes	Confusion	3–4 hours
h. Female	6	Fell in gym	0	5 minutes	Confusion	4 hours
i. Male	8	Fell while playing	0	1 hour	Confusion	2 days

All above patients had migraine before or after trauma and all had a positive family history of migraine.

signs. To this may be added confusional state, which occurred in a number of the 'somnolent, irritable and vomiting' patients (for further discussion see p. 109). The syndromes were not sharply defined, and frequently overlapped in a given incident.

In patients with multiple episodes, the clinical expression was not necessarily stereotyped; and in some patients repeat trauma induced either the same, or a different constellation of signs and symptoms. Headache, nausea and vomiting were frequent but not invariable concomitants. The duration of the episodes was usually measured in hours. In a few patients, spontaneous complex episodes occurred that were similar to those precipitated by trauma, and the incidence of vascular headache in both affected children and especially in their family was high.

These points favor the interpretation (Haas and Sovner 1969, Haas *et al.* 1975) that the basis of these reactions is a migrainic diathesis. In four patients of the Haas *et al.* series, the persistence of focal signs led to angiography. Occlusion of branches of the middle cerebral artery was demonstrated in two of these patients.

It is the patients with post-traumatic cortical blindness who have attracted the most attention in the literature (Pickles 1949, Bodian 1964, Griffith and Dodge 1968, Gjerris and Mellemgaard 1969). Haas and Sovner (1969) and Greenblatt (1973) were instrumental in linking this syndrome to migraine. The latter author also remarked upon the occasional association with seizures during the acute phase of the syndrome.

It seems probable that post-traumatic transient cortical blindness may occur in anyone with appropriate provocation, but that migrainic children are especially vulnerable. The rare adult cases required more head trauma as measured by the frequency of loss of consciousness and its duration. Also, the reaction was more severe, as measured by the duration of the blindness, the associated amnesia, and extent and duration of confusion. Adolescent boys would seem to be the most frequently affected age-group. The frequency of contact-sports injury at this age is probably the critical factor in this epidemiologic observation.

My own experience with complex migraine triggered by trauma is contained in Table XIII.

The presumption that head trauma triggers transient vasospasm is probably the most satisfactory formulation of the basis of migraine triggered by head injury. It is also possible that the stress and anxiety of trauma may call forth humoral and vaso-active substances that in turn are responsible for the vasomotor symptomatology.

Only the passage of time during the acute episode can be fully reassuring as to whether it is migraine or some more serious complication, but it is useful if the attending physician is aware of the possibility of migraine in the differential diagnosis.

Parenthetically it is of interest that seizure disorder should also occur in the described symptomatology of this group of patients. This brings to mind the patients who have a single convulsion subsequent to similar mild head trauma. Such individuals may occasionally have an 'aura' suggestive of vasomotor reaction in the immediate prodrome of their convulsion. The principal importance of this group of patients is the likely possibility of excellent outcome with regard to recurring seizure disorder.

In a recent paper by Snoek *et al.* (1984), the issue of neurological syndromes developing after a post-traumatic latent interval was analyzed in 40 children out of a total of 967 consecutive patients. Of these, only two had initial loss of consciousness, and in these the duration of immediate loss of consciousness was less than five minutes. 13 children developed post-traumatic seizures, half with status epilepticus, and only one had recurrent seizures on six months to three year follow-up. 29 children developed general or focal neurologic signs after a latent interval. In most, the latent interval was five to 30 minutes, and the duration of signs was two to 12 hours. In 23 the onset was abrupt, and 22 recovered completely, although one child died with presumed cerebral edema after a rapid deterioration. It is in the abrupt onset group that one would expect to find the patients with migrainic reaction. Unfortunately neither family history nor individual history of migraine was recorded. In contrast there was a smaller group of six children whose neurologic deterioration evolved slowly. This group contained a child with a posterior fossa extradural hematoma, and two additional patients who died of cerebral edema. In those who recovered, at least one had clinical evidence of massive cerebral edema. It is clear that the transient, benign post-traumatic syndromes are more likely to be found in those patients whose symptoms develop relatively suddenly after a variable latent interval, while those with more malignant potential develop more gradually. It is also apparent that there are several pathophysiologic entities in this group of patients, of which migrainic reaction is one, probably the most common over-all.

Migraine confusional state precipitated by trauma

CASE 40
This 14-year-old boy was well until two years before evaluation. He fell in the playground in school and struck the back of his head. Although he remembered little of the day beyond his mother taking him to school, observers indicated that he did not lose consciousness and seemed normal until about 30 minutes after the fall when he became obviously confused and disoriented. This lasted 60 minutes followed by a severe pounding headache that continued for the duration of the day. The skull x-rays were normal but the EEG was said to be 'abnormal'. An EEG six weeks later was normal.

Approximately four months later he had another period of several hours of disorientation, not associated with trauma, which required hospitalization overnight. LP and CT scans on that occasion were normal.

Subsequently he had periodic episodes of variable frequency during which he developed visual scotomata associated with a 'fuzzy feeling' in his left hand. The scotomata appeared throughout the entire visual field, and after several minutes this was followed by a throbbing headache on the right associated with nausea and vomiting. The duration of the headache was several hours or until sleep.

There was no family history of headache.

Examination revealed him to be entirely normal, both on general physical and neurological examination, with the exception of several *café-au-lait* spots over his trunk (no other member of the family had birthmarks).

It was suggested that Cafergot be used at the beginning of the aura, and on three month follow-up this had been effective in aborting any further headaches. He was returned to the care of his referring physician.

Comment: This 14-year-old boy had a migrainic confusional state and headache precipitated by trauma, and a subsequent course of periodic vascular headaches with migrainic scotomata.

Concussion

The generally accepted definition of concussion is based upon loss of consciousness of variable duration immediately following an injury. Degree is appropriately judged by the duration of immediate loss of consciousness, which in most instances amounts to a few seconds to a minute or so. Any immediate loss of consciousness signifies concussion. Unconsciousness of longer duration carries a greater risk of more malignant complications.

Amnesia is complete for the period of unconsciousness, and may extend retrograde and anterograde in more severe reactions. If a history of duration of unconsciousness can be established by an eyewitness and correlated with the patient's memory of events, useful information relating to the degree of concussion can be established. This is impossible in some patients at any age, and the problem is compounded in children.

During the period of post-traumatic confusion after awakening, a Korsakoff syndrome, *i.e.* poor immediate memory and confabulation, is very common. This may last for hours or several days. As the confusion lifts, retrograde and anterograde memory loss shrinks, and eventually reaches a steady state, sometimes requiring a period of weeks or months. Headache is almost invariable during the acute phase, and may blend into one of the sub-acute or chronic headache syndromes described below.

A point to be re-emphasized is the close time-link between injury and symptoms in concussion. A short latent period between injury and symptoms, or a period of relative recovery and then new symptoms, means that something more than concussion has occurred. In some instances this point cannot be established in the history, but when it can, it may be of considerable importance. As discussed above, a reaction in the immediate post-traumatic or post-concussion period may be a vasomotor event. These vasomotor reactions usually occur after a period of latency which is a most useful point in differentiating concussion from a migrainic reaction. More serious complications of head injury may also develop after a period of latency. These include such surgically important lesions as epidural hematoma and acute subdural hematoma, as well as post-traumatic stroke.

In many patients the period subsequent to concussion is marked by generalized headache of variable quality, postural dysequilibrium or episodes of true vertigo, and general symptoms of lethargy and irritability. The usual duration in children is a few days to a week or so.

Contusion

The diagnosis of contusion of brain tissue is based upon persistence of the period of unconsciousness, CT evidence of brain parenchymal changes including hemorrhage, and at times the confirmatory presence of persistent sequelae beyond the acute phase. Sequelae may be subtle or absent, and often outspoken neurologic signs may improve in a spectacular fashion even after many months in children when the basis is trauma, as compared with certain other brain-damaging events such as asphyxia.

The acute phase of contusion involves continuing unconsciousness, therefore headache is not a complaint. Even as the state of awareness rises, headache is usually of secondary importance to more pressing issues. The duration of coma and subsequent stupor is usually directly correlated with the degree of injury to brain parenchyma.

The pathologic basis of contusion is parenchymal hemorrhage of greatly varying size, tissue necrosis in direct or *contra coup* relation to the trauma, and edema which may be lateralized or generalized. In some instances contusion is complicated by infarction due to thrombosis of intracranial arteries or veins, or occlusion of major blood vessels in the neck.

Edema develops after a latency of hours or days, as may stroke, and either may account for relatively abrupt worsening during the course of recovery.

Other than associated surgical emergencies such as epidural, acute subdural and large parenchymal hemorrhages, the therapeutic efforts are primarily supportive together with the use of osmotic dehydrators and dexamethasone to treat edema. The value of the CT scan is obvious in analyzing the intracranial status of patients with contusion. On clinical indication, repeat CT studies can be of considerable value. The expected course is one of continuous recovery once the process has begun. Any worsening of symptoms implies an additional complication and mandates a repeat scan. Lumbar puncture gives little information beyond CT.

Skull x-rays may reveal a linear fracture, but unless the fracture line crosses the path of the middle cerebral artery or the major venous channels of the occipital bone, they are of little immediate consequence. Fracture through mastoid, paranasal sinuses and cribriform plate may be a route for meningeal infection, and warrants broad spectrum antibiotic therapy, as does any CSF leak. Depressed fracture should be elevated surgically.

Chronic post-traumatic headache and other symptoms are reasonably common among patients who have recovered from serious cerebral contusion, but probably no more so than the incidence following lesser degrees of head injury.

Acute subdural and epidural hematoma

A prime consideration of the acute period after head trauma is the recognition of acute subdural or epidural bleeding and the resulting urgent surgical implications. In general the degree of trauma is greater than in simple concussion, immediate loss of consciousness almost always occurs and either persists or deepens in the initial hours, sometimes after a period of lucency. Skull fracture may be present, the most significant being a fracture across the course of the middle meningeal artery (the basis of epidural bleeding) or the lateral venous sinus of the occipital bone. (The possibility of posterior fossa subdural hematoma should not be overlooked.) Careful and frequent clinical observations are mandatory in the early phase, with special attention to pupils, depth of stupor and coma, vital signs, nuchal rigidity and symmetrical or assymetrical long tract signs.

The CT scan is the definitive procedure to detect the presence of subdural or epidural hematomas. The radiodensity of fresh blood is easily seen. The scan may be done too early, particularly in thin acute subdural lesions where they may blend with the density of the bony calvarium. Subdural blood of this extent is inconsequential clinically unless bleeding continues, hence the need for repeat CT depending upon clinical course.

Stroke
The issue of vascular occlusion or hemorrhagic stroke bridges the period between the acute and sub-acute phase after blunt closed head and neck injury. It can occur in either period, and as such is a significant possibility in the differential diagnosis of the post-traumatic complex migraine syndromes.

The trauma which precedes the development of stroke is highly variable and ranges from motor vehicle accidents, falls and diving accidents to more esoteric trauma such as chiropractic manipulation of the neck, attempted strangling, and children falling with a pencil in their mouth with resulting trauma to the tonsillar fossa (Schneider and Lemmen 1952, Braudo 1956, Gurdjian *et al.* 1963, Morin and Pitts 1970, Schneider *et al.* 1972, Marks and Freed 1973, Zimmerman *et al.* 1978). In most, the trauma is either exclusively cervical, primarily stretch or sharp twisting, or direct blunt trauma to the region of the carotid arteries. It may be craniocervical where the exact site of injury is ambiguous. The pathologic basis is often injury to the carotid or vertebral vessel-wall with dissecting aneurysm or intima damage and subsequent thrombosis and/or embolization to smaller vessels upstream.

The initial injury need not lead to loss of consciousness. In fact, the more restricted blunt injuries to the neck seldom cause altered consciousness. In combined craniocervical injuries, initial symptoms vary from minor concussion to more serious contusion syndromes.

The full age-span is vulnerable. There is a greater frequency of this complication in middle age and older adults because of the presence of previously damaged arteries from atherosclerosis and hypertension. Perhaps other systemic risk factors (including the migrainic diathesis), increase the risk of thrombotic complication (Zimmerman *et al.* 1978). In this context, the Haas *et al.* (1975) report is of special interest in that two of the 25 juvenile migraine patients, who had focal signs secondary to head trauma that persisted beyond one week, had angiographic evidence of occlusion. The unexpected number of strokes in this group of patients supports the provocative concept that the combination of migraine with other risk factors such as trauma is more threatening than either alone. This issue is also considered in Chapter 7, with reference to other risk factors such as mitral valve prolapse.

189

The latent interval between trauma and stroke is usually six to 12 hours (Schneider *et al.* 1972). It may be immediate, or occur very soon after the trauma (Marks and Freed 1973) or delayed for one to two weeks (Gurdjian *et al.* 1963). The relationship to trauma in the delayed thrombotic and embolic episodes is more convincing in the young patient.

The symptoms in the interval between trauma and stroke are variable. They may blend with the expected symptoms of concussion or contusion in the more acute cases, to recurring headaches, vertigo and other symptoms of the post-trauma syndrome in those with longer latency. Some patients are entirely asymptomatic during the latent period. There is no clinical clue to suggest a given patient may be prone to develop this complication, except for the special vulnerability of those who have suffered blunt trauma to the neck.

The stroke itself is not distinctive. It can be sudden, which suggests embolus, or can evolve over hours and days in a gradually progressive or step-wise course. It need not necessarily be arterial, and can involve jugular vein thrombosis (see p. 243).

Sub-acute post-traumatic complications
Subdural hematoma, hygroma and pseudotumor cerebri
In the sub-acute period of the several weeks following injury, a principal concern raised by post-traumatic vascular or other headaches is the possibility of abnormal subdural fluid collection.

In the child or adolescent, subdural hematoma is quite rare, although Rahme and Green (1961) collected 15 adolescent and young adult cases from the literature and added two of their own. The symptomatology is not significantly different from that of the older adult. However, head injury is more likely to be significant and remembered. The clinical syndrome centers about headache, accompanied by gradual decline in mental competence and alertness, together with increasing fluctuating lethargy. Lateralizing signs are not prominent and focal signs such as hemianopsia are very unusual unless infarction has also occurred. If CSF is examined, the fluid may be xanthochromic and the protein content moderately elevated, but there is often little if any increase in intracranial pressure. Papilledema is not present in more than 50 per cent of patients.

CT scan will usually reveal the lesion, but the fluid may be isodense with brain parenchyma. Angiography may be necessary to demonstrate the subdural collection in such instances.

Davidoff and Dyke (1938) called attention to an interesting group of juvenile patients who apparently had subdural hematomas five to 10 years earlier in life which spontaneously resolved leaving residual membranes in place. They pointed out that relatively minor head trauma later in life, often during adolescense, led to rebleeding into the old membranes. In two of their four patients, the later head trauma occurred during boxing. This probably means that almost any patient who has had a subdural hematoma in infancy is to some extent vulnerable into adult life. Even operative membrane-stripping at the time of initial treatment leaves some membrane behind.

A more common lesion in the child and adolescent is subdural hygroma, which presumably results from an arachnoid tear with leak of clear fluid into the subdural space and a gradual build-up of pressure. Aside from headache, such patients are surprisingly free of symptoms, although most will have papilledema at the point of ascertainment. The presentation is similar to post-traumatic pseudotumor cerebri, another lesion to be considered, the pathogenesis of which is most likely to be bland occlusion of major venous sinuses or the jugular vein in the neck (see Chapter 13, p. 243).

Hydrocephalus is a known post-traumatic complication in the weeks following injury. The basis is either arachnoid blockage of fluid flow secondary to the fibrotic meningeal reaction to blood, or decompensation of a previously balanced hydrocephalus secondary to a congenital defect such as aqueductal stenosis. In the latter instance the head is usually abnormally large by measurement and the trauma may be minor. In contrast, it usually requires significant injury to produce sufficient subarachnoid bleeding for hydrocephalus to be the result of blood-induced subarachnoid fibrosis. Symptoms are similar in both varieties, consisting of increasingly frequent and severe headache, perhaps diplopia and sixth nerve palsy, ataxia and altered mental status. The CT scan is the procedure of choice to settle the question.

Sub-acute and chronic post-traumatic headache syndromes

Head trauma figures prominently among the 'red herrings' of medicine. Both the parents and the patient may be inclined to attribute chronic neurologic problems to remembered head trauma, when in fact trauma was incidental and merely an easily remembered starting point in the history. The most convincing association of continuing symptoms that are truly etiologically related to trauma are those when true concussion (*i.e.* loss of consciousness) has occurred or when even more extensive immediate symptoms and signs have developed shortly after the accident.

However, even this minimal requirement does not encompass a number of convincing post-traumatic entities, such as the acute post-traumatic migraine syndromes and instances of the chronic post-traumatic headaches that will be described below. In these situations most patients may be merely stunned by the blow and there is no loss of consciousness. In the final analysis, clinical judgement becomes the critical factor.

Headache may become the focal point of litigation. This is much less often the case in children than in adults. The reason for the difference is twofold. In children with moderate to severe injury, headache is less frequent, and is secondary in importance to other more dramatic behavioral, intellectual, and motor dysfunctions. In adults, industrial accidents produce a higher incidence of litigation than recreational or home accidents (Brenner *et al.* 1944), and for obvious reasons the exposure to industrial accidents is remote in childhood, and rare in adolescence. The rôle of motor vehicle accidents probably lies somewhere in between, and litigation is strongly associated with the issue of responsibility for the accident.

If not the chronic headache, episodic postural vertigo, irritability syndrome of adults, what is the clinical picture of post-concussion syndrome in children? In a comprehensive review of the problem based on 50 children between three and 13 years who had been referred for evaluation, Dillon and Leopold (1961) summarized their findings as follows: 'In 47 of the 50 children studied, personality changes and psychological phenomena were the outstanding post-concussion symptoms. Behavioral changes, including increased aggressiveness, regression and withdrawal, and antisocial behavior were found in 31. Sleep disturbances were extremely common, and eight children developed enuresis. . . Clinical seizures were developed by eight children'. This summary contains no mention of headache. In fact, 37 of the 50 patients did report headache, but it was generally mild and of short duration.

These observations are in accord with the general experience regarding the consequences of head trauma in children. Harris (1957), in a study of 150 patients, found that the 'typical' post-concussion syndrome of adults occurred in only 6 per cent of children, and half of these patients were over 15 years of age. On the other hand, psychological and behavioral symptoms were common and were persistent in 50 per cent. Of interest is the fact that one nine-year-old boy in this series had a chronic subdural hematoma.

In another study, Rowbotham *et al.* (1954) compared the follow-up status of children with adults. The adults had the expected 70 per cent incidence of headache, dizziness and nervous irritability, while 52 of 82 children were symptom-free in several weeks and 43 had returned to school. 30 had had transient headache and dizziness, but these symptoms were persistent in only eight cases. On the other hand, 27 of the children had prolonged changes in temperament. These consisted of nervousness, temper outbursts, memory disturbance and enuresis.

It is therefore necessary to turn to the much larger experience with adults to gain a perspective of those relatively few young people who develop the post-traumatic headache syndromes that are so characteristic and common in older patients (Brenner *et al.* 1944).

One point should be made at the outset. There seems to be no correlation between the degree of trauma (*i.e.* concussion *vs.* contusion and other major complications) and the incidence of chronic post-traumatic headache syndromes (Brenner *et al.* 1944).

The key paper with regard to chronic post-traumatic headache is that of Simons and Wolff (1946). The study dealt with 63 adult patients. The authors divided the cranial symptomatology into three types.

Type I headache was universally present in all 63 patients and 70 per cent had this type alone. It consisted of a dull aching pain together with feelings of 'pressure' and 'tightness' in a cap or band configuration. The discomfort waxed and waned with exacerbations lasting from a few hours to many days. It was worsened by coughing and sneezing and also by emotional tension and intellectual effort. Vertigo, giddiness and photophobia were occasional concomitants of the headache, but not nausea or vomiting. Electromyographic studies of these patients showed exaggerated muscle potentials during the headache. It was their conclusion that this variety of headache was directly related to low-grade muscle contraction.

Type II headache was found in about 25 per cent of patients and consisted of spontaneous aching pain and tenderness to palpation or in response to a hat, comb, *etc.* at the site of the initial injury. Sometimes the affected scalp was fixed, more often normally movable. It was believed that Type II discomfort was related to local injury to nerve endings together with reactive fibrosis. Injection of local anesthetic into the area gave relief.

Type III headache was least common of all, and affected only 7 per cent of the series. It consisted of unilateral throbbing pain which then generalized and was associated with nausea and vomiting. The headaches were periodic, several hours in duration and often associated with prostration. These patients frequently had had similar headaches of lesser frequency before the injury. Ergotamine tartrate provided relief, and the headaches were believed to be vascular.

In the post-traumatic syndromes of adults, about 50 per cent of patients have dizziness and vertigo that is strongly influenced by changes in posture (Friedman *et al.* 1945). A final element in the adult triad of symptoms is that of irritability and other behavioral complaints.

The comments of Simons and Wolff (1946), with regard to the pre-injury emotional status of their patients, are of considerable significance. Roughly four-fifths were 'psychoneurotic before they sustained head injury'. This revealing assessment was based on interview and a standard questionnaire. It may account for the significant difference in the incidence of post-traumatic syndromes in children and adults. It certainly accounts for the difference in frequency of Type I headache symptoms which are essentially a recapitulation of psychogenic tension headaches. Such headaches are relatively uncommon in children under any circumstances.

The other issue that arises is one of ascertainment. A mildly or moderately psychoneurotic adult, particularly if attracted to the possibility of reward from litigation, is much more likely than a child or most adolescents to present themselves for medical assessment for what may be a comparable degree of discomfort. Most children, and for that matter many adults, accept the Type II localized head tenderness as being a natural consequence of blunt trauma, and allow time and nature to affect a cure. It also may be true that the muscle contraction headaches occur in many children after head trauma (Dillon and Leopold 1961), but are accepted with relative equanimity and are short-lived for this reason. Similarly, vertigo and dizziness may also be quite common in children but under usual circumstances not too much is made of them.

This is not to say that post-traumatic syndromes are not 'real', but it does imply that they are peculiarly susceptible to ancillary psychologic factors and attitudes. It is certain that the very real personality and behavioral changes observed in children after head trauma are more of a problem to their caretakers, hence the frequency with which such children are presented to the physician to 'do something'.

On the other hand, the Type III variety of recurrent vascular headaches, induced or aggravated by trauma, comprises a highly significant aspect of the post-traumatic headache problem in children. There is nothing that distinguishes the post-traumatic patients from those with ordinary juvenile migraine, except for the higher incidence of muscle tension symptoms (Type I) and focal tenderness (Type II) in these patients.

TABLE XIV
Trauma-related Chronic Headache Syndromes
(16 Consecutive Patients)

Age	8–18 years.
Trauma	Auto 4 (struck by vehicle 2 patients, inside vehicle 2 patients). Sports and play 10 (contact sports 2 patients; fall in playground or other 4 patients; slipped on ice 1 patient; fell from bicycle 1 patient; fall in gymnasium 1 patient). Household 2 (struck head on shelf 1 patient; struck head on doorway 1 patient).
Initially unconscious	6 (duration 7 days—struck by car; duration 7 hours, struck by truck; duration 10 minutes, inside auto; 2–3 minutes, football; less than 1 minute, inside auto; less than 1 minute, basketball).
Chronic manifestations	Tension (Type I) alone 0 Tension (Type I) plus local pain (Type II) 1 Tension (Type I) local pain (Type II) plus vascular (Type III) 3 Vascular (Type III) alone 9 Vascular (Type III) plus local pain (Type II) 3 16

In my own personal series of 16 patients (not counting an additional eight patients where trauma-precipitated single migrainic events including those with complex syndromes such as confusional state and hemisyndromes), none had muscle tension (Type I) headache alone, three were mixed vascular and muscle tension, and nine were purely vascular. Four had concussion and were unconscious for one to 10 minutes, two had contusion and sustained continuing neurologic signs and seizure disorder. Seven of the 16 patients had local pain at the site of the injury (Type II) (see Table XIV).

Post-cerebral contusion vascular headache syndrome

CASE 41 This 11-year-old girl was struck by an automobile while waiting for a school bus in October 1974, approximately a year before her first visit. She was comatose for approximately seven days, then began to speak 14 days subsequent to the injury. Over the next three weeks she improved considerably although she had residual neurological signs.

During her convalescence she developed headaches that were frequent and severe during the six months post injury. They lessened during the summer of 1975 and then increased in frequency and severity in the early fall 1975. They were throbbing in quality, frontal in location, and of about 30 minutes duration. They were accompanied by an episodic spinning sensation, and with many of the headaches she was nauseated and vomited.

Approximately one month before her visit, she had an episode in which she fell limply to the floor and struck her head. She had no memory of this incident and within a few seconds she was awake and normal again.

There was no family history of migraine although a paternal

194

grandfather had adult onset seizures. The patient herself had had no headaches prior to the accident.

Examination revealed her to be generally healthy in appearance. Speech was slow. There was a mild intention tremor in both upper extremities, more marked on the left. The reflexes were all overactive, left greater than right, and she had bilateral extensor plantar reponses. However, she was able to walk tandem and hop, and her gait was normal.

An EEG was reported as a borderline record because of intermittent posterior slowing. There were no seizure discharges.

She was treated with phenytoin 50 mg in the morning and 100 mg at night, and she had no subsequent akinetic seizures. The headaches became much less frequent and less severe and were no longer associated with nausea and dizziness. After about two months she became headache-free, and remained free of headache for the subsequent year.

Comment: This 11-year-old girl had a cerebral contusion after being struck by an automobile. During convalescence she developed periodic headaches that had a vascular quality, and also an akinetic seizure. Treatment with phenytoin improved both complaints and by two years post injury she had only minimal neurologic signs and had been headache- and seizure-free for a period of six months.

Post-traumatic mixed vascular and muscle contraction headache syndrome
This girl was age 16 when she was involved in an auto accident in June **CASE**
1979. The car in which she was riding struck another car in the rear and she **42**
was thrown forward striking her forehead. She was probably unconscious for less than a minute and thereafter felt weird and 'dreamy' for at least an hour. There was a laceration on her forehead and both eyes were blackened.

In the three months subsequent to the accident she had been subject to headaches almost continuously. The headaches usually consisted of a pressure sensation occasionally building to a throbbing bitemporal discomfort that would last five to 60 minutes. The throbbing headache occurred almost daily.

In addition she believed she was more forgetful and certainly more nervous and tense. She tired easily, and was having difficulties in school. She complained that the left side of her forehead had a numb sensation which was particularly noticeable when it was stimulated by pressure, combing her hair, *etc.* This sensation was continuous.

Past history revealed that since age 10 she had had occasional throbbing headaches associated with photophobia and nausea. The family history indicated that her maternal grandmother had migraine and a 15-year-old brother also had migraine.

Comment: After a head injury with mild concussion, this girl developed both tension and vascular headaches plus a continuous local sensation of discomfort in the region of the injury. This was combined with the general complaints of forgetfulness and nervousness, all of which subsided during the six months following the accident, except the local head sensitivity that persisted. She had previously had vascular headaches, of which there was a family history.

Traumatic carotidynia

Vijayan (1977) has called attention to a unique headache syndrome that follows trauma to the neck. He recorded seven patients, the youngest of whom was 23 years. There is no reason to think that a similar syndrome does not develop in younger people, although it has not yet been a part of my own experience.

Direct accidental trauma to the neck, or less commonly whiplash injury, was usually followed by a period of continuous local pain for a few weeks following injury. Then ipsilateral periodic hemicranial throbbing headaches developed that were accompanied by pupillary dilatation and facial hyperhidrosis on the same side. This phase was followed by miosis and ptosis, that could last several days. Headache lasted eight to 12 hours, accompanied by nausea and vomiting. It occurred several times per month. The headache was not preceded by an aura, nor were these patients members of families with migraine, although this latter point was not fully reported as a specific negative. Another point that distinguished these patients from those with more usual post-traumatic vascular headache syndrome was the lack of response to ergot, while propranolol was uniformly effective.

In some respects these patients are reminiscent of patients who have severe headache following the 'trauma' of carotid endarterectomy (Leviton 1975, Leviton *et al.* 1975). However, the endarterectomy patients reported did not demonstrate the sympathoparetic component.

The syndrome is also somewhat reminiscent of carotidynia (Raskin and Prusiner 1977): although in this entity pain is located in the neck, is associated with more standard migraine headaches without sympathoparesis, and may respond to the full antimigrainic pharmacopeia.

It is probable that traumatic carotidynia results from damage to the carotid and sympathetic pathway in the neck. Denervation super-sensitivity may be a significant factor in the pathogenesis of the associated signs of cervical sympathetic involvement.

Summary of post-traumatic headache in juveniles

(1) In children, the subject of post-traumatic headache is in large part a variation on the theme of juvenile migraine, with the exception of those due to organic intracranial complications. The latter include the development of concussion, contusion and the surgical emergencies of acute bleeding in the epidural and subdural spaces. Post-traumatic complications also include stroke, and the sub-acute development of subdural hematoma, hygroma, hydrocephalus and the pseudotumor cerebri syndrome.

(2) The incident of trauma can precipitate, usually after a latent interval, a single episode of common, classic or complicated migraine as well as some of the alternative juvenile migraine syndromes such as cyclic vomiting.

196

(3) Head trauma can precipitate a cluster of vascular headaches. This is the commonest chronic post-traumatic headache syndrome in children, in contrast with adults, where it amounts to less than 10 per cent.

(4) In some few juveniles, the almost universal adult complaint of muscle tension headache may occur alone or occurs together with other elements of the post-traumatic vascular headache syndrome.

(5) The usual clinical expression of a post-traumatic syndrome in children is behavioral abnormality, not headache. However, the age-groups may not be as different as would at first seem to be the case. Perhaps the adult is more indirectly reacting to a similar behavioral syndrome (expressed as irritability) in their very common complaint of muscle tension headache.

11
MISCELLANEOUS HEADACHE SYNDROMES

The temporomandibular joint pain-dysfunction syndrome
Definition
This disorder has become a reasonably well-established concept in adult dentistry and medicine, although many aspects remain controversial (Guralnick *et al.* 1978, Friedman *et al.* 1983). The story begins with patients who have demonstrable anatomical lesions of the joint such as juvenile rheumatoid arthritis and tumors of adjacent bone which invade the joint. Such patients comprise only a small minority of individuals who have a generally similar clinical syndrome of hemifacial-temporal and ear pain, spasm of masseter and other jaw musculature and restricted or asymmetrical jaw opening. However, in most patients the disorder is based upon functional mechanisms which in some may relate to dental malocclusion. In other instances the pathogenesis is less clear. Primary or secondary psychological factors play an important rôle in the pathogenesis. Recently the temporomandibular joint syndrome (TMJ) has been reported in the pediatric age-group, especially in adolescents (Belfer and Kaban 1982, Holmes and Zimmerman 1983).

Epidemiology
The population incidence of the disorder is not known. In an adult headache clinic, the problem was identified in 11 of a series of 100 consecutive headache patients, mostly in young women (Reik and Hale 1981). About 10 per cent of the 400 patients diagnosed as having TMJ dysfunction in one large dental clinic over a six-year period were under age 16 years. In a pediatric headache clinic in which about 500 patients were seen in a two-year period, five patients were found, ranging in age between 15 and 18 years (Holmes and Zimmerman 1983).

Females outnumber males by 20:1 in adult series and seem to predominate in adolescents (Holmes and Zimmerman 1983). However, in a series of 40 children under age 16 (Belfer and Kaban 1982) girls and boys were almost equal in numbers (28 girls and 22 boys).

Differential diagnosis
The first concern when a patient presents with TMJ syndrome is to settle the issue of organic disease of the joint. Although mild TMJ involvement is frequent in patients with rheumatoid arthritis, the disease is usually manifest in other joints, and no serious diagnostic problem is encountered, unless one forgets that the TMJ may also be involved. The involvement is much more often serious and debilitating in juvenile rheumatoid arthritis than in the adult form.

Traumatic arthropathy is not common, but does occur in children due to direct accidental trauma to the jaw, as for example due to striking bicycle handlebars after a sudden stop. In the acute phase a hairline fracture may be found and fracture into the joint may lead to ankylosis. Fracture of the styloid process, usually in relation to dental work, may be a cause of similar symptoms.

Because of the frequency of ear pain in TMJ dysfunction, diagnostic interest often centers about the ear. The frequency of low-grade sub-acute otitis in children may lead to a misplaced focus of concern regarding middle-ear infection, and the TMJ as the actual source of the difficulty may be overlooked.

Tumors, usually benign osteomas or chondromas, may also occur in or around the joint and can be the cause of the syndrome.

Because of the typical daily occurrence of pain in TMJ dysfunction, *i.e.* the occurrence pattern of psychogenic headache, the possibility of the physician assuming that this is the appropriate diagnosis is very real. In fact, the basis of much of the discomfort would seem to be muscle contraction, and psychologic issues are an important aspect of the pathogenesis. There may be virtue in the concept that TMJ dysfunction syndrome may be best categorized as a special variety of muscle contraction headache. The treatment of TMJ dysfunction differs from the more usual psychogenic headache, and this is sufficient reason for maintaining a nosologic separation. The hemicranial distribution of the pain suggests the diagnosis of migraine, another common designation in TMJ patients prior to establishing the proper diagnosis. Aside from hemicrania, many other features of migraine, in particular the paroxysmal occurrence, are quite different. Moreover the positive objective features of TMJ dysfunction, such as limited jaw opening and palpable spasm and tenderness of masseter and ptergoid muscles, are not found in migraine.

The clinical presentation
The onset of pain is usually gradual, but may be relatively sudden. It is described as having a dull aching quality which is continuous, but may be greatly accentuated by jaw movement or chewing, at which time a pulsatile quality may be appreciated. Pain is located in the ear or in front of the ear and may extend to the temple, neck or angle of the jaw. It is unilateral in the great majority of patients. It may be present upon awakening. Nausea is uncommon and vomiting is very rare.

The additional history of bruxism, the nervous mannerism of jaw-clenching, gum-chewing or excessive yawning may be elicited.

Important supporting information can be gained by the physical examination. There may be distinctive tenderness on palpation of the masseter and temporalis muscles as well as the ptergoid muscles. Palpation may also reveal tenderness of the TMJ joint and the external ear canal. There may be restricted jaw-opening and audible clicks in the joint. In some patients the jaw may deviate upon opening. Malocclusion of upper and lower jaw may be apparent.

Anxiety and particularly depression in younger children may be obvious on presentation or becomes apparent as one gets to know the patient. Belfer and Kaban (1982) found that 35 per cent of their pediatric patients had 'primary' psychopathology and in all of them it was reactive depression.

Pathogenesis
The central feature of the genesis of the painful discomfort is contraction and spasm

of the muscles of mastication which spreads to contiguous musculature. There may also be some element of pain related to the TM joint itself. This is particularly the case if there is organic disease of bone or joint. The basis of the muscle contraction is multifactorial. Dental malocclusion plays a rôle in a number of patients, a rôle that can be the only discernible factor in the pathogenesis. However, in almost all patients there is a variable substrate of psychological tensions, which act to produce some of the habit mannerisms such as bruxism, tic-like extended jaw opening or frequent yawning. These psychologic factors also form the basis of the susceptible pathophysiologic state that perhaps leads to sustained tension in the muscles of mastication and a vicious cycle of events.

Management
Diagnostic management must include x-rays of the temporomandibular joint and consideration of systemic factors such as the possibility of rheumatoid arthritis. Dental consultation is necessary to assess any malocclusion that may be present. In many patients a bite-plate is necessary for a period of time to equalize the bite and reduce bruxism.

In addition to attention to dental factors, the therapeutic program should include a soft diet to give the masticatory system as much rest as possible. Local heat application and analgesics can be helpful, and the patient should be cautioned regarding gum-chewing, wide yawning and other habits that may have participated in the causation of the problem. Diazepam, for its muscle relaxant and other more general effects, is often recommended. Amitryptiline can be helpful, particularly if there is a depressive component to the psychological aspects. More formal psychotherapy may be required.

An important aspect of therapy is a full discussion with the patient that touches upon the several aspects of the pathogenesis. The objectives of treatment should be rationalized and explained, and both psychological and physical jaw-stress factors given appropriate consideration. With these measures, significant relief can be achieved in many patients.

Temporomandibular mandibular joint dysfunction syndrome
CASE 43
This 15-year-old girl had had occasional headaches in the left fronto-temporal region for one or two years. They were sharp, jabbing in quality and lasted for about five minutes. The pain became continuous in the month before her visit, and she became increasingly nervous and concerned. There were frequent sharp paroxysms in which the pain would radiate to the ipsilateral ear canal and jaw. A history of nocturnal bruxism was obtained. Upon opening her jaw there was slight deviation to the right and ptergoid muscles were tender. x-rays of the temporomandibular joint revealed no abnormality.

She was seen by Dr. Leonard Kaban who confirmed the diagnosis and identified a minor malocclusion. A treatment program was initiated which consisted of local heat, a soft diet and diazepam 5 mg t.i.d. This program led to significant relief and objective relaxation of the ptergoid muscles

200

sufficient to identify malocclusion. A night guard was fashioned to be worn at night, and she was also advised to carry it with her and use it during the daytime if headache occurred.

Comment: This girl presented with a characteristic history of TMJ dysfunction that was effectively managed by a combination of physical and pharmacologic measures plus reassurance about the nature of her distress.

Post-lumbar puncture headache

Headache following upon lumbar puncture, with a greater incidence following myelography and spinal anesthesia, especially in association with labor and delivery, is a common problem in adults. It is much less common in children and very rare under age 10 (Fernbach 1981). In all age-groups the patient who has migraine is especially vulnerable.

The headache is usually occipital or generalized, may have a throbbing quality and is almost exclusively related to the upright posture. It occurs within 12 to 24 hours after the spinal puncture. Associated symptoms may include nausea, nuchal rigidity and blurred vision. Diplopia is uncommon and overt abducens palsy may occur, presumably due to traction on this cranial nerve.

The presumptive etiology is a continuing CSF leak at the site of the dural puncture. Low spinal CSF pressure leads to traction on intracranial pain-sensitive dura and the larger arteries. This mechanism may be compounded by a mild aseptic meningeal reaction, especially if contrast material has been injected.

The best approach to management is prevention. The smaller the needle, the less likely is post-puncture headache to occur (Spielman 1982). When more attempted passes are made, the patient is more vulnerable, and effort should be made to pass the needle at a slight angle so that the dural and arachnoid penetration is at a slightly different point. The bevel of the needle should be directed upward in order to split the transverse dural fibres, and thereby minimize the chance of a tear. Children of 10 years and over especially should be kept supine or prone for six to eight hours following lumbar puncture. These precautions are especially appropriate in the child or adolescent with juvenile migraine.

If headache occurs, analgesics, sedatives and maintenance of bed-rest and hydration are appropriate and almost invariably successful over a few days to a week or so. In exceptional cases it may be necessary to inject autologous blood into the epidural space (Gormley 1960). The epidural blood acts as a tamponade, and the organization of the clot repairs the dural tear. The technique has apparently proved to be useful in stubborn cases in adults, but I am not familiar with its use in children, nor of a circumstance where it even required serious discussion.

Spontaneous intracranial hypotension and headache

Symptoms very similar to post-lumbar puncture headache, especially the strong postural component, can develop spontaneously in some patients (Lasater 1970). The pathophysiologic basis is mysterious, but may involve a spontaneous internal CSF leak. In a minority of patients, an incident such as a prolonged coughing spell can be implicated, as was the case in one of the five patients Lasater (1970)

201

reported. It is easier to understand in the shunt-treated hydrocephalic patient who may need a higher pressure valve. In the spontaneous cases, bed-rest and time together with the symptomatic management described above is all that is required. I can recall one such patient in my own experience, an adolescent girl who required a number of weeks before symptomatic relief occurred.

A recent case report (Murros and Fogelholm 1983) adds two important observations. The CT scan in their patient whose CSF pressure was zero showed slit ventricles and tight basal cisterns. After 24 hours treatment with IM dexamethasone the patient became asymptomatic and a subsequent CT scan was normal.

Cough headache

Almost any headache, whatever its basis, may be aggravated by coughing, sneezing, straining or bending forward. However, these maneuvers may also precipitate transient head pain, usually severe, as an isolated complaint. There has been a tendency to link these headaches with 'exertional headache', but there are significant differences sufficient to warrant clinical separation. Most exertional headaches in children are fundamentally migraine headaches triggered by sustained physical exertion (see Chapter 3). It is probably inappropriate to think of true cough headaches as migrainic in nature, since such factors as quality and duration are so different.

The pain that occurs with cough *etc.* is not characteristically of throbbing quality; rather it is sharp, stabbing, and usually measured in a portion of a minute or a few minutes in duration. It is seldom if ever hemicranial, but may otherwise have almost any pattern of distribution. It most commonly centers about the vertex or occiput. It is not particularly common at any age, but most reported examples are in adults. Males are more frequently affected than females.

Symonds (1956b) has written the definitive paper on the subject. He drew attention to the fact that this variety of headache is frequently an early symptom of intracranial mass lesions, or of structural abnormality of bone or soft tissue in the region of the foramen magnum. This was true of six of his 21 patients. He grouped the remaining patients into those who had cough headache alone, and those with both typical cough headache and spontaneous similar (but usually more prolonged) headache. Prognosis of both benign groups was variable, but the commonest tendency was for spontaneous remission to occur after a number of months or years.

All of Symonds's patients were adults in middle to late years. The benign syndrome must be relatively rare in childhood, somewhat commoner in adolescents. It is my impression that the risk of structural lesions of surgical importance of brief cough headache is even greater in the young (see case 47, Chapter 13).

With regard to the pathogenesis of the pain, it is hypothesized that it may be due to traction on pain-sensitive structures such as falx or tentorium, or perhaps a sudden passive distention of large veins or venous sinuses. No specific treatment can be offered.

Ice-cream headache

Almost everyone who has eaten ice-cream can remember the experience of the 'ice-cream headache'. It is directly related to eating a large bolus, and usually swallowing it too rapidly. The resulting pain radiates from the palate to the mid-frontal and temporal region and is associated with a feeling of pressure in the head. It is short-lived, but sharp and often brings tears to the eyes. It is probably more common in children until caution is learned, because it can be prevented by taking small quantities and letting it warm in the mouth. The mechanism may be painful vasospasm, or temperature stimulation of the glossopharyngeal nerve. Migrainics would seem to be more susceptible. One study (Raskin and Knittle 1976) indicates that 90 per cent of adult patients with migraine were susceptible while only 30 per cent of headache-free individuals were affected.

Ice-pick pain
Raskin and Schwartz (1980) have called attention to the occurrence of very sharp, jabbing pain that may be located anywhere about the head, but usually in the region of the eye or the temple. The duration of the pain is very brief and measured in seconds, usually consisting of a single jab. These authors point out that it occurs much more commonly in adult migrainics (42 per cent) than in a non-headache control population (3 per cent). In migrainics it may also occur during an otherwise characteristic headache. It is occasionally preceded by scotomata, and may be precipitated by sudden postural change, physical exertion, dark/light transition, and sudden motion of the head during a headache. The principal differential consideration is trigeminal or occipital neuralgic pain. This symptom has not been mentioned by my pre-pubertal patients, although occasional adolescents have spoken about it. No childhood study comparable to the Raskin and Schwartz (1980) survey has been done.

12
SYMPTOMATIC HEADACHE: EVALUATION AND INVESTIGATION

Introduction

The first principle to be established is that any headache in childhood may be symptomatic of underlying systemic, cranial or intracranial disease. There is no characteristic clinical expression of an 'organic' headache. However, there are clinical clues that can be used to segregate those patients who are at greater risk than the overwhelming majority of patients whose headaches are 'benign' and the expression of a migrainic diathesis or of psychologic factors and nervous tension.

The relative infrequency of headache as a complaint in children as compared with adults tends to increase the odds that the symptom in children reflects a significant disease process. This is scarcely useful because it is likely that the primary physician will see several hundred children with sub-acute or chronic headache problems before encountering a child with significant intracranial disease.

Adult patients not infrequently and usually quite correctly diagnose and manage their own headache and most are not brought to medical attention. This is less often the case when a child is the patient, so the physician must assess, and usually manage symptomatically, a relatively large number of young people with headache, always with the lurking concern about overlooking a brain tumor. The pediatrician or primary physician often has a sense of unease about his young patients with headache. Referral for headache evaluation has therefore become a significant aspect of consulting pediatric neurological practice. These remarks apply principally to sub-acute and chronic headaches in childhood. Acute problems, usually in the setting of febrile disease, are much more comfortably handled.

As a corollary to the above-stated principle that any headache may signal an organic disease process, the concept of 'symptomatic headache' should be enunciated. This means that headache with good clinical diagnostic grounds for categorization as either psychogenic or vascular-migrainic may be the symptomatic expression of intracranial disease such as tumor or arteriovenous malformation. Compare this with the other common paroxysmal neurologic symptom of childhood, seizures, where the concept of symptomatic expression of an underlying specific cerebral lesion, as opposed to an idiopathic expression, is well established and generally understood.

It follows that the clinical diagnosis of a vascular or migrainic process is only the first step, albeit important. The question must then be asked, 'Is it the expression of an inborn suceptibility to inherited excessive vascular reactivity that is almost invariably benign, or have these symptoms been set in motion by another process?' The question of a threshold of vascular reactivity also becomes an issue.

TABLE XV
Ten Reasons to Obtain a CT Scan in a Patient with Sub-acute or Chronic Headache

1. Abnormal neurological signs, including unexplained reduced visual acuity and enlarged head circumference (95% risk of tumor).
2. Suggestive general symptoms such as recent school failure, behavioral change (especially anorexia and apathy), fall-off in linear growth rate.
3. Frequent nocturnal awakening or a.m. occurrence of headache especially if the history is less than 4–6 months duration or if headaches are increasing in frequency or severity.
4. If periodic headache and seizures occur in the same individual, especially if seizures have a focal (clinical or EEG) expression or if the vascular syndrome is complex.
5. If migrainic and seizure phenomena occur in the same episode, and vascular symptoms precede the seizure (20–50% risk of tumor or AVM). If first study negative, repeat in 4–6 months.
6. Cluster headaches (migrainous neuralgia) in a child, or any child under age 5 or 6 years whose principal complaint is headache.
7. If focal neurological symptoms or signs develop *during* the headache (complicated migraine).
8. If focal neurological symptoms or signs (except classic visual symptoms of migraine) develop during the aura and there is fixed laterality, or if focal signs of the aura persist or recur in the headache phase.
9. If visual gray-out occurs at the peak of a headache as opposed to the aura.
10. Brief cough headache in a child or adolescent.

The theoretical equation becomes quite complex, but the practical issue is straightforward. Who should get a CT scan? (Table XV). The answer might be 'every young patient with a headache'. If so, this chapter could be quite brief, and limited to a discussion of when to repeat the CT scan. However, one must assume that anyone who reads this monograph accepts the professional and economic responsibility to make a judgement based on the findings of a relevant history and examination. In choosing this course, it must be acknowledged that the occasional AVM will be missed, and the diagnosis of the occasional brain tumor will be deferred. This, however, is part of the professional responsibility one accepts in becoming a doctor.

The physical examination
Consideration of the general physical and neurological examinations is placed before discussion of points of history, which usually comes first in the order of the traditional presentation. The reason is clear. The physical examination is the key to the detection of the great majority of organic processes. For example, abnormal physical signs were present in 94 per cent of a series of 72 consecutive children with brain tumor headaches when the diagnosis was made, mostly at an early point in the course (Honig and Charney 1982).

Acute illness
The examination is of prime importance in acute headache problems, especially those with more serious implications. A significant first consideration is the presence or absence of fever and other relatively non-specific signs of acute illness such as diaphoresis, flushing or pallor. The next step is to ascertain the cause of fever and assess whether the headache reflects general toxicity, or is a symptom of direct involvement of cranial structures. If the infection involves sinuses or

mastoid, point tenderness can often be elicited. Quite localized headache and skull tenderness can also occasionally be found overlying brain abscess, one of the few circumstances where sharply localized headache is meaningful.

Signs of meningeal irritation, nuchal rigidity, limitation of straight leg raising, Kernig's and Brudzinski's signs are of great importance in assessment of the possibility of meningitis, meningo-encephalitis, and aseptic meningeal reactions as well as subarachnoid bleeding, in all of which headache is usually a prominent symptom. Somnolence, stupor, agitation and confusion are significant, but non-specific indications of acute illness, and are not necessarily indicative of primary neurologic disease in a febrile setting.

Convulsions are also highly significant events, but the majority are a non-specific threshold response to fever. In the age-group where headache is a prominent complaint, meningeal signs, or focal aspects of the convulsion itself are critical factors in favor of an organic encephalopathy. Aphasia can be difficult to assess in a child in the acute setting. Young children usually merely cease attempting to talk, and lack of understanding can be misinterpreted as withdrawal or confusion. Elementary neurological signs are of obvious importance as indicators of focal, multifocal or diffuse brain parenchymal involvement, but detailed elaboration is not appropriate in this monograph.

Papilledema is uncommon in an acute process despite grossly elevated intracranial pressure. Lack of ocular venous pulsation and lack of venous compressibility to gentle ocular pressure are more sensitive during the hours required for papilledema to develop.

Sub-acute and chronic illness
Headache as the primary symptom of a somewhat more prolonged illness measured in a sub-acute course of several weeks is only slightly more likely to be monosymptomatic and occur without signs. Again, the full spectrum of general physical and neurological signs is important. Papilledema is more likely to be present and meningeal signs are less likely to be as prominent as in acute illnesses. It should be remembered that nuchal rigidity may be found in a patient with posterior fossa tumor or cervical adenitis and is not an automatic indication for lumbar puncture. Such subtle indicators as a preferential head tilt, drift of an outstretched arm or loss of ability to hop on one foot are sufficient to warrant neuroradiologic study as a preliminary step.

The findings on general examination can also be helpful indicators of the risk of intracranial pathology. For example, headache developing in a child or young adult who has congenital heart disease with right to left shunt (cyanotic type congenital heart disease), or pulmonary arteriovenous shunts usually with associated dermal or mucosal telangiectasias (Rendu-Osler-Weber disease), is highly suspicious of brain abscess and should be further investigated. Although less common in the current era, the same may be said for chronic otitis media and mastoiditis, while the patient with acute sinusitis is at risk of cerebral epidural abscess.

It is the more chronic and recurrent headaches that pose a greater problem, although the incidence of neurologic signs as a positive indicator of intracranial and other pathology remains high, and abnormal signs are the best selection criteria. The study of Honig and Charney (1982) emphasizes the importance of ocular signs. Of the 72 tumor cases examined in detail, 42 patients (63 per cent) had papilledema, while 12 had diplopia, eight had decreased visual acuity, nine had strabismus. There were fewer with nystagmus (five), optic atrophy (four), blindness (two), Parinaud's syndrome (two) and anisocoria (one). In the same study there were 11 patients with head tilt.

Truncal ataxia is probably the commonest motor sign, followed closely by hemiparesis. The relatively frequent mild hemiparesis in children that dates to a perinatal encephalopathy, and is of no significance to the newer headache problem, can be a source of confusion. Yet a mild non-progressive hemiparesis may be discovered for the first time in this context. Confusion may be alleviated by finding a concomitant growth-disturbance of the affected side, usually minimally manifest as a small thumbnail or index fingernail. This, particularly if reinforced by information that the child has always rather strongly preferred the opposite hand and chose it under the age of nine to 10 months, is a good indication of an early acquired lesion, probably dating back to the time of birth or under age two years.

Signs on the general physical examination can also be important. Small stature, especially if one can then determine a decline in the rate of growth in the past, can be an indicator of tumor about the hypothalamus, usually cranio-pharyngioma. Examination of the skin can reveal evidence of neurofibromatosis or tuberose sclerosis with their well-known associated intracranial pathology. A flat vascular or lightly pigmented naevus can also be an external indicator of vascular anomaly within the brain. This is more helpful for spinal than cerebral lesions, except in Sturge-Weber disease. The flat red mark below the external occipital protuberance, and its less common concomitant on the forehead between the eyes (the 'stork bite') is not meaningful.

Percussion of the head can be a useful maneuver and the resonance ('cracked pot') of separated sutures is a helpful sign. Auscultation for bruits more often leads to a false alarm than a meaningful clue. The frequency of soft vascular head sounds is appreciable in normal children, but a loud bruit can be indicative of intracranial pathology. To move the stethoscope from heart to head is a maneuver that seldom fails to impress the patient and parents with the ingenuity and thoroughness of the examination. It is worth doing for the sake of good physician-patient relations, especially if a CT scan is to be denied. Occasionally a meaningful bruit is heard.

General physical and neurological signs in the chronic headaches of childhood are less common, but of equal importance if they can be determined to be new. The remarks in the above paragraphs relating to examination in the sub-acute phase apply equally to chronic headache problems. There is nothing special to be said about headaches of one or more years duration except the cautionary point that one tends to be more casual about organic possibilities, and as a consequence becomes less vigilant.

Papilledema

Papilledema is a key finding in the evaluation of any headache. It is therefore appropriate to consider this important physical sign in greater depth, particularly as it relates to the pediatric age-group. The first issue is the question of whether finding blurred, obscured, and elevated optic disc margins reflects pathologic edema of the optic nerve, or a clinically unimportant aberration of the usual anatomy. The term pseudopapilledema is applied to the latter phenomenon. It is frequently familial, and on a number of occasions examination of the mother or father will reveal optic discs of very similar appearance. The question of pseudopapilledema *vs.* true edema of the optic disc can usually be resolved when necessary by fluorescein retinal angiography.

The appearance of aberrant myelinated nerve fibres that extend beyond the disc is sufficiently characteristic that once seen, will not be confused with papilledema. The disc is not elevated and myelinated fibres produce a feathery irregular margin with a linear quality radiating from the disc.

Some children may have high-grade refractive errors such as myopia or astigmatism, in which the optic nerve head is difficult to bring into focus. This can be confusing, usually clarified by examination of visual acuity. The combination of severe refractive error plus papilledema is of course possible. It can be useful to leave the patient's glasses in place and use their artificial lenses to aid the clinician and the standard ophthalmoscopic examination.

Optic neuritis is a traditional point of differential diagnosis, and not usually a serious issue if it is remembered that loss of vision is profound whether the inflammatory process is retrobulbar or at the nerve head. The minor visual changes that result from papilledema, such as an enlarged blind spot, are not recognized by the patient, even when the swelling and accompanying hemorrhages are gross. In the usual patient with optic neuritis, the inflammatory process is principally retrobulbar and the only visible change is slight erythema of the nerve head, or nothing at all. In the occasional young optic neuritis patient, swelling of the disc may be of several diopters and accompanied by hemorrhage. However, the differential point of visual loss remains the key issue whatever the appearance of the disc. A confounding possibility is papilledema superimposed upon optic atrophy. This is very rare, but can occur despite the well-known resistance of the atrophic optic nerve to edema. The clue is in the color of the nerve which remains dead white even if edematous, as opposed to the expected exaggerated pink of either papilledema or papillitis.

Providing the observed disc changes are not due to papillitis or central retinal venous thrombosis, the appearance of the ocular veins gives one a moment-to-moment indicator of intracranial pressure. Edema of the nerve head takes at least hours to develop and usually develops over days or weeks. After pressure returns to normal, it will require days to recede. Venous engorgement and some tortuosity is the easiest detectable observation, but in low-grade papilledema it is minimal and often ambiguous. Lack of the expected pulsation of veins in a normal intracranial-ocular pressure relationship can be most helpful. It is often difficult to assess, especially in young children, because the eyes are not held motionless.

In a study of adult patients, Levin (1978) established that almost 90 per cent of normal people will show spontaneous venous pulsations on routine ophthalmoscopic examination, and that most of those who failed to show pulsations were males in the fifth and sixth decades. In a smaller group of of nine patients with elevated intracranial pressure, it was found that pulsations tended to disappear at pressures of 180 to 190 mm CSF.

It can also be useful to compress the globe lightly with a fingertip and simultaneously observe the compressibility of ocular veins during this maneuver. This procedure requires patient co-operation, but with experience one can make a rough estimate of intracranial pressure on this basis. At normal pressures, veins are easily compressed and the change is quite dramatic. At pressures of 180 to 200 mm CSF the veins become resistant to light eyeball pressure. These observations can be helpful in initial diagnosis, as well as in follow-up assessments of the status of intracranial pressure before edema of the nerve head can be expected to subside.

In polycythemia and cardiac decompensation, the status of ocular veins is more difficult to evaluate. The cyanotic fundi of the patient with congenital heart disease can look like papilledema with engorged, tortuous veins and hyperemic discs. Perhaps it is somewhat dangerous to be aware of this fact, in view of the frequency of cerebral abscess in these patients and the tendency to pass off the appearance of the fundus as the expected appearance of cyanosis when it is really early papilledema. These issues are becoming less of a problem. Few children with congenital heart disease remain deeply cyanotic because either definitive or palliative operations are done in infancy.

The danger of prolonged papilledema is loss of vision. Fortunately this is currently a rare occurrence. There is a general correlation of risk with duration of papilledema but this is more a guideline than a rule. This risk applies to all patients, including those with pseudotumor cerebri. Visual loss with or without secondary optic atrophy may occur with a latency of months or years after the initial symptoms and occasionally after the intracranial hypertension has long since subsided (see case 49). The highest risk would seem to be in adults with concomitant systemic arterial hypertension (Corbett *et al.* 1982).

History
There is something to be said for a relatively undirected history, and 'letting the patient or parent do the talking', at least at the outset. However it soon becomes necessary and appropriate to direct the process with specific questions that relate to points of clinical information relevant to the judgements that must be made. Most parental historians are much more interested in relating the sequence of physicians seen, and what they said or did in the way of diagnostic and therapeutic interventions, than in a rendition of the description of the headache and associated symptoms.

A few points can help to indicate an organic bas s for the headache:
(1) The *duration* of the headache problem is probably the most significant historical factor. Most organic intracranial pathology, especially tumor, will declare itself by two to four months (Honig and Charney 1982), usually by the development

of abnormal neurologic signs. Often the headaches become more frequent and more severe in a rising crescendo. Occasionally in younger children, there is relative or even complete temporary remission after a few weeks, presumably at the time when sutures separate.

(2) Another feature of sufficient frequency to be of considerable value is *nocturnal awakening* or presence of headache on *arising*, a phenomenon known to clinicians for many years. Neither occurs at all commonly in psychogenic headache. Around 10 per cent of my patients with juvenile migraine have had occasional headaches that awaken them at night or are present upon awakening. It is usually not a frequently recurring pattern in any particular migraine patient. My own series would also indicate that onset on arising occurs only occasionally in the vascular headache group. On the other hand, in children with brain tumor headaches, 67 per cent had headaches that awakened them at night or were present on arising, the morning headaches characteristically tending to recur repeatedly (Honig and Charney 1982).

Nocturnal or morning headaches tend to correlate with raised intracranial pressure and posterior fossa mass lesions. The pathophysiologic basis of association with the recumbent posture and sleep is not precisely known. Intracranial vascular dynamics, vasodilatation, increased cranial blood volume, and the relationship of these factors to plateaux of increased pressure play a crucial rôle. Continuous ventricular pressure readings in children with low-grade hydrocephalus reveal that during sleep there are significant increases in mean intracranial pressure, with concomitant increases in pulse pressure (DiRocco *et al.* 1975). There is a general rise in mean pressure during sleep, with dramatically exaggerated plateaux of increase during REM sleep.

These observations are relevant to the nocturnal and early morning onset of headache caused by obstructing tumors. The factors that induce these changes are not fully understood. After shunting, REM sleep continues to induce elevations of mean pressure and wider pulse pressures, but both are much less marked (DiRocco *et al.* 1977). It is possible that these less dramatic sleep-related pressure changes that are presumably observed in sleep in normal individuals are sufficient to trigger occasional vascular headaches in the migrainic patient.

(3) *Lack of a family history* of vascular headache in a child with periodic throbbing headaches is a point of relative concern in view of the high incidence of family expression in juvenile migraine. On the other hand, children who have inherited the migrainic diathesis are especially prone to react with symptomatic vascular headache to a wide variety of intracranial abnormalities such as low-grade hydrocephalus, tumors, arteriovenous malformations, systemic processes such as vasculitis, and metabolic disorders. This point is well illustrated in the case reports in Chapter 13. The association of a family history of migraine in patients with tumor or AVM, and the resulting vasomotor phenomenology including headache, lends credibility to the concept of the structural lesion triggering vasomotor symptoms in individuals with inherited predisposition and a lower 'threshold'.

(4) There are several *miscellaneous* factors relating to the headache itself that can be significant. Although visual symptomatology is relatively common in the

prodromal phase of migraine, alteration of vision at the peak of a headache is not. Visual gray-out or black-out at the peak of a headache may reflect retinal ischemia secondary to a surge of intracranial pressure and should be taken seriously. It is a rare event and almost invariably associated with papilledema.

(5) Headache that is persistently *lateralized* to the same side may be the clue to organic disease. Most patie ts with lateralized migraine will have m re, or even most, headaches on the same side. Close questioning will usually unveil the rare headache on the opposite side, even in those who initially insist that it is always on the same side. Persistent lateralization is most frequent in headaches that have the characteristics of migrainous neuralgia (cluster headaches). This headache syndrome is rare in children and may be sufficiently characteristic as to be reassuring, but head and face pain clinically reminiscent of cluster headache can be symptomatic of structural lesions (see Chapter 13, case 52).

(6) *Cough headache*, which is described in Chapter 9, is also associated with a high incidence of organic intracranial pathology.

(7) Nausea and vomiting are the commonest *associated symptoms* of juvenile migraine. They are also among the most frequent concomitants of headache related to organic intracranial disease. In some tumors of the posterior fossa, particularly ependymoma, vomiting may precede the appearance of headache by several weeks or longer, presumably due to direct irritation of the floor of the fourth ventricle by the tumor itself (see case 11). Vomiting in young children for any reason is frequently explosive and 'projectile' in quality. Projectile vomiting is not a particular characteristic of tumor or raised intracranial pressure from any cause.

(8) *Change in behavior* is a frequent early symptom of organic neurologic illness. It may include the entire gamut of behavioral disorders of childhood. Irritability associated with lethargy is common. Minimal degrees of lethargy or apathy can be misinterpreted. The child is regarded as being unusually 'good' in contrast with the previous ebullience of childhood. Any change in behavior may be an important clue. Less effective school performance is closely linked to general behavioral changes, but may also reflect altered intellectual ability.

(9) *Seizure disorder* is another symptom of importance if associated with headache. This relationship is discussed extensively in Chapter 7. The duration of the seizure problem may be very prolonged and encompass a number of years and even much of the lifetime of the young patient (Page *et al.* 1969). The recent development of headache, even in chronic convulsive disorder, can be of special significance. With regard to the seizures *per se*, focality, unexplained break in control, persistent difficulty in control, or a change in character of the attacks all provide clues of possible tumor or AVM. The occurrence of seizures in a patient with neurofibromatosis carries at least a 10 per cent risk of brain tumor, whether headache or other symptoms and signs are present or not. Finally, as indicated in Chapter 7, there is a high risk of tumor or AVM in patients in whom migraine and seizure phenomena are both present in the same episode.

(10) All of the *complex and complicated* migrainic syndromes imply a greater risk of an organic lesion than common or classic migraine. They are considered individually in the chapter on complicated migraine and will not be discussed

further at this point, except to reiterate that complex phenomena that are always lateralized to the same side are a special concern (see case 50).

(11) There are a number of miscellaneous symptoms that mandate attention whether they occur in isolation or in the context of headache. Prominent among them are indicators of decreased visual acuity if not corrected by lenses. Excessive thirst, nocturnal enuresis and daytime frequency may be the first signal of the presence of a dysgerminoma. Decrease in the rate of linear growth may be the first symptom of craniopharyngioma. A full recitation of all the possible provocative symptoms is beyond the scope of this monograph.

(12) The elementary factor of *age* can be a significant issue in the evaluation of headaches in childhood. The younger the child, the greater the risk of an organic etiology, whether the headache be acute or more chronic in occurrence. All varieties of benign headaches are very unusual under age five or six, and all children under this age should probably have a CT scan if a leading complaint is headache. A child of four or five years or younger who complains of headache has a tumor until proved otherwise, although migraine is a possible alternative explanation (Vahlquist and Hackzell 1949). The migrainic syndromes of abdominal pain and cyclic vomiting are less provocative but nevertheless warrant careful assessment at the earlier ages. The occurrence of the syndrome of cluster headache in any pre-pubertal child and probably in adolescent girls as well also warrants CT investigation (Vannucci *et al.* 1974, Herzeberg *et al.* 1975, Mani and Deetor 1982).

Diagnostic management and neuro-radiologic and other laboratory examinations
The appropriate examinations usually follow quite naturally upon the results of a careful history and physical examination. Most patients with headache, whether it be common or classic migraine, or related to psychologic factors, will require no further study. They all require careful and repeated follow-up assessment at intervals appropriate to the nature of the problem. The 'appropriate' interval depends upon the acuity of the symptoms, and ranges from several times a day in some acute illnesses to once or twice a year in more stable situations. The most sensitive period in the sub-acute or new headache is the first two to four months.

There is no routine test to be applied to every child with headache or related disorders. This section consists of a consideration of various laboratory options that are particularly pertinent to the evaluation of cranial and intracranial disease. The investigation of the related syndromes of abdominal migraine and cyclical vomiting which involve studies of the gastro-intestinal system, and syndromes which suggest metabolic-endocrine disorders, are considered in the sections dealing with those problems.

x-rays of the head and neck
Prior to computerized tomography (CT), standard skull x-rays were very frequently made in children with headache despite the low yield of useful information. It came very close to becoming a routine in consulting practice and was often anticipated by the referring pediatrician. My own practice, at an earlier period, was to obtain regular skull films in an estimated nine out of 10 patients. It is difficult to remember

an instance when it was unexpectedly abnormal.

As I write this, I have trouble remembering the last patient with headache in whom regular skull x-rays were requested as a screening procedure. The reason for the change is obviously the availability of cranial CT scan. I suspect that my experience is shared by most physicians, and many fewer studies are now done in patients whose chief complaint is headache. There is also more careful assessment of indication. Skull x-rays are as capable as ever of demonstrating parenchymal calcification and separated sutures, eroded clinoids and the inner table markings of raised intracranial pressure. However in practice these occasional advantages are refinements, and relegate skull x-rays to a status secondary to CT.

Regular x-rays remain advantageous for certain specific questions such as skull fracture in head injury, for assessment of sinusitis and mastoiditis, questions of metastatic calvarial involvement or of bony extension of adjacent tumors or granulomatous process especially at the base of the skull. For most of these purposes, special views and tomography are either better or necessary as the case may be. Regular x-rays are also useful in assessing the possibility of platybasia, basilar impression and the integrity of the odontoid process. A widened upper cervical spine, especially in the sagittal diameter, can be a helpful clue to mass lesions of the high cervical region and foramen magnum.

Computerized tomography

The real decision to be made in patients with headache is when to request a CT scan and upon what indication (Table XV). The content of much of the chapter on symptomatic headache deals directly or indirectly with the CT issue. My own rate of CT requests is probably about one in 15 to 20 patients presenting with vascular or psychogenic headache. This represents an over-all economy in the medical economics of headache management, despite the fact that the cost of CT scan is two to three times the amount of a regular skull series.

Another issue that arises if a CT scan is to be done relates to the need for a contrast enhancement study. Part of the problem of making all these decisions is the as yet incomplete information of the value of CT, enhanced or not, as a screening procedure for various specific disease entities. Moreover, the technology has advanced so dramatically in the past decade, and resolution has so improved in the process, that the published series of patients studied in the past with older instruments are now out of date.

However it is possible to predict one outcome. Some CT scans will be done too early in some patients in the course of certain disorders, especially tumors. One must be careful not to be falsely reassured by a negative study, and be prepared to repeat the scan when the clinical course of the patient warrants it. Certain clinical situations are sufficiently provocative that one may as well begin with the notion that a repeat study will be appropriate if the first is a negative study. For example it is my own teaching principle that the combination of vasomotor and seizure symptomatology in a single episode warrants not one, but two CT scans because of the frequency with which structural lesions will eventually be found to be responsible.

The CT scan without contrast can be depended upon to reveal the enlarged ventricular system of hydrocephalus. It can help greatly in the additional judgement as to the degree of activity of the process by showing the relative decreased attenuation in the zone of periventricular white matter adjacent to the frontal horns of the lateral ventricle.

Most tumors will be distinguished on CT scan by focal increased or decreased attenuation, or by the presence of calcification. Many will show surrounding edema and will displace and compress ventricles. Certain more chronic lesions will quite frequently cause dilation of a portion of the adjacent ventricle. This finding can confuse the issue. Such lesions are more prone to produce seizure disorder than headache syndromes. Contrast enhancement will increase the tumor yield on CT scanning, but the increment of additional positive studies may be quite low.

The CT scan is highly effective in detecting intraparenchymal hemorrhage because of the high attenuation of blood, the limits of which are only the size of the clot (approximately 0.3 cm diameter) and the distance between the sweeps. Subarachnoid bleeding is detected with less certainty unless it is fairly extensive, but this issue can be settled by subsequent lumbar punctures. The demonstration of acute hydrocephalus in subarachnoid hemorrhage is simple, convenient, and can be important information in management.

Most subdural hematomas will be revealed as crescentic lesions of greater or lesser density than brain parenchyma with a sharp smooth inner margin. The ipsilateral ventricle is usually compressed and shifted and there may be swelling of the hemisphere. If the convexity subdural is bilateral, shift is less likely. At some stage in its evolution, the chronic subdural hematoma is isodense with brain. At this point, bilateral lesions, and some unilateral lesions will be overlooked. Subdural hematomas may also occur in the interhemispheric fissure and in the posterior fossa. Both are unusual sites in children, the latter usually occurring in association with acute trauma to the back of the head with fracture through the transverse venous sinus. Epidural hematoma develops acutely after head injury associated with fracture through the course of the middle meningeal artery. It is usually of sufficient size, density and location to be easily seen.

Most arteriovenous malformations are of sufficient size to be easily visible on CT scan, and contrast enhancement increases the yield. In a small series of 15 young patients reported in 1977, Kelly *et al.* (1978) noted CT abnormality in 13. Newer generation scanners have surely improved these results, but an extended series has not been reported. There may be uncertainty from CT appearance alone whether the lesion is tumor or AVM, but this can be resolved by angiography. Unless of large size, berry aneurysms will not be seen.

Brain infarcts are subject to considerable variability from the perspective of CT demonstration. The variables relate to timing of the study, size of the lesion, the associated feature of edema (which is directly related to lesion size), and the degree of tissue loss. Lesions in the first few days often do not show at all. After several days to a week one sees lucency of tissue which should relate to a vascular territory and may have a wedge shape with the larger end at the surface of the hemisphere. Weeks and months later, shrinkage or cystic cavitation may be found. The relatively small amount of blood in a hemorrhagic embolic infarction or in a venous infarct usually does not show on CT. Many small or incomplete infarcts never become visible. Contrast enhancement probably has only marginal advantage in the study of infarction.

Finally, it should be recalled that the CT may be abnormal even in what may seem to be uncomplicated migraine. Mathew *et al.* (1977) studied 29 migrainics within four to seven days of their attacks and found six with CT evidence of parenchymal low density, that had disappeared on re-examination in three months. All patients were relatively young (28 to 36 years) and all but one had had complicated migrainic episodes. Three patients had more than one lucent area. The authors concluded that the most likely explanation was that the lucent areas represented foci of cerebral edema.

Cerebral abscess
Cerebral abscess is a lesion in which the CT scan is clearly superior to all other diagnostic tests. Many of these lesions were not revealed by arteriography and pneumography in the past. In the pre-CT era the combination of radio-isotope scan with TC99 and EEG had the best record. The use of contrast enhancement with CT is indicated, and a ring density lesion is the characteristic expression. Abscess may have other characteristics, and other lesions such as tumor and granulomas may show the ring of contrast-enhanced density about a more lucent center.

CT is not only useful in making the initial diagnosis, but is of great value in following the course of the abscess. It has given one the confidence to treat occasional abscesses with antibiotics alone, especially when they are in relatively inaccessible locations, although surgical drainage remains the preferred treatment.

CT may be less definitive in the early diagnosis of epidural abscess. The layer of pus may be quite thin and is more likely to be isodense with brain than subdural hematoma. The chief asset of CT in purulent meningitis is in the detection of complications such as subdural effusions, infarction and hydrocephalus.

CT combined with intrathecal contrast material is another aspect of this extraordinary technique that has much to offer in selected patients. It can be particularly advantageous when combined with myelography in examining the difficult region of the cervical-medullary junction for tumor or Chiari malformation. By timing studies, the flow of the contrast material can be assessed, a technique which can be of occasional value in the study of hydrocephalus. Similarly intraventricular placement of contrast material may add an additional body of informative detail.

The technique of coronal scanning or coronal reformating has added a significant measure of detail in the visualization of the anatomy of lesions throughout the brain, but is of particular value in lesions in and around the pituitary fossa.

Cerebral angiography
This procedure as done *via* femoral catheterization with direct visualization of the placement of the injection material has very low morbidity in children in

215

experienced hands. Yet angiography is distinctly more invasive than CT, and its use has declined markedly. In children it is almost always done as a second-stage diagnostic procedure subsequent to CT scanning. In considering its purely diagnostic use, as opposed to its value in surgical planning, its current value is principally related to the assessment of intrinsic disease of blood vessels such as abnormality of vessel walls, occlusion of arteries and major venous channels, the Moya-Moya collateral flow phenomena, and congenital berry aneurysm. It can be helpful in predicting the nature of certain parenchymal lesions and separating tumor from AVM.

The degree to which angiography is superior to the CT scan in detecting AVM is uncertain as yet, but it is likely to have some continuing advantage in this regard. In the face of a negative CT scan, the clinical indication to proceed to angiography must be quite strong, such as the presence of unexplained subarachnoid blood, headache with focal neurologic signs, mixed vasomotor-seizure episodes and certain of the complex hemisyndromes of migraine, such as those of long duration which develop during the course of the episode rather than have transient expression in the prodrome. Finally, there is occasional ambiguity about subdural collections of fluid when angiography can be crucial in demonstrating unnatural space between calvarium and brain. The rare isodense subdural lesions are the chief issue in this regard. Perhaps this problem comes up more frequently in subdural abscess than in subdural hematoma, for reasons previously stated. A thin effusion or hematoma would be insignificant clinically, a situation which is not the case with pus.

The incidence of thrombotic stroke in children as a complication of angiography must be very low in the current era. There is an almost certain slightly increased risk when this procedure is carried out in patients with migraine, especially when done during or shortly after an attack. There are several recorded instances in the literature in which angiography precipitated a transient hemiplegic episode in patients with complicated migraine (Blau and Whitty 1955, Ross 1958, Jensen *et al.* 1981). There are other reports in which permanent neurologic deficits were the result (Alpers and Yaskin 1951, Rowbotham *et al.* 1953, Patterson *et al.* 1964).

Most studies date to an earlier era of angiography and the technique of direct carotid puncture. For example, Patterson *et al.* (1964) reported a 19 per cent complication rate in 27 migrainics. Three of the five complications resulted in permanent hemiparesis. The authors pointed out that the complications occurred if the arteriogram was done during or soon after a headache.

It would seem that infarction precipitated by angiography is a definite but rare possibility in adults, although probably much less common with modern techniques of femoral catheterization. The risk can be assumed to be less in children. Nevertheless there are occasions in which the procedure must be done, usually in close time proximity to a complicated migraine incident.

In view of this issue it has become customary in a number of centers, including our own service at CH Boston, to pre-treat patients with corticosteroids when migraine is recognized prior to angiography. Unfortunately there is no data available to assure one that steriod pre-treatment is effective in preventing either transient vasospasm in these patients or the more serious complication of infarction.

Pneumoencephalography

This procedure now has very limited uses, perhaps confined to the detection of abnormality in and around the floor of the third and fourth ventricles in the assessment of small lesions. Tomography of the area in question is a necessary adjunct on essentially all occasions when it is done.

Clinical neurophysiologic studies

The value of the standard EEG in relation to juvenile migraine is considered in an earlier chapter. Furthermore, the use of EEG in the detection of organic lesions of brain is quite generally known and does not require repetition here. The usual question to be asked in assessing a headache problem requires an anatomical answer, and anatomical approaches such as the CT scan are supreme. When a question of function arises, electrophysiologic methodologies are now the best method with wide clinical availability, although PET scanning is clearly of great interest as a potential clinical tool, and has already indicated its value. Its practical disadvantage is the need for an available cyclotron, which seriously limits its general use.

Computer averaging techniques have made it possible to analyze the integrity of the visual, auditory and somatosensory systems as well as the auditory conducting pathways of the brainstem. In some patients, especially those who cannot co-operate for neurological or neurophysiological assessment, these electrophysiologic techniques can provide information about the functional integrity of those systems. Further computerized analysis as in the Brain Electrical Activity Mapping (BEAM) technique devised by Duffy et al. (1979) represents a significant advance in functional electrophysiologic analysis that may have particular value in assessing the course of illness in certain patients.

Radio-isotope scanning techniques

CT scanning, especially with contrast enhancement, has had negative impact on the frequency of use of radionuclide procedures for headache investigation. They can have value on indication as secondary studies to help resolve specific questions. Early 'flow' studies after systemic administration may provide indication for angiography in some instances where infarction is suspected, but are not likely to preclude angiographic study. This technique may have some advantage over CT early in the course of infarction. Timed intrathecal radionuclide studies provide a dynamic assessment of CSF flow in hydrocephalus. Ventricular reflux and slow movement over the convexity surface can provide pathophysiologic information in questionable cases. Galium bone scans can be valuable in detecting inflammation and tumor of cranial bones. Radionuclide scanning techniques have little value in the common issue of screening for tumor or AVM in patients with headache.

217

Lumbar puncture

Examination of cerebrospinal fluid (CSF) is a key method of obtaining crucial information about neurologic disorders that may present with headache as a prominent symptom. This is particularly true of acute problems where infection may be the basis of the disorder. The CSF is the only way to make a specific diagnosis, and the urgency to initiate appropriate treatment makes lumbar puncture necessary at an early stage of the investigation of acute meningeal syndromes, especially if associated with fever. The analysis of cells, glucose, protein and particularly smear and culture of the fluid usually settles the question as to whether the process is infection, as well as to indicate the infectious agent. Although CSF pleocytosis is usually indicative of an infectious process it can be a manifestation of tumor and rarely can be found in complex migraine, as exemplified by Symonds's report (1931) and in rare patients in my own experience (for example a child with hemiplegic migraine who had 8 wbc-35 per cent polys). Rossi *et al.* (1984) described four children who had CSF pleocytosis ranging from 34 to 145 cells (both lymphocytes and polymorphonuclear leucocytes) during episodes of complex migrainic hemisyndromes. These children had no clinical evidence of an infectious process. In other instances symptomatic vascular headache and other phenomenology can be triggered by a low-grade meningeal infectious process and the CSF cells then reflect the primary pathology. The presence of fever and other signs of systemic infection is the usual distinguishing feature in these patients.

CSF examination is equally definitive if the process is hemorrhage, or in the rare instances of meningeal neoplasm. In differentiating subarachnoid hemorrhage from a traumatic tap, the presence of xanthochromia in the supernatant fluid can be crucial in making this judgement. The opportunity to make this critical observation is frequently overlooked, and is lost if the fluid is not centrifuged and carefully examined for color. Most febrile acute meningeal syndromes in childhood require LP as the first stage of the investigation.

In most other situations requiring CSF examination in children, LP should be deferred until a CT scan has been obtained, a delay of only a few hours. This is especially the case if there is papilledema, or if there are focal or lateralizing neurological signs. One must be particularly cautious in a clinical setting in which cerebral abscess is a possibility, such as congenital heart disease with right to left shunt, chronic mastoiditis or chronic purulent pulmonary disease. The same reservations apply to clinical circumstances in which cerebral epidural abscess is a possibility, *i.e.* acute sinusitis, meningeal signs, seizures or lateralized neurological signs in a patient who is too ill for the clinical status to be easily attributable to sinusitis alone.

The danger of herniation subsequent to lumbar puncture is greatest in subdural abscess and brain abscess, followed by brain tumor, especially in the posterior fossa (except for brainstem glioma). It is significant in those conditions in which there is gross generalized brain swelling such as in lead encephalopathy and Reyes syndrome. This means that LP should not be done when these conditions are possibilities until reports of emergency ammonia levels are received, or the possibility of lead intoxication has been assessed, usually most rapidly done by x-ray of the long bones. The milder degrees of cerebral edema of pseudotumor cerebri or hypertensive encephalopathy do not pose a threat, nor is there a significant problem in acute meningeal syndromes such as purulent meningitis or subarachnoid hemorrhage (where the removal of fluid can be therapeutic) or in communicating hydrocephalus.

Perhaps one of the most effective advantages of the readily available CT scan is its use in the management of acute neurological problems. When there is any doubt, CT before LP. If, as sometimes will be the case, the LP shows grossly elevated pressure and CT or other laboratory results then indicate a lesion which may provoke herniation, it is reassuring to remember that herniation is seldom an immediate event following LP, and that two to 12 hours are usually available in which to initiate osmotic dehydration, dexamethasone or ventricular drainage.

The measurement of CSF pressure (after CT scan) is of critical value in the diagnosis and management of pseudotumor cerebri, and can be useful in evaluating the status of some patients with hydrocephalus. There is little value and some danger in jugular compression for the evaluation of competence of the jugular vein. Children, in their struggling, demonstrate the patency of the system which may be the only real value in abdominal compression and jugular compression in the assessment of cerebral disease processes. Careful manometrics with cervical sphygmomanometer cuff can be of some value in assessing partial spinal block, but this technique can be applied to very few children. In any patient in whom there is indication of spinal block, the more definitive myelogram should be performed.

Elevation of CSF protein can provide the clue to an active CNS process in the absence of any other abnormality of ancillary testing. This can range from the hypothyroid state and low-grade meningeal disorders, to small and CT invisible tumors. Severe and prolonged juvenile migraine headache, especially if combined with complex symptomatology, may produce modest elevations of CSF protein in the range of 50 to 80 mg per cent (in children the normal value rarely exceeds 25 mg per cent). However, the flux of protein into CSF should last no longer than the period of vascular permeability during the acute phase. Re-examination three days later should reveal a return to normal values if there is not some other reason for the elevated CSF protein.

13
CAUSES OF SYMPTOMATIC HEADACHE

Causes of symptomatic headache

For the sake of a relatively complete review of etiologic possibilities, it is appropriate to survey the major categories of disease and to consider those in which headache is a prominent symptom. It is the traditional construct of a full differential diagnosis, although in actual practice it is seldom necessary and usually grossly inefficient in terms of time and effort.

(1) *Trauma*. Both organic and 'functional' headaches associated with trauma are considered in Chapter 10.

(2) *Tumor*. Much of the focus of this chapter and a number of other sections of this monograph deal with headache as a symptom of brain tumors of various kinds and in various locations. Most of the time the clinical problem is straightforward, but on some occasions it can be difficult, as exemplified by certain of the case reports appended below (p. 247). The specific presenting symptom of headache has been carefully analyzed in the Honig and Charney (1982) report, and many of the major distinguishing features of these headaches have been described above.

The frequency of headache as a prominent symptom of brain tumors in childhood is generally conceded to be high. It leads the list of symptoms of supratentorial (80 per cent) and is a close second to vomiting in infratentorial tumors (82 per cent) in the 164 children under 16 years with brain tumor reported by Odom *et al.* (1956).

Meningeal neoplasm is rare in children, as compared with adults in whom carcinomatosis of the meninges is more frequent. This is particularly the case now that the development of leukemic meningeal infiltration has been anticipated and prevented by cranial x-irradiation and intrathecal methotrexate at an initial stage of treatment. Meningeal leukemia still occurs during relapse but it is less common in the current era. Very rarely, the initial presentation of lymphatic leukemia consists of meningeal symptoms and signs due to leukemic 'meningitis'. Glial tumors and meningeal sarcoma are other examples of malignant disease that may invade meninges without any indication of parenchymal mass lesion. In some instances tumor in childhood may declare itself by acute subarachnoid bleeding, at times in repeated episodes prior to the discovery of the true cause. Wong *et al.* (1983) found tumor to be the cause in 26 per cent of a series of 15 children who presented with subarachnoid hemorrhage.

In the consideration of tumor as a cause of head and face pain, one should not overlook the possibility of localization in the nasopharynx, paranasal sinuses, and in cranial bones, especially at the base of the skull. Local tenderness can be a significant clinical finding, especially if the lesion is within frontal or maxillary sinuses. Enduring signs of involvement of upper and middle cranial nerves are an unequivocal indication to pursue the investigation aggressively. As an example, mucocele of the sphenoid sinus has been reported as a cause of a syndrome

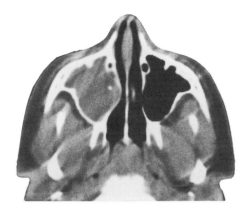

Fig. 13. This CT scan shows relatively uniform opacification of the right maxillary sinus with bulging of the inner wall into the nasal cavity. The lesion proved to be a hamartoma (case 44).

reminiscent of ophthalmoplegic migraine syndrome (Herman and Hall 1944, Hayes and Creston 1964, Norman and Yanagisawa 1964).

Benign maxillary sinus tumor causing unilateral headache
This boy of 13 years* first presented with a history of right upper facial pain **CASE** of six weeks duration. Past history revealed that he had had right maxillary **44** sinusitis two years before. Family history was negative for migraine.

His illness began with pain and fever of 101°F (38°C) associated with cervical adenopathy and right face and head pain. It was interpreted as a recurrence of maxillary sinus and treated with antiboitics. The fever subsided but the pain persisted.

The pain was continuous and located in the right forehead to the vertex. It was present in the morning upon awakening and he eventually required chloral hydrate for sleep. He lost seven pounds. A number of medications were tried, but none gave relief.

Examination was negative except for slight erythema over the right cheek. There was hyperesthesia to pin and touch that was sharply confined to the first and second divisions of the trigeminal nerve from mid-face to vertex. Corneal reflexes were normal.

CT scan showed an expanding lesion in the right maxillary sinus that left the bony margin of the sinus intact (Fig. 13). At operation, an irregularly shaped firm mass was removed from the maxillary sinus. Histologic examination showed it to consist of cavernous tissue with multiple sites of thrombosis and infarct necrosis. It was believed to be a hamartoma.

Comment: This boy's continuous lateralized headache proved to be due to a benign tumor of the maxillary sinus. Past history revealed sinusitis and findings consisted of hyperesthesia sharply confined to the first and second divisions of the trigeminal nerve.

*Patient seen courtesy of Dr. Paul Chervin.

ARACHNOID CYSTS

In the context of the discussion of tumor as a cause of headache it is appropriate to mention a group of benign cysts of the meninges that occur in a number of sites within the cranium. Perhaps the most extensively reported are those of the middle fossa and Sylvian fissure. Cysts in this location have been referred to as 'temporal lobe agenesis' which is a misnomer because the result of the cyst is to displace and compress the underlying temporal lobe, not to replace it (van der Meche and Braakman 1983). Cysts are also found over the cerebral convexity, in the interhemispheric fissure, around the base of the brain and in the posterior fossa.

They ordinarily contain clear fluid of low protein content, the origin of which is not fully understood. A number of histopathologic reports have described the presence of ependymal cells as well as glial elements in the cyst wall (Jakubiak *et al.* 1968). These cells probably account for the elaboration of fluid, which in turn promotes the slow expansion of the cyst under low-grade pressure. Other cysts seem to represent splits in the arachnoid membrane (Dyck and Gruskin 1977).

Most of these lesions represent a congenital fault, although some may develop secondary to inflammatory or hemorrhagic arachnoiditis, or form in relation to abnormal metabolic products as in the mucopolysaccaridoses. When they become symptomatic they have the general characteristics of a low-grade tumor, and indeed represent a mass lesion. They frequently cause local external cranial expansion, a clinically visible external expression of their presence. This finding is especially useful in lesions of the middle fossa, where the subtle asymmetrical bulge of the temporal bone is most distinctive.

Meningeal cysts may become symptomatic at any time of life. In infancy the usual presentation of both supratentorial and infratentorial cysts is as hydrocephalus, which is indeed the usual result of cysts in the posterior fossa at any age. During childhood and beyond, the clinical presentation is usually consistent with a slow-growing tumor. More acute symptoms due to secondary bleeding into the cyst or in the overlying subdural space are relatively common (van der Meche and Braakman 1983). Convulsive disorder is prominent among the symptoms of supratentorial cysts. Headache is less common (Drew and Grant 1948), but occurs in both chronic presentations and especially in patients with bleeding as a complication. The development of lateralizing or focal signs is unusual at an early stage despite the presence of a large cyst. The definitive study is the CT scan.

Benign intracranial cysts of another category develop within brain parenchyma. They are pathogenetically quite different, and relate to tissue destruction at an earlier age with necrosis and porencephalic cyst formation. Most connect with the ventricular system and are under no tension. For some unaccountable reason, in the occasional patient, the cysts are under tension and gradually expand (Handa and Bucy 1956). They act like very slow-growing tumors, and usually present in infancy, less commonly in childhood. Headaches are a prominent complaint in older children.

(3) *Vascular disease*
Arteriovenous malformations—Congenital vascular malformations constitute a

222

significant fraction of vascular disease in childhood. The commonest and most important group consist of the parenchymal arteriovenous malformations (AVM) especially as a cause of chronic periodic headache, either with the quality of common migraine or with classic or complex symptomatology. Although headache and associated symptoms may be the only clinical manifestation of AVM for many years, the most common presentation is as an acute illness with subarachnoid or parenchymal hemorrhage spilling into the subarachnoid space (40 to 50 per cent). Of the less catastrophic consequences, convulsions (25 to 30 per cent) are more common than headache (15 to 20 per cent) (MacKenzie 1953, Paterson and McKissock, 1956, Lees 1962, Kelly *et al.* 1978).

Roughly 45 to 50 per cent of AV malformations will become symptomatic under the age of 20 years (MacKenzie 1953, Paterson and McKissock 1956). This incidence does not include about 5 to 10 per cent of the total childhood group who present in infancy with cardiac failure or hydrocephalus due to AVMs which drain into the vein of Galen (Lagos and Riley 1971, Kelly *et al.* 1978).

From the perspective of this discussion, interest centers upon those patients whose first symptoms consist of headache with onset in childhood. Although uncommon over-all in the clinical picture of AVM, they occur in sufficient numbers to be meaningful. They are of special importance because early recognition prior to bleeding may be therapeutically advantageous. In the MacKenzie series (1953) all of the seven patients who presented with migrainic symptoms had their first symptoms between 11 and 17 years. Although the natural history of AVM is not known in detail, the patients who present with seizures and/or headache are less likely to bleed. The danger of re-bleeding is greater when the initial presentation is hemorrhage. Kjellberg *et al.* (1983) have reviewed the literature and compiled their own data, which indicates that if the presentation of AVM is hemorrhage there is a 6 to 7 per cent per year chance of further bleeding. If the symptoms or signs were other than hemorrhage, then the rate of bleeding is 1 to 2 per cent per year. The headache of AVM has a throbbing quality and is indeed a vascular headache. It may be indistinguishable from common or complex migraine.

In the majority of cases, unequivocally suspicious characteristics usually develop either early in the course, or as time passes. The most common troublesome features are the development of seizures or subarachnoid hemorrhage. As indicated earlier in this chapter and in Chapter 7, the occurrence of migrainic phenomena and seizure in the same episode is especially likely to indicate a lesion. This is well illustrated in the Pearce and Foster (1965) report which deals specifically with the AVM and complex migraine. The two patients discovered to have AVM in this series of 40 patients had the seizure-migraine symptom complex.

There are also more subtle features which provide clues that the 'migraine' is atypical. They are all mentioned in the context of warning signs elsewhere in this monograph, but deserve the emphasis of repetition. They are based on points extracted from the actual case histories of three large series of patients (MacKenzie 1953, Paterson and McKissock 1956, Lees 1962). In all patients, if the headache was lateralized, it repeatedly occurred on the side of the vascular malformation, and was what Lees (1962) referred to as 'fixed' migraine. Similarly, complex symptoms of numbness, hemiparetic weakness or aphasia were equally 'fixed' in their laterality. Moreover, complex symptomatology tended to persist beyond the aura, or appear during a well-developed headache. In some patients there were persistent abnormal neurologic signs that were detected on initial examination.

As an illustration of the close imitation of a known headache syndrome, the case report of a young woman is pertinent (Mani and Deetor 1982). She had entirely typical migrainous neuralgia (cluster headache) with hemicrania (always on the left side) associated with lacrimation, nasal congestion and rhinorrhea on the same side over a 14-year period. CT scan demonstrated an AVM of the left posterior inferior occipital lobe. Removal totally relieved the headaches.

A similar patient was described by Herzeberg et al. (1975). This woman had had 'fixed' headaches with features of migrainous neuralgia (cluster), for 17 years. They were accompanied by ipsilateral ocular and nasal symptoms and were relieved to some extent by ergot. She was found to have a large AVM on angiography.

The definitive neuro-diagnostic procedure is angiography. The reliability of the CT scan is only slightly less, and certainly improving with the resolution possible with new generation scanners. Closely related to arteriovenous malformations, but much less likely to present as headache, are the congenital venous and capillary angiomas that are occasionally the cause of symptoms, usually parenchymal and/or subarachnoid hemorrhage. These lesions are frequently asymptomatic until they bleed.

Arteriovenous malformation

CASE 45 This nine-year-old girl had had about two generalized throbbing headaches per year for the preceding three years. They were accompanied by abdominal pain and were severe enough for her to remain home from school. During the headaches she was photophobic but there was no nausea or vomiting and no aura. Family history included a paternal uncle with throbbing headaches that were diagnosed as migraine, and her mother also had severe headaches associated with menses.

On the day before admission, while playing in the yard, she developed a headache that had the usual quality. After a short period she developed weakness of the left leg with lesser involvement of the arm on the same side. She was hospitalized at a local hospital and transferred to the Children's Hospital Boston on the following day. By that time her arm had improved significantly but the leg remained persistently weak.

On examination, she was found to be mentally alert, comfortable and no longer complaining of headache. The blood pressure was 90/70 and other vital signs and general physical examination were normal. On neurological examination she had a left hemiparesis with the leg more affected than the arm.

The cerebrospinal fluid was grossly bloody. An EEG showed a slow wave focus with reversals in the right parietal area, and an arteriogram (Figs. 14a,b) revealed an arteriovenous malformation in the right posterior frontal parasagittal region that consisted of a cluster of pathological vessels

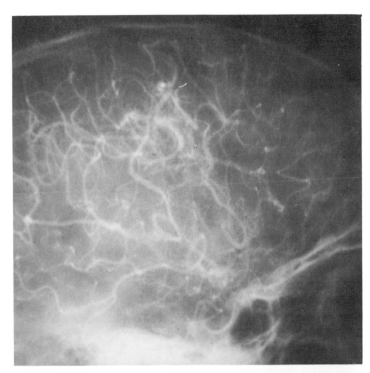

Fig. 14a. This right carotid arteriogram in a late arterial phase demonstrates an arteriovenous malformation in the fronto-parietal region (case 45).

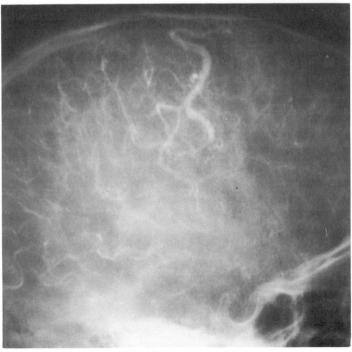

Fig. 14b. At a slightly later phase, the venous drainage of the lesion is well illustrated (case 45).

with early venous filling, associated with an avascular mass posterior to the lesion. There was spasm of the main branch of the pericallosal artery which was dilated proximal to the spasm.

On the fourth hospital day she developed low-grade papilledema, and treatment with dexamethasone was begun. On the 10th day in hospital she underwent right craniotomy with excision of a right frontal arteriovenous malformation.

When seen for follow-up examination approximately four years later she had minimal neurological residual, her strength and gait were normal. Plantar response was bilaterally flexor although she had slightly more active reflexes in the left lower extremity. She had had no subsequent headache.

Comment: This girl had practically no warning of the presence of her arteriovenous malformation beyond occasional vascular headaches. In the setting of a family history of migraine, they were not considered of particular significance until the episode of parenchymal and subarachnoid hemorrhage. Fortunately the location of the AVM was favorable and complete operative removal was possible.

Note. For additional patients with AVM, see cases 29 and 30 in Chapter 7.

Berry aneurysm

Symptomatic congenital berry aneurysm is generally considered to be rare in childhood, although it amounts to about 30 per cent of vascular malformations in this age group (Matson 1969). Its manifestations are not significantly different in childhood from the presentation in adults. Because of the frequency of oculomotor nerve involvement in aneurysm, the chief differential concern relates to ophthalmoplegic migraine (see p. 115). Ophthalmoplegia with headache under age 10 is more commonly due to other conditions such as tumor or migraine.

An exceptional patient was a woman reported by Reinecke (1961) who had a subarachnoid hemorrhage from a ruptured aneurysm at age 43 after a history of vascular headaches dating back to age five years. She did not have ophthalmoplegia with her periodic headaches, which were, however, preceded by a 20-minute aura of serrated flashes of light, always in the right visual field, followed by headache and the atypical additional feature of right mid-face pain.

The usual presentation of berry aneurysm in childhood is acute subarachnoid hemorrhage without a prior history of headache. However, even subarachnoid hemorrhage and its accompanying symptoms of severe headache, meningeal signs and altered consciousness is more commonly due to AVM or tumor (Wong *et al.* 1983).

Congenital berry aneurysm with rupture

CASE 46 This 12-year-old boy was in excellent health until 14 days before admission when he presented with the complaint of a 20-hour history of throbbing frontal headache, vomiting and low-grade fever. He was found to have

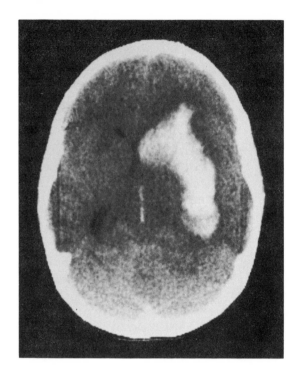

Fig. 15. This CT scan shows massive parenchymal and intraventricular hemorrhage in the left hemisphere with shift of the midline structures (case 46). The cause proved to be a ruptured berry aneurysm.

nuchal rigidity and referred to the emergency room. He was alert and afebrile and found to have slight meningismus, an injected pharynx and right tonsillar exudate. He had tender right cervical adenopathy and no other abnormal signs. The family history was positive for migraine.

Spinal fluid examination was interpreted as a 'traumatic tap'. There were 58,000 rbcs, 72 wbcs and a protein of 130 mg per cent. The supernatant fluid did not show xanthochromia. The peripheral wbc was 13,000 with 86 per cent polys and four bands. He was believed to have a viral syndrome with a question of streptococcus pharyngitis. Culture of the throat subsequently revealed no growth and two days later on telephone conversation he was symptomatically improved.

On the day of admission, he complained of a sudden onset of headache and then collapsed. When seen in a local emergency room he was unresponsive, vital signs were unstable and his pupils were fixed and dilated. He was intubated, hyperventilated, given mannitol and dexamethasone and transferred to the Children's Hospital. He was deeply comatose with decerebrate posturing to painful stimuli. He had no spontaneous respirations and shortly thereafter the corneal reflexes and gag response were absent. A CT scan revealed a large left parenchymal and intraventricular hemorrhage with midline shift (Fig. 15).

Subsequent postmortem examination showed the cause of the cerebral hemorrhage to be a ruptured aneurysm at the junction of the left anterior and middle cerebral artery with hemorrhage into the subarachnoid space, adjacent brain, and left lateral ventricle. In addition, there was cerebral edema and cerebellar tonsillar herniation. On microscopic examination there was indication of a previous episode of bleeding in that there were hemosiderophages in the meninges adjacent to the aneurysm. This finding was believed to be consistent with the event two weeks before the fatal rupture.

Comment: Unlike most cerebral congenital berry aneurysms in childhood that present for the first time with subarachnoid hemorrhage, this boy had an episode of minor leakage from the aneurysm two weeks before his fatal hemorrhage. Studies at the time of the initial incident led to misinterpretation of the CSF findings as a 'bloody tap' rather than pathologic subarachnoid hemorrhage.

Acute subarachnoid hemorrhage

As discussed above, acute bleeding into the subarachnoid space is a common initial clinical declaration of both AVM and congenital berry aneurysm. It warrants further discussion at this juncture, although it is far less common in childhood than the usual infectious causes of the meningeal syndrome in children.

The clinical presentation of subarachnoid bleeding is dominated by sudden development of severe headache. The headache is not localized, but may be more prominent at the back of the head. Nausea and vomiting are common as are changes in the mental status. There may be rapid progression from irritability and agitation to stupor and coma, decerebration and death.

The signs consist of nuchal rigidity and other evidences of meningeal irritation. Additional neurologic signs that may indicate the nature of the lesion such as lateralized cerebral signs (AVM) and upper cranial nerve signs (berry aneurysm) may be present.

The CSF is grossly bloody and under elevated pressure. In some cases there may be uncertainty as to whether the findings are artefacts of a struggling child and a traumatic tap. The former may not be soluble, but an attempt to quiet the child and get an accurate measure is worth a trial. Xanthochromia of supernatant fluid is the best way to differentiate a traumatic tap from pathologic subarachnoid bleeding. If the bleeding has been present for longer than about six hours, a yellowish tinge to the centrifuged supernatant fluid should be seen. It is always surprising to me how often this opportunity is lost in pediatric practice. The fact that CSF blood is often traumatic, and pathologic subarachnoid bleeding is rare in childhood, is not really an excuse.

In current practice, lumbar puncture should usually be preceded by CT scan unless meningeal infection is the likely cause (as evidenced primarily by fever). The very sudden onset and absence of fever are prime clinical clues that the process is bleeding rather than infection.

The causes of subarachnoid bleeding in children are quite different from adults, primarily due to the lesser incidence of hypertension and berry aneurysm in children. AVM and berry aneurysms are the leading cause and account for over 50 per cent of childhood cases, while tumor accounts for 25 per cent and in about the same number the cause is not determined (Wong *et al.* 1983). Subarachnoid bleeding has been reported in adults in the context of a paroxysm of migraine (Pearce and Foster 1965). This must be very unusual in children, and to my knowledge has not been reported in this age-group.

Connective tissue disease
Patients with systemic connective tissue disease, especially those with 'mixed connective tissue disease', have vascular headache as a frequent complaint, 35 per cent in a recent series (Bronshvag *et al.* 1978). Several of the patients reported in this series were children. The spectrum of headache varied from common to classic migraine. All of the children had the common type. Similar observations of vascular headache associated with lupus erythematosis and other connective tissue disorders have been made.

Vascular headache does not seem to predict cerebral complications in these patients. It is probably best regarded as an epiphenomenon of the disease. Incidence is not much greater than the expected incidence in the population and may represent migraine provoked by a systemic disease process. Perhaps the vasculitic component of the connective tissue disorders acts as a special irritant to inherited vasomotor instability in these patients.

Hypertension and hypertensive encephalopathy
Malignant hypertension and encephalopathy are now uncommon in adult patients, and have always been exceedingly rare in children. The usual etiology is chronic renal disease in children although other lesions such as coarctatin of the aorta and pheochromocytonia may occasionally be the cause. By the time encephalopathy develops, evidence of renal dysfunction such as elevated BUN is almost invariable whatever the etiology.

The premalignant phase may be asymptomatic or marked by the relatively non-specific symptoms of the underlying disease (Chester *et al.* 1978). Headache is uncommon and is usually mild. It may assume the character of either vascular or muscle contraction tension headaches. There is a tendency to occipital localization and morning occurrence.

An accelerated phase then ensues that is characterized by greater hypertension, vessel changes, exudates, and hemorrhage in the retina without papilledema (Chester *et al.* 1978). In this phase the patient develops more overt neurological symptoms. Headache becomes more severe and persistent, with episodes of transient visual disturbance and confusion. Convulsions may occur in younger children. Successful treatment of hypertension is effective in reversing the symptomatology.

In the final phase of acute encephalopathy papilledema develops, the *sine qua non* of the diagnosis. Episodes of distorted consciousness are more prominent, marked by agitation, transient focal or lateralizing neurological signs and eventually coma. Headache is prominent and convulsions are more frequent (Chester *et al.* 1978). At this stage aggressive treatment of hypertension may result

TABLE XVI
Some Risk Factors of Stroke in Childhood

Thrombosis (arterial and venous)	*Emboli*
Congenital heart disease	Cardiac surgery
Meningitis	Subacute bacterial endocarditis
Sickle cell disease	*Prolapsed mitral valve
Infantile dehyration	Myxoma
Homocystinuria	
*Trauma (head and neck)	*Hemorrhage*
Radiotherapy (head and neck)	AVM and berry aneurysm
Amphetamine abuse	Mycotic aneurysm
Arteriosclerosis	Amphetamine abuse
Arteritis—idiopathic	Trauma
Connective tissue disease (Lupus, periarteritis)	Moya-Moya revascularization
Auto-thrombin III deficiency	Bleeding diathesis
*Fibromuscular dysplasia	
Kinks and coils of major arteries	
Neurofibromatosis	
*Birth-control pills	
L. Asparaginase	
Migraine	

*Indication that concomitant migraine may represent an added risk factor.

in transient improvement, but the development of hypertensive encephalopathy heralds death from either cerebral or renal causes.

The key issue in the diagnosis is the measurement of blood pressure, which should be done on each visit in all pediatric patients with headache. It will rarely be abnormal, but if it is, the implication of significant disease is clear whether relevant to the presenting complaint of headache or not.

The differential diagnostic problem usually consists of the ascertainment of the cause of the hypertension. An occasional concern is the differentiation from brain tumor because of papilledema in both conditions. The combination of other changes in the fundus such as arteriolar changes and hard exudates, and the fact that elevation of blood pressure to compensate for raised intracranial pressure is a late change in tumor, make the clinical differentiation quite straightforward in children, especially if there is elevated BUN, *etc.* Cranial CT will settle the issue. Other acute encephalopathies such as lead encephalopathy and Reye's disease may come into the differential consideration. They can be identified by specific laboratory investigation, but the elevated blood pressure, BUN, and changes in the fundi are usually the distinguishing features in favor of hypertensive encephalopathy.

Childhood stroke
Previous recurring headache is not a common history in children who develop stroke, although headache as part of the acute event is reasonably common. The chief point of differential diagnosis comes about in the consideration in the complex migraine syndromes, especially the various hemisyndromes associated with migraine.

Stroke in childhood and adolescents, sometimes alternatively expressed as 'acute hemiplegia', may be caused by a large number of different conditions (Table XVI), and it is appropriate to deal with the subject only as it relates to the problem at hand (Isler 1971, Strand 1976). Among the pathologies other than vascular accidents, one must consider focal encephalitis (viral, or bacterial as for example in association with thrombophlebitis in meningitis), acute hemorrhagic leuco-encephalitis, and occasionally tumor. A large group of disorder, especially the acutely developing hemiplegias in patients under two years, are caused by a poorly understood process that evolves in the setting of prolonged hemiconvulsions (Aicardi *et al.* 1969, Isler 1971).

Among the true vascular events one must consider causes related to any of the three major varieties, *i.e.* hemorrhage, embolus, and thrombosis (Table XVI).

Hemorrhagic stroke
Hemorrhage resulting from trauma and from hemorrhagic diathesis hardly ever causes differential diagnostic confusion because the clinical circumstances are usually obvious. On the other hand, arteriovenous malformation is frequently first manifested as acute intracerebral hemorrhage, and as described above, a significant number of these patients may have a periodic vascular headache, seizure disorder or both prior to hemorrhage.

Amphetamine abuse is now recognized a a common cause of intracranial hemorrhage in the young adult and adolescent (Delaney and Estes 1980). Almost all patients who develop hemorrhage on this basis have severe headache as a prodromal symptom of the acute event perhaps as a result of a surge of hypertension, but prior headache is not mentioned as a rule. Recently it has become apparent that oral or nasally administered amphetamine is capable of causing cerebral hemorrhage as well as the more commonly reported intravenous administration (Harrington *et al.* 1983).

The increased collateral vascularity of the 'Moya-Moya' lesion may also bleed, and a number of patients give a history of prior periodic headaches. Finally, a significant cause of cerebral hemorrhage is myocotic aneurysm in the setting of sub-acute bacterial endocarditis. Fortunately the availability of the CT scan expeditiously answers the question of hemorrhage, although not necessarily the basis for the bleeding.

Embolic stroke
A reasonable attribution to embolus requires a source, which is usually the heart in childhood. The most common basis is those emboli which develop during or subsequent to cardiac surgery. This circumstance poses little diagnostic difficulty. Sub-acute bacterial endocarditis is also reasonably common, and can be occult in terms of systemic manifestations. Myxoma is a rare cause, as are transient arrhythmias. Embolic stroke is not associated with prior headache as a rule.

The place of prolapsed mitral valve as a cause of emboli, either *via* transient arrhythmia or *via* bland vegetation on the valve, has yet to be fully assessed (Barnett *et al.* 1980). The frequency in the population is such that this lesion may be

231

a significant basis for stroke in the young patient. The relationship to migraine is discussed in Chapters 2 and 7.

Thrombotic stroke

Many strokes in childhood can be attributed to *in situ* thrombosis of major vessels in the neck or of intracranial arteries or veins (Strand 1976). Headache may occur as a prior symptom or at the time of the acute event, but it is not common, except perhaps in the acute phase of cortical venous thrombosis.

Cyanotic congenital heart disease is still an important risk factor, but early surgery and treatment of occult iron deficiency has resulted in a most favorable amelioration of risk in these patients (Phornphutkul *et al.* 1973). Probably the commonest current cause of thrombotic stroke in childhood is the arteritis or thrombophlebitis associated with meningitis. However, even if the meningeal infection is of low grade, the diagnostic problem is not too difficult because the clinical picture is usually dominated by meningeal signs, fever and other systemic signs of infection. Cerebral thrombosis is also a well-documented and reasonably common consequence of sickle cell disease (Portnoy and Herion 1972) and thrombosis may be a complication of homocystinuria. A nitroprusside urine test is necessary in all juveniles with ischemic stroke, although most patients with this condition will have characteristic body habitus, dislocated lenses, *etc.*

Prior trauma to the neck and head or the tonsillar fossa is the basis of some instances of thrombosis (Frantzen *et al.* 1961, Bickerstaff 1964*b*, see also Chapter 10). The late effects of radiotherapy as a cause of large as well as small arterial occlusions have become better appreciated recently (Painter *et al.* 1975, Wright and Bresnan 1976).

Amphetamine abuse may cause thrombosis as well as hemorrhage, and the same can be said of the Moya-Moya lesion. Instances of stroke related to inherited antithrombin III deficiency have been recorded (Ambruso *et al.* 1980), and it is likely that instances of stroke related to other clotting factors will be found. The addition of L-asparaginase to the induction therapy of leukemia has been associated with a 1 to 2 per cent incidence of hemorrhagic infarction, probably related to changes in blood coagulation factors (Cairo *et al.* 1980, Priest *et al.* 1982). Recent personal experience with three such patients who also had juvenile migraine has raised the question of enhanced risk when the patient also has migraine. Cerebral arteriosclerosis has also been associated with stroke in children. Daniels *et al.* (1982) recorded eight such children, who had abnormal cholesterol, triglyceride and lipoprotein levels in blood.

A significant number of pediatric patients with stroke are diagnosed as having 'arteritis', on angiographic grounds for the most part. Occasionally in this group a systemic disorder such as lupus erythematosis or peri-arteritis nodosa can be found, but this is very rare. More commonly there is no evidence of systemic disorder, and sedimentation rate, antinuclear antibodies, gamma globulin, *etc.* are all normal. The process may affect one or multiple cerebral arteries. The basis of the diagnosis is irregularity of the lumen of vessels that may or may not demonstrate occlusions more distal in their course. The radiologic diagnosis of arteritis may be generally correct, but some caution is in order. The visualized changes may in some instances relate to an artefact of abnormal flow in the arteries and not inflammation (Serdaru *et al.* 1984). The most convincing examples of arteritis are those where the demonstrated arterial changes or occlusion are in the segment of the carotid artery adjacent to tonsillar infection.

Miscellaneous structural abnormalities of the blood vessels have also been associated with childhood thrombotic stroke, such as agenesis or hypoplasia of arteries and 'kinks and coils' of the vessels. One must also consider the mysterious process of fibromuscular dysplasia, which is more common in the older female, and where the angiographic appearance of 'a string of beads' is considered to be characteristic. Mettinger and Ericson (1982) found that approximately 30 per cent of their patients with fibromuscular dysplasia had had unilateral throbbing headaches prior to infarction.

In a somewhat similar context is the report of Hilal *et al.* (1971) in which vascular occlusion associated with tortuosity and ectasia of arteries was demonstrated in seven patients with phakomatoses including neurofibromatosis. A complicating feature of the Hilal *et al.* (1971) patients was the fact that all three of the young people with neurofibromatosis had had radiation therapy for optic nerve glioma in the past. In view of more recent information about radiation induced changes in large vessels (see above) it is possible that this treatment played a rôle in the pathogenesis of the thrombotic stroke. The case report of Vannucci *et al.* (1974) is more straightforward. They described a boy of three and a half years with neurofibromatosis who had migrainous neuralgia for one year prior to a thrombotic stroke.

Despite the relatively numerous causes of stroke in children mentioned above, and other causes not mentioned in this discussion, it is important to emphasize that a large number, perhaps even the majority, of strokes in childhood and adolescents cannot be assigned a specific etiology (Strand 1976).

It is upon this background that consideration of migraine induced stroke must be placed. Both problems, especially migraine, are sufficiently common in childhood that some overlap is expected. Even when the relationship to a typical vascular headache is clear, it is important to consider the other factors relevant to stroke in childhood. The subject of migraine as a cause of stroke, and the relationship of the migrainic diathesis as a risk factor in stroke from other causes, are discussed in Chapters 2 and 7.

Summary—vascular disease as a cause of headache in childhood
The following points can be made:
(1) Headache may be a significant aspect of the acute presentation of any lesion that produces stroke in children. It is much more likely to be prominent in the acute phase of hemorrhagic stroke, whether from ruptured AVM or congenital berry aneurysm, and in cerebral hemorrhage from other causes. Headache as part of the acute presentation is less common in infarction from embolus or thrombosis, except in cortical venous thrombosis.
(2) Periodic or continuous headache is not commonly part of the symptomatology

in the weeks and months prior to the stroke. The disorders in which this occurs with any regularity are few, and the incidence of headache is relatively low.

(3) The lesions in which chronic recurring headaches are most prominent include AVM, congenital berry aneurysm, fibromuscular dysplasia, and perhaps in other related anomalies of vessel wall such as those which occur in the phakomatoses. Although not discussed in this section of the monograph (see Chapter 3), the exacerbation of migraine in young women taking birth-control pills is a clear warning of the possibility of cerebral vascular thrombosis.

(4) Headache is quite frequently a prominent aspect of the symptomatology of 'mixed connective tissue disease' without any implication of impending stroke.

(5) Any of the complicated migraine syndromes may be symptomatic of structural vascular disease. The risk is greater than in common or classic migraine, but is nevertheless quite low.

(6) Some strokes in childhood can be said to occur as a result of migraine (see Chapter 7), in others migraine may constitute an additional risk factor.

Congenital malformation and hydrocephalus

Malformations other than those related to blood vessels can cause recurring headache as a prominent symptom. These malformations share with some very slow growing gliomas the potential of prolonged chronicity. The resulting headache is usually the headache of low-grade hydrocephalus although some malformations such as a Chiari I may also produce local mass effect at the foramen magnum.

The commonest issue in this context is hydrocephalus that has 'arrested' or compensated during the first years of life, and then decompensates at some point during childhood. This is most common between three and six years of age. The precipitating incident may be trauma or febrile illness, but frequently no specific event can be identified. The most significant clue is an enlarged head circumference that has usually been noticeable for much of the child's lifetime.

In addition to headache, which has no special identifying features beyond those that have already been mentioned as providing clues to the presence of raised intracranial pressure, symptoms may include vomiting, diplopia and unsteadiness of gait. Neither these symptoms nor the signs that attend them (e.g. papilledema, abnormal cranial percussion, abducens weakness or mild truncal ataxia) provide clues to the specific nature of the pathologic process. Except for enlarged head circumference, the clinical picture is similar to other causes of hydrocephalus such as midline or posterior fossa tumor, or low-grade meningeal infectious process.

Although delayed onset of symptoms for several years is perhaps most characteristic of congenital lesions at the acqueduct of Sylvius, other anatomical reasons for hydrocephalus may be found. Such lesions as posterior fossa cysts, or outlet obstruction of the foramina of Lushka and Magendie combined with midline defect in the cerebellum (Dandy-Walker syndrome) are occasionally responsible. All share the feature of having caused some degree of hydrocephalus in the past, with the process having 'arrested' or being of low-grade activity, *i.e.* low-pressure hydrocephalus.

At times the low-pressure hydrocephalus syndrome may present in childhood as it does in adults in a setting with little or no headache. In these patients, the most prominent symptoms are behavioral disorder, usually overactivity and shortened attention span, school failure and non-specific gross and fine motor disability consisting primarily of clumsiness. A large head and perhaps occasional periodic headaches may provide a clue that something is unusual in this group of patients. Vigilance is necessary to segregate those for further study from the overwhelming numbers of patients with similar complaints who are referred for behavioral and learning disability assessment. The difficulty in recognition is compounded by the relatively frequent juvenile migraine headaches that are found in these hyperactive learning-disabled children. In the final analysis, it is the enlarged head which provides the crucial clue.

The Chiari I malformation, an abnormality that consists of caudally situated lower brainstem and midline cerebellum as opposed to the much more common similar malformation that is associated with meningomyelocoele (Chiari II), requires separate consideration. Overt clinical symptoms and signs characteristically develop comparatively later in life as a rule, *i.e.* anytime during childhood into early and middle adult life. The symptomatology is primarily due to hydrocephalus with obstruction at the level of fourth ventricle and outflow foramina. There is also the mass effect of aberrant cerebellar tissue within the foramen magnum. This may be responsible for the periodic occipital headache that is frequent in these patients.

The headache may have the sharp lancinating quality of occipital neuralgia, but it more often consists of posterior periodic throbbing headaches or those reminiscent of occipital muscular tension headaches. Cough headache may also be recognized in these patients (see case 47 reported below). The resulting hydrocephalus may cause more generalized headache, often periodic and occasionally associated with migrainic visual symptoms, vertigo or light-headedness.

The signs are frequently quite subtle. The most localizing consist of evidence of dysfunction of lower cranial nerves, wasting of suboccipital musculature which may be asymmetrical, nuchal rigidity, low hairline and short neck together with cerebellar or corticospinal signs. Papilledema or other signs of increased intracranial pressure may develop and make the evaluation straightforward, but they are frequently absent at an early stage.

Another possible clinical presentation that is recognized with increasing frequency in recent years is the syndrome of syringomyelia based on the Chiari I malformation in which the pressure dynamics of the obstruction are directed caudally and force the opening of central cavities in the spinal cord. The syringomyelic syndrome is not usually associated with headache.

Many of the above remarks also apply to slow-growing tumors of the region of the foramen magnum and to congenital anomalies of upper cervical spine and base of the skull, *i.e.* platybasia, and basilar impression, whether primary anomalies or secondary to specific disease processes.

Although the later manifestations of congenital malformations are probably the commonest cause of low-grade hydrocephalus and later decompensation, other entities can behave in a similar fashion. The most prominent include post-meningitic and post-hemorrhagic arachnoiditis that obstructs CSF flow in the basilar cisterns or over the convexity. The story of the initial infectious or hemorrhagic incident is usually well documented in the history. More threatening than a single incident are repeated episodes, particularly episodes of low-grade subarachnoid bleeding whch are notorious for eventually causing hydrocephalus. Parenthetically, the usual cause of repeated episodes of bleeding is tumor or a small hamartoma with a vascular component.

In massive subarachnoid hemorrhage that has resulted from AVM, ruptured congenital aneurysm, or from any cause, a significant aspect of the immediate problem may be acutely developing hydrocephalus. CT scanning allows one to follow this process, and intervene with external drainage if necessary.

Chiari I malformation

CASE 47 This young man was 21 years when first seen with a complaint of headache that dated four to five years prior to his visit. The headaches were occipital in location and consisted of a very intense pressure sensation of two to three minutes duration. It was usually sufficiently severe that he ceased all activity and sat down. On occasion he observed silver speckles of light throughout his visual field at the peak of the headache. He also felt light-headed and unsteady during the paroxysm. The headaches were of variable frequency but in the several months prior to presentation they had begun to occur several times per day.

They were first noted during the stress of playing baseball, and over the years it was quite clear that these were either aggravated or initiated by coughing, laughing, sneezing or bowel movement. An additional complaint was a feeling of stiffness in his neck which was present all the time. Occasionally he experienced the visual phenomena without associated headache. He also noted that quick head movements would frequently make him lose his balance for a minute or two. The problem had become sufficiently severe that he limited all physical activities. He became depressed and made an abortive suicide attempt five months prior to his initial visit. There was no family history of headache. Past medical history was uneventful.

The general physical examination was normal aside from a depressive demeanor. Examination of cranial nerve function revealed transient nystagmus to the right after quick postural change and after extreme extension of his head. Stretch reflexes were symmetrically overactive and there were a few beats of clonus at both ankles. There was minimal intention tremor on the left, and the plantar response was bilaterally flexor. A pneumoencephalogram demonstrated a normal ventricular system and displaced cerebellar tissue down to about the upper limit of the arch of C1, accompanied by downward displacement of the entire brainstem and fourth ventricle.

Dr. John Shillito performed a suboccipital craniectomy and laminectomy of C1 together with a subtotal laminectomy of C2. Cerebellar tonsils were found to be flattened and displaced downward to C2. A dural

236

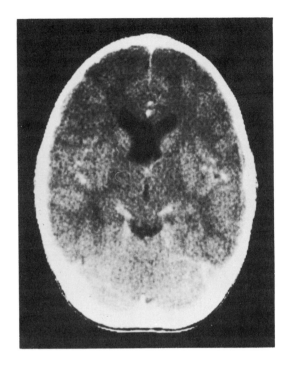

Fig. 16. This CT scan shows asymmetrical low-grade hydrocephalus with dilated lateral ventricles with a third ventricle of normal size. The right ventricle is considerably more dilated than the left (case 48).

patch graft was placed to allow for more freedom in the area.

Within a week or so of the operation, neck stiffness and episodic headache were relieved. On follow-up evaluation four years later he continued in good health, without symptoms and without depression. Examination revealed no abnormal signs.

Comment: In addition to the eventual development of mild but definite neurological signs, there were several features of the headaches themselves which were suggestive of structural disease. Brief headaches provoked by cough or straining are always suggestive, as is visual phenomenology at the peak of headache rather than in the prodrome or aura.

Hydrocephalus

This boy was age eight when first seen in November 1982. Since February and March in the same year he had experienced periodic headaches. They consisted of a frontal throbbing sensation during which time he became pale and inactive. They were of 20 minutes duration and occurred as often as two to three times a day, with occasional intervals of several days. Headaches occasionally awakened him in the middle of the night and were sometimes present on awakening in the morning. There was no accompanying nausea or vomiting.

The family history indicated that his mother developed migraine while

CASE 48

237

taking birth-control pills, but had otherwise not experienced headache; nor were there other members of the family with vascular headaches.

Examination in the hospital approximately six weeks after the onset of headaches revealed slight blurring of the optic discs bilaterally with no venous pulsations. Otherwise all aspects of the neurological examination were normal.

A CT scan showed asymmetrical dilated lateral ventricles (Fig. 16) and a ventriculogram showed a small nodule anterior in the third ventricle. In late March Dr. Kenneth Winston performed a transcolossal craniotomy for excision of the 'tumor' which was found to be an enlarged choroid plexus in the third ventricle extending into the foramen of Monroe. This tissue was removed.

Postoperatively, he did well throughout the summer but beginning in October began to have headaches again of a quality and frequency similar to his initial trouble. In addition to being bifrontal and throbbing there now was occasional associated nausea and light-headedness. Duration was five to 25 minutes. The CT scan at that point showed no change in the size of the ventricular system from its postoperative status, and it was decided to treat with various antimigrainic medications on a trial basis, and to observe the results.

There was no response to propranolol, cyproheptadine, and amitriptyline. By early January 1983 the CT scan showed very slightly increased ventricular size. There were no neurological signs or evidence of increased intracranial pressure on funduscopic examination. Then in mid-January 1983 he began to have periods during which time he was lethargic and inattentive, associated with slight confusion which would last 30 to 40 minutes but with no accompanying headache. However, the headaches occurred independently and increased in frequency. He showed some indication of reduced competence in school.

Despite the lack of dramatic change on the CT scan it was decided to re-admit him for a ventriculo-peritoneal shunt. On admission, he was found to be neurologically normal although there was lack of venous pulsation on fundoscopy.

Ventricular catheter was placed over a period of several days which showed normal pressure measuring 100 to 110 mm of water, but with increased pulse pressure. In early February he was treated with a ventriculo-peritoneal shunt with a high pressure Hakim valve that had a closing pressure of 104. Shortly after this was done, the headaches were much improved, and he had no further episodes of lethargy and confusion.

Comment: This boy had low-grade hydrocephalus with periodic vascular headaches as the principal manifestation. Initial studies indicated a possible third ventricular tumor which turned out be redundant choroid plexus in the foramen of Monroe and third ventricle. This was removed with temporary relief, but headaches recurred at a time when his ventricular size was improved leading to ambiguity as to cause of headache. It was uncertain whether they were migraine (family history positive), or symptomatic vascular headaches based on a low-grade hydrocephalus. After several months the development of periodic lethargy and increased frequency of headaches led to further assessment including continuous intraventricular pressure-monitoring which showed normal resting pressure, but greater than normal pulse pressure. A ventriculo-peritoneal shunt was done which relieved the periodic headaches and other symptoms.

Infectious processes
In order to keep the principal focus of this monograph on sub-acute and chronic headache problems, no effort will be made to deal in detail with infectious causes of acute headache syndromes such as purulent meningitis and viral meningo-encephalitis. However, acute and chronic sinusitis and several relatively less common acute problems will be considered in somewhat more detail.

Paranasal sinusitis
Headache is a prominent symptom of acute sinusitis, which usually develops as an extension of an immediately preceding upper respiratory infection. Another pathogenetic mechanism is infection secondary to underwater swimming and diving.

Sinusitis tends to be a problem of the older child and adolescent. Both ethmoid and maxillary sinuses are of sufficient size in infancy to be clinically significant but infection is not common. The sphenoid sinus is present at birth, but usually does not become clinically important until three to five years, while the slowly developing frontal sinuses do not assume clinical significance until age six to 10 years.

Simultaneous infection of more than one sinus is common, and the vulnerability to clinically significant infection among the various sinuses varies considerably. Kogutt and Swischuk (1973) analyzed the findings in 100 consecutive infants and children and reported that in 96 per cent there was involvement of maxillary, while ethmoids were involved in 37 per cent, frontal in 13 per cent and sphenoids in 7 per cent.

The commonest organisms are H influenza and S pneumoniae in acute infections (Wald *et al.* 1981), while the bacterial agents of chronic infection include a wider array of organisms, mostly gram-negative organisms and various staphylococci (Lew *et al.* 1983).

In the usual patient, clinical indication of the onset of sinus infection merges almost imperceptibly with the upper respiratory infection from which it arises. The acute phase of the URI may clear to leave persistent rhinorrhoea (in 77 per cent), post-nasal drainage and cough (in 44 per cent) as the principal evidence of continuing infection (Wald *et al.* 1981). Sinus infection secondary to underwater activity may be more abrupt and not follow URI. Fever is usually present in the acute phase, but may be low-grade, especially in older children and adolescents.

Headache is not one of the commoner symptoms. It was a leading complaint in only 13 per cent of the Kogutt and Swischuk (1973) series, and all of these patients were over 12 years. The incidence varies with the sinus involved and is apparently more common in maxillary disease where it was described as 'common' in older children by Wald *et al.* (1981), but these authors also remark that headache is seldom encountered as a symptom under age five. Headache may be a localized dull and constant pressure sensation, sometimes with more intense and sharp exacerbations.

Its localization may give some indication of the specific sinus involved. Frontal sinus infection is distributed in the ipsilateral fronto-temporal region of the head, associated with tenderness of the region of the sinus itself; while in maxillary infection, face and ear may be involved in the painful discomfort together with sensitivity of ipsilateral teeth as well as tenderness on direct percussion over the sinus. Sphenoid sinus headache may be unilateral, frontal, temporal and/or occipital or be centered in the peri-orbital region. It may also affect nose, cheek, teeth and gums (Lew *et al.* 1983). Ethmoid disease leads to pain about the eye and may extend to any region innervated by the trigeminal nerve.

The distribution of the headache is not nearly as definitive as objective signs of tenderness over the frontal or maxillary sinus. Tenderness may be accompanied by visible erythema and edema of the overlying skin. The deeply situated sphenoid and ethmoids cannot be palpated but close observation for clues in the skin can be rewarding, with ethmoid sinusitis producing edema and erythema of eyelids especially in younger children. Either ethmoid or sphenoid may produce slight erythema near the bridge of the nose. These observations apply to the acute and sub-acute infections, and as the process tends toward chronicity only focal tenderness may be found and this is inconstant.

x-rays of the sinuses are usually the definitive confirmatory examination, 96 per cent of which will show clouding or mucosal thickening, while only 5 per cent show air-fluid levels (Kogutt and Swischuk 1973). At times these findings can be misleading and reflect under-developed sinus or asymptomatic disease. The demonstration of x-ray changes does not necessarily mean that a headache syndrome is related to sinusitis. The total clinical picture, including examination of the nose and throat, must be taken into account.

Complications of acute sinusitis consist of aseptic meningeal reactions secondary to the parameningeal focus, and much less commonly purulent meningitis and epidural abscess (see below). Recurrent acute sinusitis can rarely cause third and sixth cranial nerve palsy or be an indicator of a lesion within the sinus such as a mucocoel (see Chapter 6, p. 115), but is more commonly an expression of allergic rhinitis or other systemic disease such as alpha 1-antitrypsin deficiency.

Chronic sinusitis symptoms are highly variable, and certainly include headaches that are variations on the theme of the acute expression. Tenderness to palpation or percussion over the accessible sinuses is an important sign. The sensation is usually of lower grade and more often described as fullness and pressure than pain. However, the leading symptoms are nasal discharge, post-nasal drip and mouth breathing (adenoids are the alternate possibility in this regard), paroxysmal sneezing and bronchitic cough, and not headache as a rule.

When periodic headache develops, it is often a sinusitis-triggered juvenile migraine as discussed in Chapter 3.

The therapeutic approach to acute and chronic sinusitis is beyond the scope of this monograph. It quite naturally depends on antibiotics and drainage. The promotion of drainage with nasal decongestants can be used as a therapeutic trial in some cases. Surgical drainage is occasionally necessary, and almost always indicated when complications arise such as epidural abscess.

Epidural abscess
Epidural abscess almost invariably results from extension of paranasal sinus infection in older children or otitis media in infants and younger children. Headache is severe, meningeal signs are common and systemic signs and laboratory evidence of sepsis are prominent. Convulsions and lateralizing signs point to cerebral involvement. The layer of subdural pus may be quite thin and can be isodense with cortex on CT scan. Therefore a high index of suspicion is important, and if appropriate antibiotics do not succeed in a suspicious clinical situation, repeat CT scan is indicated. This may show cerebral swelling and shift unless the process is bilateral. If the CT scan is ambiguous, angiography may be in order.

Cerebral abscess
In contrast, parenchymal brain abscess may have a sub-acute to chronic course especially if the expression has been modified by antibiotic treatment. There need be no systemic indicators of infection such as fever and leucocytosis. The sedimentation rate is more likely to be abnormal, but can be in the normal range.

The chief asset to the discovery of brain abscess is an index of suspicion based on the requisite systemic risk factors. This is most commonly a history of cyanotic congenital heart disease with right to left shunt. The patient will be over age two years and may no longer be cyanotic to any significant degree because of previous surgery. It is important to remember that the surgery may not have corrected the shunt so that vulnerability to transient systemic bacteremia (probably often related to teeth and ostensibly the reason that the child of age two or older is vulnerable) remains.

Any cerebral syndrome in these patients, which most often includes headache at an early stage, makes one highly suspicious of abscess. The headache in abscess may be sharply localized to the cranium external to the lesion. Part of the management must include the deferral of any temptation to examine the CSF. Of all the clinical situations in which lumbar puncture is dangerous, it is most apt to cause trouble in cerebral abscess. The CT scan is a non-invasive, safe and definitive examination, and it should be done as the first step in evaluation. If an abscess is demonstrated, then an LP should not be done.

A similar approach is appropriate in Rendu-Osler-Weber disease or hereditary hemorrhagic telangiectasia (Román *et al.* 1978). This condition is an autosomal dominant disorder defined by multiple dermal, mucosal, and visceral telangiectasias, the latter including brain. Pulmonary arteriovenous fistulas set the stage for cerebral abscess, a complication that develops in 13 per cent of patients. The incidence of neurologic complications secondary to vascular malformations of brain and cord is higher, about 35 per cent. The combination of threat of cerebral abscess and other complications of pulmonary arteriovenous fistula is sufficient that when these lesions are recognized in the lung, they should be removed (Roman *et al.* 1978).

Any pericranial chronic infection, primarily mastoiditis but occasionally frontal sinusitis, is another significant risk factor for cerebral abscess. Such infections are a somewhat lesser threat than heretofore, but still significant. Cerebral abscess from mastoiditis occurs in the ipsilateral temporal lobe or in the cerebellar hemisphere. In the temporal lobe it may be relatively silent of focal findings if in the non-dominant hemisphere. The same may be said of the frontal-lobe localization that results from frontal sinus disease. Metastatic abscess may occur anywhere in the brain. Although unusual in the posterior fossa, it may even occur in the brainstem.

In the final analysis, the chief clinical issue in assessing the possibility of cerebral abscess is an assessment of risk based upon systemic factors. The most important of these is the potential for right to left shunt and chronic and sometimes acute pericranial infection, especially mastoiditis. Without these factors the chance of abscess is remote, even in such provocative situations as sub-acute bacterial endocarditis due to streptococcus viridans where it is in fact very rare if it occurs at all. Brain abscess, often multiple, is common as a late event in acute bacterial endocarditis due to staphylococcal infection.

With the basic risk factor present, especially right to left shunt in congenital heart disease, any cerebral symptom—especially the development of headache—is a brain abscess until proved otherwise.

Granulomatous meningitis
Brief reference should be made to the possibility of granulomatous meningitis in the consideration of infectious causes of headache. The process is usually sub-acute, but may be relatively chronic. Headache, perhaps associated with some degree of disordered mental status, is the leading symptom. Meningeal signs, usually so dependable in more acute meningeal infections in children over age six to eight months, are less prominent but usually present to some degree. Cranial nerves are often involved, especially abducens and oculomotor. Some degree of hydrocephalus usually results, and is a frequent basis of headache in these patients, although headache can result from meningeal involvement alone.

A large variety of infectious agents can present in this fashion. The most prominent of these is tuberculosis, but possibilities also include cryptococcus, echinococcus and sarcoidosis. Each may display some suggestive feature of the presentation such as exposure opportunity, details of the CSF formula and systemic involvement, but they are more alike than different. Certainly the headache syndrome is similar.

All depend upon laboratory demonstration of the organism or in some instances CSF or serum antibody for a precise diagnosis, which is the essential requirement for definitive therapy. On a number of occasions it is appropriate to initiate the most logical treatment, usually anti-tuberculous therapy before a definitive diagnosis is made.

The CSF formula is generally quite similar in this group of diseases. It consists of mild to moderate pleocytosis, usually predominantly lymphocytic, elevated protein, and either normal or low glucose levels.

The possibility of opportunistic infection with this group of organisms is especially prominent in immune deficiency states. The immune incompetent patients are also vulnerable to infection with cytomegalovirus, candida, and aspergillus.

Pseudotumor cerebri

When listing the basic processes underlying any symptomatic expression of disease, there always seems to be some entity that defies the usual classification into 'tumor-trauma-infection'. When discussing headache it is the syndrome of benign intracranial hypertension or pseudotumor cerebri that qualifies for the rôle of maverick. Headache is the leading symptom, and the problem is reasonably frequent.

The central feature of the illness is the observation of true papilledema which is usually discovered in the course of investigation of a presenting complaint of headache, sometimes with nausea and vomiting, diplopia or some other visual complaint (Rose and Matson 1967, Weisberg and Chutorian 1977). Rarely, papilledema is discovered on routine examination in an otherwise asymptomatic child. A key feature of the clinical presentation is the remarkable preservation of neurologic function and general well-being. This is perhaps especially noteworthy with regard to mental status and behavioral changes, which are usually fully normal in this illness, as contrasted with almost any other cause of elevated intracranial pressure.

The essential criteria for inclusion within the syndrome, beyond signs and symptoms of elevated intracranial pressure, include documentation of an essentially normal or small ventricular system (it may be slightly enlarged) and a CSF that is normal in all respects except for elevated pressure (CSF protein may be lower than average).

The headache of pseudotumor cerebri is not distinctive. The course is usually under two months. In most respects it conforms to the clinical features of any headache related to raised intracranial pressure in that it is intermittent, accentuated by straining and coughing, and may have nocturnal or morning occurrence. There may be a throbbing quality. Older patients, who may also have migraine, are usually able to distinguish this new headache from their more usual vascular headache. At times, however, it would seem that the new development consists of a noteworthy increase in frequency and severity of their chronic vascular headaches. Nausea and vomiting occur, but are not particularly common. These symptoms are more prominent in the younger children.

Ocular symptoms, especially diplopia and variable demonstrable abducens nerve palsy, are common as a non-specific reflection of elevated intracranial pressure. The presence of other neurologic signs is fundamentally inconsistent with

243

the diagnosis, although very rarely minimal ataxia or a weak extensor plantar response are discovered in an otherwise typical case.

A wide variety of more specific diseases have been associated with the syndrome. In practice, the two commonest circumstances are corticosteroid withdrawal after use in a wide variety of illnesses, and in association with otitis media. The latter led to the concept of 'otitic hydrocephalus' (Symonds 1931), which is only a partial misnomer as will be discussed further below. In any series of children (Rose and Matson 1967, Weisberg and Chutorian 1977) the majority of patients are 'idiopathic', although a number may be related in time to infectious illnesses other than otitis media. Another significant group is associated with trauma to the head or neck. Exogenous intoxication with a number of agents has been implicated etiologically, the most prominent of which are tetracycline, vitamin A in gross excess, and birth-control pills in adolescents and young adults. Vitamin A deficiency has also been responsible for the syndrome.

Endocrine dysfunction has been implicated in a number of cases. One of the commonest identified causes is the iatrogenic use of corticosteroids, usually in the period shortly after withdrawal. It may also occur during treatment, usually in high dosage. Both hyperadrenalism and hypo-adrenal states are also rare causes. It occurs in hypoparathyroidism, whether congenital or acquired. Considerable interest has centered about a possible endocrine relationship in women, the only pediatric aspect of which relates to association with menarche (Green 1964).

Amongst the miscellaneous and rare associations are examples occurring in lupus erythematosis and polyneuritis. A full listing of occasionally reported examples is beyond the scope of this discussion. If the reader wishes to pursue this further, an impressive listing with references is available in the paper by Buchheit *et al.* (1969).

The usual course of the illness in children is from a few weeks to a few months. Whatever is done in the way of treatment, there is a tendency to spontaneous recovery. The only serious hazard is visual failure secondary to elevated intracranial pressure and papilledema (Corbett *et al.* 1982).

In those patients in whom corticosteroid withdrawal is at fault, re-instituting the drug at the previous highest dose followed by more gradual withdrawal is appropriate and usually successful. In many other patients, CSF withdrawal daily or every other day is effective. It may be necessary in the corticosteroid withdrawal patients as well. Only one or two such treatments may be required, although most require periodic lumbar drainage for a week or so, and in some patients a prolonged series of treatments over months is necessary. Frequency of lumbar puncture can be titrated in the more chronic patients and spaced at greater intervals.

Medical measures such as treatment with corticosteroids (Weisberg and Chutorian 1977), or osmotic dehydrating agents (Jefferson and Clark 1976) and acetazolamide also have their proponents.

In those patients in whom CSF pressure does not subside in a few weeks, and in some who seem to respond and then recur, there is always the lurking possibility that a tumor was overlooked in the first round of studies. It is probably a wise

244

clinical posture to accept the principle that the first point in the differential diagnosis of pseudotumor is tumor, and to remain alert to this possibility for some months beyond the initial phase of the illness. This is especially true if corticosteroids have been a part of the therapeutic plan, because of the well-known effect of these agents in ameliorating brain tumor symptoms and signs. Nevertheless, rare patients with pseudotumor cerebri run a very prolonged course of a year or more, usually with some remission and exacerbation (see case 49 below).

The pathogenesis of pseudotumor remains a mystery to some extent although certain key issues are clearer now. It has been shown in human studies that the intracranial vascular compartment (blood volume) is expanded, but that this is insufficient to account for the problem, and that tissue swelling must also be part of the process (Raichle *et al.* 1978). Cerebral edema is probably a central feature in the pathogenesis of the disorder in all patients and may account for the considerable diversity in the associated provoking causes. This variety of edema, however, is unusual in clinical practice because it is essentially free of associated symptoms of parenchymal involvement. This leads to the speculation that it may be truly 'interstitial' as opposed to the 'vasogenic' edema that is associated with tumor, abscess and infarction, or the 'cytotoxic' edema of lead encephalopathy or Reye's syndrome (Fishman 1975). A final pathophysiologic abnormality that can be demonstrated in most patients with pseudotumor is abnormal resistance to the movement of CSF out of the system (Johnson and Paterson 1974).

These findings of increased cerebral blood volume, a peculiarly asymptomatic brain edema which is probably interstitial and caused by hydrostatic pressure, together with abnormal resistance to the outflow of CSF, all point to venous hypertension or occlusion of major veins or venous sinuses as a possible unifying factor in the syndrome.

Since Symonds's second paper on the subject (Symonds 1937) the group of patients whose pseudotumor syndrome was associated with otitis have been consistently shown to have thrombosis of major cerebral venous sinuses. It begins with the contiguous lateral sinus and extends to the torcula and beyond (Greer 1962). It has also been known for some time that the pseudotumor syndrome is associated with mediastinal lesions which obstruct venous return from the head (Walsh 1958) as well as rare examples of cardiac decompensation associated with papilledema (Beaumont and Hearn 1948). When one examines the cerebral venous system systematically, with retrograde venography as well as cerebral arteriography, it is possible to demonstrate that 80 per cent of children with pseudotumor have venous outflow obstruction, whatever the presumed etiologic condition, including one example of corticosteroid withdrawal pseudotumor (Bresnan *et al.* 1973, Strand 1976).

If one reviews the list of causes of the disorder from the perspective of whether jugular vein or venous sinus thrombosis may not be an occasional complication, it is impressive how frequently this is the case. Cerebral venous hypertension or obstruction is probably the potentially unifying pathogenesis of the syndrome and accountable for the majority of cases. For those remaining, a benign, probably interstitial brain edema on another basis, is the likely mechanism.

There is little to be gained from systematic investigation of these patients by invasive procedures such as angiography and retrograde venography. Prognosis for recovery is excellent due to the development of collateral outflow (Strand 1976) or re-canalization, and neither anticoagulant therapy nor venous ligation to prevent venous embolization is necessary.

Pseudotumor cerebri—chronic course

CASE 49 This girl was first seen at age 12 and a half years. For the previous year she had had periodic bifrontal throbbing headaches without associated nausea and vomiting. They tended to occur in the afternoon on school-days. Pediatric evaluation led to the conclusion that they were probably related to psychological tensions. Approximately nine months before admission, with the beginning of the school year, they became more frequent and somewhat more severe. She had been examined on several occasions by her pediatrician and then one week prior to admission was seen by an ophthalmologist who found papilledema. The family history indicated no history of headaches.

Examination on admission revealed a normal general physical examination including a blood pressure of 100/70. Head circumference was at the 40th percentile. Funduscopic examination revealed early papilledema without venous pulsations. Mental status was entirely normal as was general neurological examination.

Skull films and a Technetium-99 brain scan were within normal limits. A bilateral carotid and left vertebral arteriogram were done which showed no abnormality except significant delayed clearance through both lateral and sigmoid sinuses. There was some opacification of the internal jugular vein seen on both sides. Spinal fluid revealed an opening pressure of 250, two lymphocytes and a CSF protein of 21.8 mg per cent. She was begun on acetazolamide 250 mg b.i.d. On repeat lumbar puncture after 48 hours, pressure was 60 mm CSF.

Shortly after discharge she no longer had headaches. Acetazolamide was continued for two weeks and then stopped. When seen approximately one month subsequently, she showed only mild nasal blurring without venous distention, and at two months the only abnormality recorded was slight gliosis of the disc margin.

Approximately six months after her initial hospitalization, she developed a mild upper respiratory infection associated with recurrence of headache of thirty minutes to one hour duration. They were quite severe, occurred daily for two weeks and then continued at lesser intensity with a frequency of two to three times per week. Optic discs showed indistinct margins and acetazolamide was instituted again. Within a week she was much better, and had no headaches after approximately one month. Acetazolamide was discontinued and she did well for the remainder of the year.

Then at age 14 she had a recurrence of periodic headache and was

246

readmitted for evaluation because of recurrence of low-grade papilledema. Spinal fluid on this occasion showed an opening pressure of 310, one lymphocyte and protein of 22.4 mg. Fluorescein angiography showed a small amount of staining of the nerve head. Venogram was performed which revealed no jugular venous block but the patency of the lateral sinus and sigmoid sinuses could not be demonstrated either from below or above. A pneumoencephalogram showed no abnormalities.

Subsequent to her second admission she was again treated with acetazolamide 250 mg b.i.d. She did well thereafter, although on occasions when she was irregular about medication there was a tendency for recurrence of headache. In six months the papilledema had totally subsided. Acetazolamide was discontinued and she subsequently did well.

She was watched closely from an ophthalmological point of view and for the first time in October 1974 (age 15), approximately a year after her most recent bout of trouble, she was found to have an inferior temporal field cut in the left eye. This subsequently improved and by a year later was no longer found.

Comment: The pseudotumor syndrome in this girl was the result of bland and unexplained venous occlusion. It was unusually persistent, although it pursued a remitting, exacerbating course. After a two-and-a-half-year course she developed a monocular visual field defect as a result of chronic recurring papilledema (Corbett *et al.* 1982).

Patients with tumor who had headache and other periodic symptoms on presentation

Migraine with tumor

This boy was age 10 when first seen in December 1971. He was born after a **CASE** normal pregnancy and delivery, and his early development was normal. **50** Family history revealed that his mother had periodic throbbing headaches, and a paternal aunt had classic migraine. Beginning February 1971 he began to have a series of episodes of visual disturbance and headaches. The episodes began with the hallucination of a ragged square in his right field of vision which exhibited variable colors. After about two minutes, he became dysarthric and confused and was usually amnesic for events during this period which lasted about five minutes, followed by a throbbing headache of approximately three hours duration. During the period of confusion his father noted that he was clumsy and unable to recognize faces and objects.

During the period between February and December 1971 he had approximately 20 such episodes, a number of which consisted of the visual hallucination alone. Shortly after the onset, a diagnosis of juvenile migraine was made and he was treated with phenytoin and later with acetazolamide. However, the episodes persisted and this led to an EEG which showed left posterior quadrant slowing, and a radio-isotope scan which showed an area of abnormal permeability in the left occipital lobe

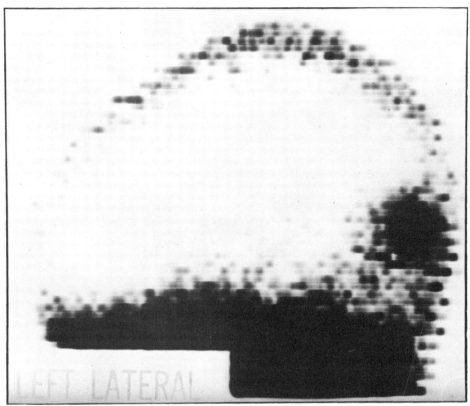

Fig. 17. This Technetium-99 brain scan shows a circular area of abnormal permeability at the left occipital pole (case 50).

(Fig. 17).

He was then referred to Children's Hospital Boston. On examination, there were no general physical abnormalities and the neurological examination was entirely normal as well, with particular attention to the fundi and visual fields. Studies included a normal skull x-ray and an electroencephalogram that showed slowing and poor background over the left posterior quadrant. A computer-averaged evoked potential visual field study showed a right upper quadrant visual field defect. The arteriogram indicated a 3 cm spherical mass in the occipital lobe with a vascularized periphery with prominent venous drainage (Fig. 18)

Dr. John Shillito removed the lesion which on histologic examination was a grade II to III glioma. He was given a course of 5000 rad radiotherapy subsequent to the operation and did well. Postoperatively the visual fields were normal.

There were no subsequent symptoms until January 1979 at age 18 when he developed left-sided throbbing headaches. CT at that time was negative for recurrence. Also in December 1979, he had right scintillating

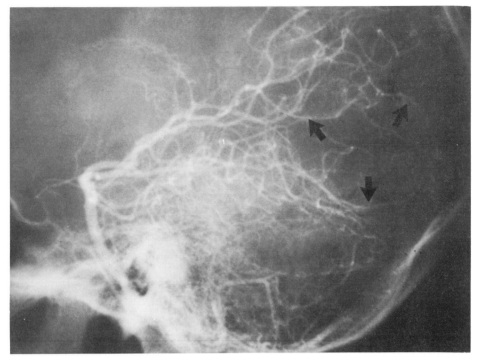

Fig. 18. This vertebral arteriogram demonstrates an avascular mass with a vascularized periphery that displaces the distal branches of the posterior cerebral artery. The lesion proved to be a grade 2 to 3 glioma (case 50).

scotomata of five to 10 minutes followed by a throbbing headache, and in March 1980 he had an episode of 'tunnel vision' followed by severe headache with essentially no trouble in the meantime. The most recent CT scan was in January 1982 which showed no change in the cystic postoperative defect.

Comment: The 'aura' preceding the throbbing headache was quite consistent with migraine, yet it always lateralized to one side and was associated with greater complexity and alteration in mental status than is usual. It is of interest that subsequent to complete eradication of the tumor, he has continued to have rare migrainic episodes. In view of a family history of migraine, this is probably not unexpected, and it also raises the question of the contribution of inherent vascular reactivity to the tumor symptomatology at the beginning.

Migraine with tumor
This boy was first seen at age seven years in July 1964. He was born after an uneventful pregnancy and normal labor and delivery. There were no problems in the neonatal period. Family history revealed that his father suffered from severe 'splitting' headaches associated with nausea.

CASE 51

249

At age three he began to have a periodic problem consisting of nocturnal awakening with repeated vomiting and on the following day he was listless and irritable. At age four the frequency had increased and at this point he was able to complain of his head hurting. The episodes lasted several hours. He was evaluated medically and found to have a mildly abnormal EEG and was treated with various anticonvulsants including phenobarbital and phenytoin. During the period of treatment, he had distinctly fewer episodes and by September 1964 medication was gradually reduced and discontinued. Shortly after the medication was stopped the headaches recurred, again primarily nocturnal. Anticonvulsants were resumed with good effect.

On initial examination there were no neurological abnormalities except for a mild congenital strabismus. He was somewhat poorly co-ordinated and left-handed (father was left-handed as well).

Then in mid-summer 1964 he developed a number of episodes which consisted of one to two minutes of confusion and relative unresponsiveness during which time he fussed with his clothes. With the development of seizures it was decided to re-evaluate his medical status with a skull x-ray that showed multiple loci of calcification in the left posterior parietal region and the EEG showed almost continuous epileptigenic activity in the same general region associated with background slowing. The lesion was removed by Dr. Donald Matson in July 1965. On histologic examination it proved to be low grade glioma-hamartoma. Postoperatively he had a hemianopsia and cortical sensory disturbance on the right side of his body.

Subsequent to the operation he was maintained on phenytoin and had no subsequent seizures and only very occasional headaches. Follow-up to 1975 indicated no recurrence of tumor, the EEG continued to show a discharging focus and anticonvulsants were maintained. The neurological signs were unchanged.

Comment: This boy had a long history of paroxysmal nocturnal episodes consistent with juvenile migraine. There was a family history of probable migraine in the father. After four years he developed complex partial seizures, and examination revealed the presence of a left parietal brain tumor. Subsequent to the removal of the tumor, although he continued on anticonvulsant medication, he had no seizures and very few headaches.

Atypical face pain caused by brainstem tumor

CASE 52 This boy was almost five years old when first seen in March 1979, with the complaint of episodic left-face and head pain which had been occurring over the previous seven months. The episodes were initiated by an excruciating painful sensation which centered about the left ear and mid-face. They were of about one hour in duration. Shortly before the episode occurred, he became noticeably tired and lethargic. Associated symptomatology consisted of photophobia and nausea. He vomited with

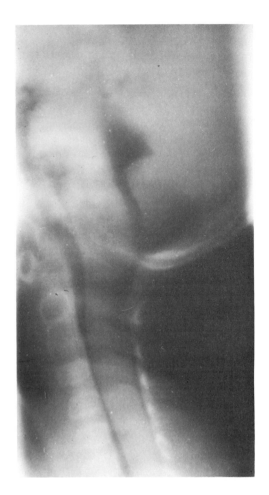

Fig. 19. This lateral tomographic view of a gas myelogram demonstrates expansion of the medulla and upper and middle cervical cord. The expected flat floor of the fourth ventricle is convex from an intrinsic lesion (case 52).

the more severe episodes. On occasion the left side of his face became noticeably flushed and sometimes puffy. Headache was associated with lacrimation and nasal discharge but inasmuch as he invariably cried it was impossible to ascertain whether this was part of the phenomenology, or secondary to crying. The frequency increased from approximately once per month to two or three times per week.

The family history was of interest in that his father had suffered from classic cluster headaches, and several other members of the family, *i.e.* a paternal grandmother and two paternal cousins, had migraine.

Examination revealed him to be generally healthy in appearance and there were no abnormal general physical signs. The neurologic examination was also negative, although there was some asymmetry of the face and a slight difference in the posture of his outstretched left hand. Facial sensation was entirely normal.

He was admitted to the hospital for evaluation, which included a number of negative examinations including a CT scan. When contrast material was injected, a typical headache was produced accompanied by an erythematous flush which involved the anterior left ear and mid-face, in the general distribution of the second division of the trigeminal nerve. An arteriogram of posterior and left cerebral circulation showed no abnormality.

At that point it was believed that he had an atypical migraine syndrome, *i.e.* lower facial migrainous neuralgia. Treatment with phenytoin 50 mg twice a day was initiated with the intent to proceed with propranolol or methysergide if this did not prove advantageous.

In the two months following discharge he had four episodes of left-sided facial and head pain, and was readmitted during a particularly troublesome episode during which the new symptom of blanching and blotchy erythematous change occurred in the skin of the left arm, accompanied by unsteadiness and left-sided weakness.

On the occasion of this second hospitalization he was found to have a mild facial weakness on the left involving both palpebral fissure and mouth. He had a mild but definite left hemiparesis. The hemiparesis cleared after approximately two days hospitalization.

CT scan was repeated and was normal while a lumbar puncture revealed as its only abnormality a protein of 50 mg per cent. X-rays of the neck showed a widened AP diameter of the spinal canal and a gas myelogram was abnormal and demonstrated expansion of the spinal cord from C2 up to the region of the pons (Fig. 19).

A diagnosis of tumor of the brainstem and upper cord was made. He was treated with dexamethasone and radiation therapy.

Subsequently he was operated upon by Dr. Fred Epstein of New York University Medical Center. The procedure was carried out under the operating microscope using the ultrasonic surgical aspirator. The tumor resection was carried up to the obex from its spinal site and then discontinued. Pathologic examination revealed this to be a ganglioglioma of low grade.

He ceased having pain on the day following the operation. His left hemiparesis improved to the point where approximately two years following surgery he was running, riding a bike and having remarkably few functional symptoms.

Comment: Before the development of neurologic signs this boy was believed to have migrainous neuralgia based on the history of his attacks reinforced by the history of migrainous neuralgia (cluster headaches) in his father. This concept was further substantiated by negative cranial CT and angiography. The development of neurological signs led to further study that included a myelogram which demonstrated the lesion. The vasomotor reactivity during episodes, and subsequent to injection of contrast material, is of particular interest.

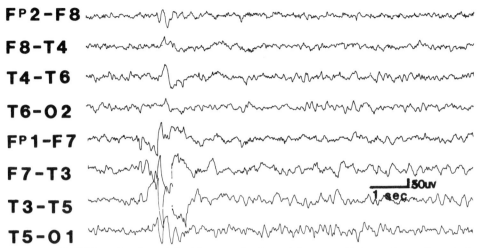

FP2-F8

F8-T4

T4-T6

T6-O2

FP1-F7

F7-T3

T3-T5

T5-O1

Fig. 20. This EEG tracing shows left mid-temporal spike and slow wave discharges in a patient who is slightly drowsy. The background in this region exhibits troublesome polymorphic, irregular theta and delta slowing (bipolar recording illustrating temporal lobe leads, right over left) (case 53).

Migraine, seizure and tumor

This boy was seven years of age when first seen in October 1981. At that time there were two complaints both of about one and a half years in duration. He had had headaches about two or three times per week. They would last two to three hours or as long as all day. The headaches were not localized. He would tend to hold his head and indicated that they had a throbbing quality. Usually he wanted to lie down, was noticeably pale, and complained of nausea but did not vomit. They had not changed significantly over the year and a half. The family history revealed a maternal grandmother who had classic migraine. Other members of the family were not affected.

CASE 53

A second problem consisted of episodes of about 20 seconds during which he would lose consciousness. On occasion they were accompanied by automatic activities, such as lip-licking, mumbling and on one occasion he placed his hand in a pail of paint. He was confused for a few minutes after the episode. They occurred irregularly and rarely in the beginning, but by July 1981 they had become more frequent. During the three-month period prior to his evaluation he had 12 episodes. An EEG done in August 1981 was abnormal indicating left temporal slowing with some sharp wave and spike activity (Fig. 20). A CT scan at that point showed a low-density lesion in the left post-temporal region without mass effect (Fig. 21).

Examination on initial evaluation showed him to be a bright and alert right-handed boy with an entirely normal general physical and neurologic examination, including a close assessment of visual fields and language.

He had been treated with phenytoin 50 mg three times a day during the month and a half prior to his initial visit. During this period he had two

253

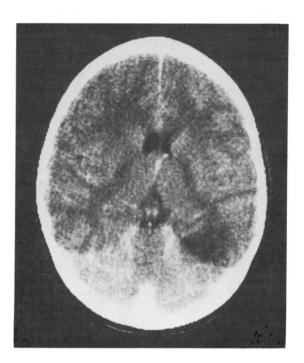

Fig. 21. This contrast-enhanced CT scan demonstrates a low-density lesion in the left posterior temporal region. There is no distortion, midline shift or abnormal permeability. Biopsy demonstrated an oligodendroglioma (case 53).

partial complex seizures and no headaches. He was hospitalized for further assessment. A CT scan showed no change in the left temporal lobe lesion. There was no midline shift. Spinal fluid revealed a pressure of 84, protein of 14 and an EEG continued to show a discharging focus and slow waves in the left temporal region.

Because of the left temporal lobe location of the lesion, coupled with total absence of neurologic signs and no evidence of growth between August and October, it was elected to observe him closely on anticonvulsants. Seizures continued despite numerous adjustments of medication. In addition to increasing phenytoin, he was given a trial of phenobarbital, sodium valproate, ethosuximide, and carbamazepine, none of which achieved control of the seizures. Headaches were not a particular problem. Repeated examinations showed no change in his entirely normal general physical and neurological examination. CT scan was repeated on several occasions at periodic intervals and it showed no change.

Computed analyzed EEG (BEAM) was done on two occasions, the first in April 1982 and the second five months later. This second study showed an increase in slow wave activity and was taken as an indication of progression. On this basis he was admitted to the hospital in October 1982 with the plan to biopsy the lesion. Wada testing indicated speech to be located on the left, so surgery was limited. The biopsy tissue was an oligodendroglioma. He then received radiation therapy. During the period

254

subsequent to the biopsy and radiation therapy, he had no seizures while maintained on carbamazepine and phenytoin. CT in January 1983 showed 'only very subtle left posterior temporal findings, considerably less than preoperatively'.

Comment: The clinical problem presented was one of periodic vascular headaches and complex partial seizures that occurred in separate episodes. This led to the definitive evidence of tumor on CT scan.

Hemangioblastoma

This boy was first seen in March 1975 at the age of nine and a half with a two-month history of dizzy spells. The episodes consisted of a spinning sensation accompanied by disequilibrium followed by a throbbing headache. The vertigo was sufficiently severe that he fell from a chair during one episode, but was brief, lasting less than a minute. The headache that followed lasted up to 15 minutes. Examination revealed exaggerated reflexes in the lower extremities, but his gait was normal and all other findings were negative including a normal EEG.

CASE 54

His father had severe throbbing headaches with associated nausea when he was a boy that continued to age 20.

On the basis of a diagnosis of juvenile migraine, he was begun on phenobarbital 30 mg b.i.d. and seemed somewhat better at first. Then approximately one month prior to admission in September 1975, he developed increasingly severe pounding frontal headaches associated with increasingly prominent vomiting. On the day of admission to the hospital, he awakened with a particularly severe headache and complaint of diplopia.

Examination revealed a boy in acute distress from headache which he localized to the right temple and right eye. Fundi showed flat discs but no spontaneous venous pulsation. He complained of diplopia without obvious ophthalmoplegia and he did not have nystagmus. There was hyperreflexia in the lower extremities, with a few beats of ankle clonus bilaterally, although both plantar responses remained flexor. He had mild bilateral intention tremor and truncal ataxia. CT scan showed mild hydrocephalus of the lateral and third ventricle and a cystic mass behind the fourth ventricle and to the right (Fig. 22).

He was operated on by Dr. Gary Fischer who removed a cystic tumor in the right cerebellar hemisphere involving tonsils and vermis. The neuropathologist reported that the lesion was a hemangioblastoma.

Postoperative course was uneventful and he was subsequently asymptomatic and neurologically normal until March 1977 (two years later) when he developed persistent hiccups, dysarthria and ataxia. He complained of occasional headache during the previous month. A CT scan was not revealing and he was admitted for further study. Examination at that time showed dysarthria, truncal ataxia and right palatal and tongue weakness. Stretch reflexes in the legs were hyperactive, more so on the left

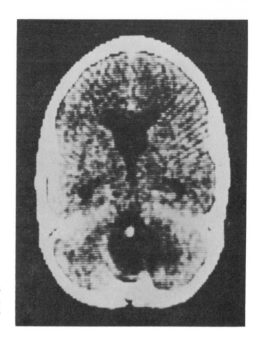

Fig. 22. This CT scan shows a cystic mass lesion in the region of the fourth ventricle with secondary hydrocephalus. The lesion proved to be a hemangioblastoma (case 54).

with an extensor plantar response on that side.

A pneumoencephalogram showed asymmetric expansion of the medulla indicative of persistent or recurrent tumor, and a subsequent angiogram showed expansion with vascular blush in the areas of brainstem abnormality demonstrated on the pneumoencephalogram. The tumor was believed to be sufficiently separate from the site of the original lesion to indicate a second site of tumor formation. Also it was believed to be inoperable, and he was treated with radiation therapy and dexamethasone.

After one month he was much improved, and by September 1977 he was asymptomatic. On examination, he was comfortable and without complaints. Cranial nerve function including the palate and tongue were all normal and his speech was clear. The legs had good strength, but continued to show overactive reflexes with clonus and flexor plantar responses. He walked somewhat carefully but was able to hop and walk tandem. He was seen at periodic intervals subsequently.

In early 1979 he developed periodic frontal throbbing headaches of about one hour in duration associated with nausea but no vomiting. Examination showed no abnormalities and a CT scan was normal. Shortly thereafter the headaches subsided. When seen in July 1980 at age 15 years, he had had no complaints and the neurologic examination was normal.

Comment: The original headaches were suggestive of basilar artery migraine and this was the working diagnosis at first in this boy whose father had had migraine as a boy. However, the development of increasingly severe headaches and persistent neurological signs led to the correct

256

diagnosis of tumor. This patient reaffirms the occasional multiplicity of site in hemangioblastoma.

Migraine seizures and lymphomatoid granulomatosis
This girl was entirely well until age 11 and a half, when one day she noted **CASE** scintillating spots before her eyes, felt nauseated and was unsteady in her **55** walking. Her speech was slurred and inappropriate. She walked home, did not seem to recognize family members and vomited on several occasions. There was no mention of headache. At the emergency room of a local hospital she developed a lateralized right body clonic seizure accompanied by postictal weakness on the right side. She then gradually improved over a six- to eight-hour period.

The EEG showed intermittent delta-slowing in the left hemisphere, and a radio-isotope scan showed no abnormality. A diagnosis of complicated migraine was made and she was treated with Bellergal on a regular basis.

A second episode occurred eight months later when she again saw spots, speech became slurred and within minutes she had developed a generalized headache with nausea. These episodes were repeated over the ensuing months on a number of occasions, always simply handled by rest and aspirin.

Approximately six months later (three months before admission in May 1978) she suddenly lost vision in a right hemianopsic pattern, accompanied by silvery spots. Her speech became slurred and she developed a mild headache, followed by an episode during which her head turned to the left associated with clonic movements of the neck.

Subsequently she had several episodes which lasted several seconds up to a minute during which her head turned to the left, all accompanied by twitching but with no alterations of consciousness. In addition, she had multiple severe generalized headaches which usually seemed to be precipitated by emotional conflict, sometimes preceded by visual phenomena.

Her schoolwork deteriorated during the three- to four-month period during which time she seemed to be working harder but achieving less. These symptoms led to medical re-evaluation which included an EEG which showed bilateral posterior slow wave and theta activity and a CT which showed a low-density area in the right frontal lobe with some displacement of the midline to the left.

Past history was not contributory. The family history revealed a grandfather who had had brain surgery in earlier life for a 'leaking blood vessel' and periodic headaches in both parents. Two brothers aged 18 and 11 also had headaches.

Examination at Children's Hospital in Boston in March 1978 revealed no general physical abnormalities. Her neurological examination showed no overt alterations of mental status. Her visual fields to confrontation were full, and the fundi were normal in appearance. Her outstretched left arm displaced a bit more readily than the right, and it was easier to depress the elevated left leg accompanied by a suspicious toe on that side, otherwise it was entirely normal.

The low-density lesion was confirmed on repeat CT scan. Cerebral angiography disclosed an avascular expansion in the right frontal area with no abnormal vessels or blush. She was seen by Dr. Keasly Welch who did a right frontal craniotomy and partial frontal lobectomy. Pathologic examination by Dr. Ana Sotrel showed mature lymphocytes, lymphomatoid cells, plasma and plasmacytoid cells with 'immunoblasts', histiocytes and macrophages along with changes of the blood vessels and extensive parenchymal necrosis suggestive of lymphomatoid granulomatosis.

She was discharged to be treated with phenytoin. Two months later she had an episode of decreased vision, slurred speech, then nausea and vomiting followed by a two-minute seizure involving arms and neck with no loss of consciousness. For a year subsequently she did relatively well except for a few headaches some of which were preceded by visual scotomata. She also had occasional seizures requiring medication readjustment. At age 15 she had an episode in which she saw spots before her eyes, then had a seizure affecting the left facial muscles and arm and leg with postictal weakness of the left face. The following day she saw spots all day long from the left eye, and that evening experienced a very bad headache. Propranolol was added to the anticonvulsant medication which had no particular advantage.

During the period between age 15 and 18 she continued to have various kinds of episodes. They usually began with multicolored spots in her central field of vision which progressed to a generalized decrease in vision, followed by an abnormal smell and taste which on some occasion progressed to a 'flashback' of visions of events in her past followed by loss of awareness and what observers report as twitching of the left side of the face and occasionally the left arm lasting about one to two minutes. After the spell she was somewhat confused and lethargic for about an hour, during which time she usually had a generalized vice-like vertex headache without throbbing or associated symptoms. On occasion, the headache preceded the spell, but could also occur without a spell. In the month or so prior to her re-evaluation, she had had behavioral modification instructions and learned that on most occasions she was able to abort the episode at the stage of visual disturbance.

An incident occurred in April 1982 in her 18th year during which she lost vision in the left eye. This was treated with a one-month period of high-dose corticosteroids without benefit. The vision remained grossly deficient.

At the time of her most recent evaluation in Boston in January 1983, general physical examination showed nothing of consequence. Neurological evaluation indicated some mild alterations of intellectual functioning, particularly in calculations and pencil constructional tasks. She was essentially blind in the left eye, and on fundoscopy there was optic atrophy. Pupillary light reaction was not well maintained on the left. There were no other cranial nerve abnormalities, and no abnormalities on general neurologic examination.

The CT scan showed the old surgical changes in the right frontal lobe and two contrast-enhancing nodules which measured about 5 mm each in the right occipital lobe surrounded by an area of hypodensity. On review of the 1978 CT scan there was indication of a lesion in this area but the changes were now more prominent and multiple.

Spinal fluid was under normal pressure. There were three cells and all were lymphocytes. CSF protein was 42 mg per cent and glucose 48 mg per cent. CBC revealed 17 per cent eosinophils. Formal psychometrics indicated a full-scale IQ of 73, verbal 81, performance 67, with the over-all impression that there was diffuse involvement with deficits associated with the left and right frontal and left and right posterior brain areas. Based on parental report of earlier abilities and developmental history, it was believed that these neuropsychological observations represented a progressive change.

In view of the multifocal and disseminated nature of the process it was recommended that cranial irradiation in a dose of 5000 rad be carried out. The results of this therapeutic effort are not at present known.

Comment: The chief clinical provocation of the early course was the combination of migrainic and seizure phenomenology in the same event. The nature of the lesion, *i.e.* lymphomatoid granulomatosis, is distinctly unusual, but whether granuloma or tumor, the clinical expression is the point of particular interest in the context of this monograph.

Endocrine-metabolic-intoxication

This category of illness is not prominently represented among the causes of headache, except as endocrine-metabolic and toxic factors are implicated in the pseudotumor syndrome, a relationship that has been discussed in the preceding section. Even in pseudotumor cerebri the occurrence is rare with the exception of the corticosteroid withdrawal patients. However, these entities are of disproportionate importance because recognition of the endocrine or toxic basis of the problem can lead to specific treatment of the basic cause.

If one includes clinical syndromes reminiscent of some of the less usual manifestations of migraine in children such as periodic vomiting, confusional states and other complex symptomatology, then several endocrine-metabolic entities assume importance in differential considerations. In this context, it is more appropriate to emphasize those disorders which have paroxysmal expression over a period of months or more, rather than acute monophasic illness. Reye's syndrome, viral encephalitis, a number of exogenous intoxications, and *petit mal* or temporal lobe status epilepticus can be reminiscent of the complex migraine syndromes in the early hours of their manifestations, but the situation is usually clarified quickly by the course of the illness, and laboratory investigations.

259

Pheochromocytoma

This tumor, which derives from cells of the adrenal medulla and sympathetic nervous system tissue elsewhere, is rare at any age and very rare in children, although Stackpole *et al.* (1963) were able to record 100 cases from the literature and include nine patients of their own. The clinical effect of this endocrine tumor is directly related to the elaboration of excessive amounts of the catecholamines norepinephrine and epinephrine. The measurement of the excretion product of these substances (VMA or 3 methoxy 4-hydroxymandelic acid) in the urine is an important aspect of the diagnosis. The tumor itself is usually in the adrenal gland, and often bilateral and multiple in children. When outside the adrenal it may be found at widely dispersed sites, usually near large arteries in the abdomen such as at the bifurcation of the aorta. Although mostly sporadic in occurrence, familial examples are known (Cone *et al.* 1957) and there is increased incidence of this tumor in neurofibromatosis and von Hippel-Lindau disease. In all familial cases, the incidence of multiple tumors is particularly high.

Although the classic expression of pheochromocytoma is paroxysmal hypertension with its associated symptoms, in children sustained hypertension is the rule and occurs in almost 90 per cent of patients (Stackpole *et al.* 1963). Signs of systemic illness are often present, the most consistent being excessive sweatiness (in two thirds) including night sweats, weight loss (one third), failure of growth, and occasionally polydipsia and polyuria.

However it is the paroxysmal symptoms which provide the best clinical clue and bring the problem into the differential diagnosis of juvenile migraine. Periodic headache occurs in 75 per cent of patients (Lance and Hinterberger 1976). They are usually severe, have some tendency to occipital location, but are more often generalized. They frequently have a throbbing quality, and in some instances they are indistinguishable from migraine. In most cases, the headaches are of only a few months duration and of increasing severity and frequency. They may be accompanied by pallor, visual disturbance (usually blurred vision), nausea and vomiting and occasionally seizures or altered consciousness (Lance and Hinterberger 1976).

Associated diaphoresis is prominent, and perhaps represents the clinical feature that distinguishes the paroxysm from the usual patient with juvenile migraine, unless the migraine is triggered by a hypoglycemic stimulus. Hypertension is the rule during an episode but only occasionally is the physician at hand to measure it. Many of these patients have red-violaceous mottling of the skin of the hands with increased local sweatiness, a finding which some adolescent and adult migrainic patients also exhibit to a lesser degree.

In summary, there are usually sufficient clues in the systemic evaluation of the clinical problem, including the measurement of blood pressure, that even if an analysis of the periodic symptoms suggest migraine, these patients tend to stand out as unusual in some respect. No patient with juvenile migraine should fail to have his blood pressure measured. Parenthetically, other causes of sustained and periodic hypertension such as renal disease can also be a cause of periodic, migrainoid headaches.

Carcinoid syndrome

This disorder is caused by the release of serotonin from carcinoid tumors of argentaffin cells in the intestinal mucosa, bronchi and rarely in teratomas. They are rare at any age, and although they are most often found in adults, they have been known to occur in adolescents. The characteristic clinical syndrome is directly related to the quantity of serotonin released and it usually implies metastasis.

The symptomatology of interest in this connection consists of paroxysmal flushing of the face which extends over the upper body. This may be accompanied by abdominal pain, watery stools, tachycardia, orbital edema, and wheezing. Episodes are measured in minutes as a rule and usually occur daily or several times a day. Headache is an unusual feature, but episodes have vasomotor implications and can be confused with migrainic phenomena. Diagnosis is established by measuring 5 hydroxy indol acetic acid (5-HIAA) in the urine, which is present in marked excess. Treatment is principally surgical.

Ketotic hypoglycemia

The predominant symptom of hypoglycemia in childhood is convulsions. Lesser degrees of hypoglycemia on any basis may lead to headache as part of the symptom complex, usually associated with diaphoresis, confusional state and/or lethargy. The mild hypoglycemic state may also trigger migraine in susceptible individuals as had been discussed in an earlier section of this monograph.

However, one hypoglycemic syndrome, *i.e.* ketotic hypoglycemia (Colle and Ulstrom 1964) deserves special mention because of its similarity to migrainic cyclic vomiting in certain respects. It is also an entity in which 'migraine' and seizure in the same episode does not carry an implication of the high incidence of structural central nervous system disease.

Onset is usually between one and a half and five years of age with spontaneous remission by age 10. Susceptible children are small with little subcutaneous fat. Episodes are usually associated with intercurrent respiratory illness or food deprivation. Fever is inconstant, may be low-grade, and some patients are hypothermic when CNS symptoms are manifest in sharp contrast with febrile convulsions. Early-morning convulsions are the commonest presenting complaint. Less frequently, but more appropriate to the diagnostic differential with migrainic cyclic vomiting, onset is marked by anorexia, then nausea and vomiting and finally lethargy proceeding to stupor. At any point a generalized major convulsion may supervene.

Ketosis is manifest at an early state in the paroxysm and is demonstrable hours before hypoglycemia is detectable. The symptoms may be reproduced by less than 24 hours of ketogenic diet in these patients and hypoglycemia is more marked and occurs earlier in ketotic hypoglycemia patients (Colle and Ulstrom 1964). The time of onset of ketosis is the same in both patients and controls, but the development of symptomatic hypoglycemia occurs after several hour in patients, but is delayed for 24 to 48 hours in controls who may not become symptomatic at all.

The metabolic defect is not precisely known but according to Colle and Ulstrom (1964) 'the timing . . . suggests that the failure of homeostasis takes place after the glycogen initially present in the liver would have been utilized, and therefore represents a failure of mechanisms for adaptation from a carbohydrate to a fat burning economy'.

Treatment is symptomatic and consists of oral or IV administration of glucose. Parents are advised to test urine for acetonuria whenever the child is indisposed and maintain a good carbohydrate intake during critical periods.

Ornithine transcarbamylase (OTC) deficiency and other hyperammonemias
OTC deficiency is an x-linked disorder (Short *et al.* 1973) of the urea cycle that leads to hyperammonemia, early neurological impairment and death in the affected male infant. Symptoms begin in the first few days of life and are linked to protein intake. The inherited defect is due to profound deficiency of the of the enyzme ornithine transcarbamylase (OTC) (Russell *et al.* 1962).

Some carrier females have periodic symptoms due to partial defect in the enzyme, usually precipitated by an unusual dietary protein intake (Glasgow *et al.* 1978). The female carriers are normal except for an early acquired aversion to high-protein foods such as meat and milk.

Periodic symptoms usually develop between two and four years of age. The resulting symptoms consist of nausea and repeated vomiting accompanied by disordered mental status. Lethargy is common, but a confusional state has also been described. The duration of symptoms varies from several hours to several days. The clinical picture is reminiscent of either migrainic 'cyclic vomiting' or of confusional migraine.

In a particularly interesting family described by Russell (1973) the syndrome in carrier females included ophthalmoplegia and ataxia in one and blindness in another in association with what was regarded as 'migrainous' headache. Of additional interest was the fact that the mother's migrainic symptomatology was greatly exaggerated during the pregnancies that resulted in an affected male infant, as if the additional ammonia load tipped a precarious balance in the mother. In the two affected families, female siblings, mothers, maternal grandmothers and great grandmothers all had migraine. The migraine syndrome, which included headache, was reproduced in severe form in the mothers by oral ammonium chloride. The symptoms were correlated with abnormal elevations of blood ammonia.

The same author then proceeded to study 15 cases of severe cyclic vomiting with oral ammonia loading. Eight showed abnormal ammonia tolerance, six of whom had symptomatology produced by the test. Three of these patients proved to have OTC defect, and a patient who was studied later was found to have a carbamyl phosphate synthetase defect, another enzyme related to the urea cycle, that has similar consequences in carriers with a partial defect.

Although dietary management is ineffective in preserving neurologic function in the affected male infants, treatment with low-protein diet plus oral keto-acid supplementation can be effective in managing the paroxysmal symptoms of carrier females (Glasgow *et al.* 1978).

In addition to OTC and carbamyl-phosphate synthetase, there are several other disorders of the urea cycle, all potentially capable of producing a similar clinical syndrome in carriers of the trait or in individuals with sufficient enzyme to manage under usual circumstances.

Amino acid disorders

Certain of the inborn errors of amino acid metabolism have been reported to produce periodic symptoms. In some instances it may be those patients who would ordinarily be regarded as carriers of the trait, while in others it is the principal expression of the disease. The resulting periodic symptomatology is not ordinarily suggestive of either classic or common migraine, but comes into the differential diagnosis of either cyclic vomiting, usually severe, or some of the complex migraine syndromes, particularly those in which ataxia is a principal expression.

Hartnup disease

Hartnup disease is an autosomal recessive disorder of the intestinal, renal and probably also of cellular transport of neutral amino acids. Excessive quantities are excreted in the urine, but blood levels are not elevated. Some of the clinical symptomatology probably relates to the metabolism of tryptophane. A result of this intracellular deficiency state of tryptophane is lack of endogenous nicotinamide, which is probably responsible for the pellagra-like symptoms.

Symptomatic expression of the Hartnup fault is rare when diet is adequate, and usually occurs only in mildly malnourished children. The classic photosensitive pellagra-like rash is inconstant, and then usually late in appearance. The chief expression is periodic symptomatology consisting of disordered mental status, ataxia, and may include vascular headache with nausea and photophobia. Episodes vary from hours to days in duration. The similarity to complex juvenile migraine is obvious. Even the effect of sun exposure in precipitating the headache and other symptoms of some patients with true migraine is mimicked, as exemplified by a report of two patients in whom exposure to sun induced reddening and burning of the skin, headache and nausea (Pomeroy *et al.* 1968).

Maple syrup urine disease

The biochemical expression of this autosomal recessive disorder consists of elevation of the branched chain amino acids, leucine, isoleucine and valine in plasma, and the excretion of the keto-acid metabolic products in the urine. The fault lies in the enzymatic decarboxylation of these compounds. The usual clinical expression is a rapidly progressive fatal neurological illness of early infancy. Of interest in the context of the differential diagnosis of migraine are reports where a lesser decarboxylase defect resulted in intermittent symptoms (Dancis *et al.* 1967).

Although most such children become symptomatic in association with acute infection between one and two years, the first episode may be delayed as late as eight years and beyond. Symptoms are usually precipitated by some incident, usually infection, but in one reported example intestinal bleeding and transfusion seemed to be responsible. Symptoms are variable and include headache, vomiting, ataxia, irritability and disordered awareness. More severe episodes lead to coma, and convulsions. Death can result. In most respects the more severe syndrome is suggestive of Reye's disease or 'toxic encephalopathy', but in lesser expression there is a similarity to patients with juvenile migraine and its variants.

In any patient, the urinary odor of maple syrup is a prime clue. Recognition of these patients is of considerable therapeutic importance. The threat of death or impairment in acute episodes may be prevented by the administration of intravenous glucose and reduction of the intake of branched chain amino acids.

Organic acidemias

In addition to maple syrup disease, there are several other disorders where inherited enzymatic deficiency leads to the accumulation of relatively specific organic acids, for example isovaleric, methylmalonic and proprionic acidemias. The biochemical details of these conditions can be pursued by referring to excellent summaries that are easily available (Menkes 1980). In most, the principal clinical syndromes consist of devastating neurologic disease with onset in early infancy. In addition, there are periodic fluctuations of enhanced severity precipitated by infection or protein intake that are marked clinically by vomiting, convulsions and disordered consciousness. Mental deficiency and/or early death are the expected consequences.

Experience with the disorders of the urea cycle and maple syrup urine disease have been recapitulated with regard to lesser degrees of enzyme deficiency in some of these disorders, and it is predictable that more will be discovered. A common clinical feature of diagnostic importance in all of the organic acidemias is the development of metabolic acidosis and resulting tachypnea and respiratory distress.

Isovaleric acidemia is a well-documented example of a disorder in which periodic symptoms occur (Budd *et al.* 1967) The distinctive clinical feature is an odor of 'sweaty feet', that is intensified during infection or dietary protein-precipitated bouts of severe vomiting and lethargy which may last hours to days. The usual onset is in infancy, but episodes may continue to occur with lessening severity during the years of childhood. Aversion to protein-containing foods is a frequently observed feature in otherwise developmentally normal children.

Miscellaneous disorders

Pyruvate decarboxylase deficiency

A particularly interesting group of patients with elevated pyruvate who present clinically with periodic ataxia and other movement disorders have been found to have pyruvate decarboxylase deficiency (Blass *et al.* 1970, 1971). The initial patient was described at age nine and had episodes since he was 16 months of age. Some episodes were preceded by irritability and pallor, or voracious hunger. He then became overtly ataxic, complained of double vision and weakness, was dysarthric and had some minor choreiform-dystonic movements. Attacks varied considerably in severity and were of several hours to several days in duration. Pyruvate levels were consistently elevated, slightly more during attacks. Muscle biopsy showed droplets of oil red-o positive material. Treatment with dexamethasone was therapeutically useful, thiamine in high doses was not. The striking similarity of this patient to those with basilar artery migraine is apparent.

Systemic carnitine deficiency

A clinically similar patient with episodes of ataxia, oculomotor palsy and confusion was found to have carnitine acetyltransferase deficiency (DiDonato *et al.* 1979). Since this report, other patients have been reported by Cruse *et al.* (1984) and others (Chapoy *et al.* 1980, Engel *et al.* 1981, DiDonato *et al.* 1982) where it is clear that abnormalities of carnitine metabolism can cause episodic neurologic symptoms in some patients, as well as a clinical syndrome of progressive myopathy in others. In some patients both are manifest. The paroxysmal clinical expression may be ataxia, but is usually dominated by altered consciousness and hyperventilation. There is laboratory evidence of keto-acidosis and significant hypoglycemia on occasion. Lactate, pyruvate and ammonia may be elevated. The clinical expression of a single incident is reminiscent of Reye's syndrome. Treatment with oral carnitine or prednisone can be useful in individual patients, although the effect is variable and unpredictable.

Biotin-responsive multiple carboxylase deficiency

Patients with a biotin-responsive disorder based upon inherited multiple carboxylase deficiency have been described (Sander *et al.* 1980). The disease leads to lactic acidosis, ketosis, hyperammonemia and takes two clinical forms. In one the onset is early in infancy and runs a rapidly progressive course, while in others, onset is later and takes the form of intermittent ataxia, combined with immunodeficiency and seizures. The therapeutic response of the intermittent ataxia to biotin in large doses (10 mg/day) is an important observation that gives urgency to the recognition of the problem, although the consequences of the immunodeficiency are apparently not prevented.

Acetazolamide-responsive intermittent neurologic syndromes

A particularly interesting and important group of patients has been identified by Evans *et al.* (1978). These patients have episodic weakness and unsteadiness, ptosis and ocular movement disorders with dysarthria and dysphagia precipitated by intercurrent infection, stress, or glucose loading. The biochemical abnormality consisted of a 'diabetic' glucose tolerance curve with elevation of blood lactate and pyruvate. The pyruvate-lactate levels were abnormal during episodes and also may be elevated in asymptomatic intervals. The enzyme defect was not identified but it was discovered that continuous use of acetazolamide was capable of preventing recurring episodes in these patients.

In several additional reports (Griggs *et al.* 1978, Donat and Auger 1979, Zasorin *et al.* 1983) the similarity to juvenile migraine, especially the basilar artery variant, becomes even stronger. Episodic clinical symptoms more clearly relate to the central nervous system and emphasize ataxia sometimes with nystagmus, and headache is also described. In these latter reports there is a less clear relationship to abnormal lactate-pyruvate metabolism, but all were dramatically responsive to acetazolamide.

265

TABLE XVII

Clinical Clues to the Presence of Metabolic Encephalopathy as the Basis of Periodic Disorders

General
1. Severe cyclic vomiting with lethargy and/or confusional state, especially if it leads to metabolic acidosis.
2. Periodic ataxia.
3. Lethargy deepening to coma.
4. Convulsions associated with episodes.
5. Episodes precipitated by infectious illness and fever.
6. Episodes precipitated by unusual protein intake.
7. Onset of paroxysmal symptoms in the first two years of life.
8. Aversion to meat, milk, and other protein-containing foods.

More specific
1. Tachypnea and respiratory distress—(organic acidemia, Leigh's disease).
2. Unusual body or urinary odors—especially during episodes (maple syrup urine disease, isovaleric acidemia and probably other organic acidemias).
3. Female siblings or relatives in families where male infants died in infancy with neurologic disease (ornithine transcarbamylase deficiency).
4. Elevated blood pressure and diaphoresis (pheochromocytoma).
5. Flush, asthma and diarrhea—(carcinoid).

Leigh's disease

This disease usually presents as a progressive neurologic disorder with predilection for the brainstem. The neuropathologic changes are similar in a number of respects to thiamine deficiency. Its metabolic basis is unknown although thiamine triphosphate inhibitor substance is found in the urine in many patients. Lactic acidosis is detected in some patients.

A relapsing remitting course with acute exacerbations has been occasionally recorded in milder forms of the disease. The longer duration of the episodes and residual signs between, set this disorder apart from migraine unless the migraine patient develops an infarct in the basilar-vertebral vascular territory.

Summary

Neither the pediatric generalist nor the pediatric neurologist can be expected to have a detailed knowledge of the group of metabolic disorders considered in the latter part of this section. The range of clinical expression has gradually expanded in recent years and new biochemical entities are being added with consistent regularity. However, the general principle is clear. Even in well-known lethal enzymopathies, there are periodic clinical expressions in some patients based on lesser degrees of enzyme defect, sometimes as found in the heterozygote and in other instances based on a variable individual capacity for compensation by alternate metabolic pathways. The resulting intermittent symptomatology is quite similar to certain of the clinical expressions of juvenile migraine, especially the syndrome of cyclic vomiting and of confusional and basilar artery migraine or of migraine complicated by seizures. Throbbing headache is less commonly recorded in these patients, but certainly does occur, perhaps primarily in those patients from families who already have some degree of migrainic neurovasomotor instability.

The important issue in current practice is the recognition of the presently definable metabolic disorders with therapeutic potential (Table XVII). Some symptoms are substrate-dependent, and protein restriction for both the intermittent hyperammonemias and of branched chain amino acid disorders (organic acidurias) can be beneficial. In certain disorders more specific therapy can be useful. For example, addition of oral keto-acids in ornithine transcarbamylase deficiency, B12 in large quantity in methylmalonic aciduria, oral carnitive or corticosteroids in certain of the periodic ataxias from carnitine deficiency and pyruvic decarboxylase deficiency, biotin in multiple carboxylase deficiency and acetazolamide in other less well-defined dysmetabolism syndromes.

The clinician is confronted with the usual dilemma of how far to go in a routine laboratory search for the several rare metabolic entities that have been mentioned above. The major indications would seem to be periodic syndromes where the predominant symptomatology is repeated vomiting, lethargy, and disordered mental status. If convulsions or coma occur, the indication is even stronger. Another prime indication are the periodic ataxias that may also be accompanied by other signs of brainstem dysfunction. If the history indicates an association with febrile illness, poor food intake, or a relationship to unusually high intake of high-protein foods or glucose loading, there is further indication to pursue metabolic possibilities. The same may be said for a history of life-long aversion to meat, milk and other high-protein foods. It is fascinating how often this runs through the history of children with periodic syndromes due to the hyperammonemias and organic amino-acidemias. There are a number of additional, somewhat more specific clinical clues that relate to specific disorders to be found in Table XVII. Headache is not usually a central feature of the presentation, but it does occur, and when it does it frequently has the quality of migraine.

Clinical suspicion should then lead to a series of laboratory measurements. They follow naturally from an awareness of the various biochemical disorders that have been discussed. This is especially appropriate when one is presented the opportunity for study during an acute episode. Measurement of blood glucose, ammonia, pyruvate and lactate, blood and urine amino acids together with assessment of electrolytes and liver function is indicated. Particular attention should be paid to blood pH, CO_2 and the possibility of a significant anion gap. If indicated by these results, more specific enzymatic studies can be arranged.

REFERENCES

Abroms, I. F., Yessayan, L., Shillito, J., Barlow, C. F. (1971) 'Spontaneous intracerebral hemorrhage in patients suspected of multiple sclerosis.' *Journal of Neurology, Neurosurgery, and Psychiatry,* **34,** 157-162.

Adler, C. S., Adler, S. M. (1976) 'Biofeedback psychotherapy for the treatment of headaches.' *Headache,* **16,** 189-191.

Aicardi, J., Amsili, J., Chevrie, J. J. (1969) 'Acute hemiplegias in infancy and childhood.' *Developmental Medicine and Child Neurology,* **11,** 162-173.

Allan, W. (1930) 'The inheritance of migraine.' *Archives of Internal Medicine,* **13,** 590-599.

Alpers, B. J. (1960) 'Epileptic vertigo.' *Laryngoscope,* **70,** 631-637.

—— Yaskin, H. E. (1951) 'Pathogenesis of ophthalmoplegic migraine.' *Archives of Ophthalmology,* **45,** 551-569.

Ambruso, D. R., Jacobson, L. J., Hathaway, W. E. (1980) 'Inherited anti-thrombin III deficiency and cerebral thrombosis in a child.' *Pediatrics,* **65,** 125-131.

Anthony, M. (1976) 'Plasma free fatty acids and prostaglandin E1 in migraine and stress.' *Headache,* **16,** 58-63.

—— Lance, J. W. (1971) 'Histamine and serotonin in cluster headache.' *Archives of Neurology,* **25,** 225-231.

Apley, J., Naish, N. (1958) 'Recurrent abdominal pains: a field survey of 1000 school children.' *Archives of Disease in Childhood,* **33,** 165-170.

Appenzeller, O. (1972) 'Altitude headache.' *Headache,* **12,** 126-129.

Barabas, G., Ferrari, M., Matthews, W. S. (1983a) 'Childhood migraine and somnambulism.' *Neurology,* **33,** 948-949.

—— Matthews, W. S., Ferrari, M. (1983b) 'Childhood migraine and motion sickness.' *Pediatrics,* **72,** 188-190.

Barlow, C. F. (1978) 'Migraine in childhood.' *Research and Clinical Studies in Headache,* **5,** 34-46.

Barnett, H. J. M., Boughner, D. R., Taylor, D. W., Cooper, P. E., Kostuk, W. J., Nichol, P. M. (1980) 'Further evidence relating mitral valve prolapse to cerebral ischemic events.' *New England Journal of Medicine,* **302,** 139-144.

Barr, R. C., Levine, M. D., Watkins, J. B. (1979) 'Recurrent abdominal pain of childhood due to lactose intolerance.' *New England Journal of Medicine,* **300,** 1449-1452.

Basser, L. S. (1964) 'Benign paroxysmal vertigo in childhood.' *Brain,* **87,** 141-152.

—— (1969) 'The relation of migraine and epilepsy.' *Brain,* **92,** 285-300.

Bayless, T. M., Huang, S. S. (1971) 'Recurrent abdominal pain due to milk and lactose intolerance in school aged children.' *Pediatrics,* **47,** 1029-1032.

Beaumont, G. E., Hearn, J. B. (1948) 'A case of reversible papilloedema due to heart failure.' *British Medical Journal,* **1,** 50.

Belfer, M. L., Kaban, L. B. (1982) 'Temporomandibular joint dysfunction with facial pain in children.' *Pediatrics,* **69,** 564-567.

Berenberg, W. (1983) *Personal communication.*

Bickerstaff, E. R. (1959) 'The periodic migrainous neuralgia of Wilfred Harris.' *Lancet,* **1,** 1069-1071.

—— (1961) 'Basilar artery migraine.' *Lancet,* **1,** 15-17.

—— (1962) 'The basilar artery and the migraine-epilepsy syndrome.' *Proceedings of the Royal Society of Medicine,* **55,** 167-169.

—— (1964a) 'Ophthalmoplegic migraine.' *Revue Neurologique,* **110,** 582-587.

—— (1964b) 'Aetiology of acute hemiplegia in childhood.' *British Medical Journal,* **2,** 82-87.

Bille, B. (1962) 'Migraine in school children.' *Acta Paediatrica,* **51,** Suppl. 136, 1-151.

—— Ludvigsson, J., Sanner, G. (1977) 'Prophylaxis of migraine in children.' *Headache,* **17,** 61-63.

Blass, J. P., Avigan, J., Uhlendorf, B. W. (1970) 'A defect in pyruvate decarboxylase in a child with intermittent movement disorder.' *Journal of Clinical Investigation,* **49,** 423-432.

—— Kark, R. A. P., Engel, W. K. (1971) 'Clinical studies of a patient with pyruvate decarboxylase deficiency.' *Archives of Neurology,* **25,** 449-460.

Blau, J. N. (1980) 'Migraine prodromes separated from the aura: complete migraine.' *British Medical Journal,* **281,** 658-660.

—— Whitty, C. W. M. (1955) 'Familial hemiplegic migraine.' *Lancet,* **2,** 1115-1116.

—— Davis, E. (1970) 'Small blood-vessels in migraine.' *Lancet,* **2,** 740-742.

268

Blitzsten, N. L., Brams, W. A. (1926) 'Migraine with abdominal equivalent.' *Journal of the American Medical Association*, **86**, 675-677.

Blodi, F. C., Gass, D. M. (1968) 'Inflammatory pseudotumor of the orbit. *British Journal of Ophthalmology*, **52**, 79-93.

Bodian, M. (1964) 'Transient loss of vision following head trauma.' *New York State Journal of Medicine*, **64**, 916-920.

Boudin, G., Pepin, B., Barbizet, J., Masson, S. (1962) 'Migraine and EEG disturbances.' *Electroencephalography and Clinical Neurophysiology*, **14**, 141-142.

Bradshaw, P., Parsons, M. (1965) 'Hemiplegic migraine, a clinical study.' *Quarterly Journal of Medicine*, **34**, 65-85.

Braudo, M. (1956) 'Thrombosis of the internal carotid artery in childhood after injuries in the region of soft palate.' *British Medical Journal*, **1**, 665-667.

Brenner, C., Friedman, A. P., Merritt, H. H., Denny-Brown, D. E. (1944) 'Post-traumatic headache.' *Journal of Neurosurgery*, **1**, 379-391.

Bresnan, M. J., Strand, R., Rosenbaum, A. (1973) 'Jugular venous block associated with benign intracranial hypertension.' *Paper presented at American Academy of Neurology Meeting, April.*

Bronshvag, M. M., Pyrstowsky, S. D., Traviesa, D. C. (1978) 'Vascular headaches in mixed connective tissue disease.' *Headache*, **18**, 154-160.

Brott, T., Leviton, A. (1976) 'Headache rounds: violence.' *Headache*, **16**, 203-209.

Brown, J. K. (1977) 'Migraine and migraine equivalents in children.' *Developmental Medicine and Child Neurology*, **19**, 683-692.

Brumback, R. A., Staton, R. D., Wilson, H. (1980) 'Neuropsychological study of children during and after remission of endogenous depressive episodes.' *Perceptual and Motor Skills*, **50**, 1163-1167.

Bruyn, G. W. (1968) 'Complicated migraine.' *In:* Vinkin, P. J., Bruyn, G. W. (Eds.) *Handbook of Clinical Neurology. Vol 5: Headaches and Cranial Neuralgias.* Amsterdam: North Holland. Ch. 6.

—— (1983) 'Epidemiology of migraine: "A personal view".' *Headache*, **23**, 127-133.

Buchheit, W. A., Barton, C., Haag, B., Shaw, D. (1969) 'Papilledema and idiopathic intracranial hypertension.' *New England Journal of Medicine*, **280**, 938-942.

Budd, M. A., Tanaka, K., Holmes, L. B., Efron, M. L., Crawford, J. D., Isselbacher, K. J. (1967) 'Isovaleric acidemia, clinical features of a new genetic defect of leucine metabolism.' *New England Journal of Medicine*, **277**, 321-327.

Burke, E. C., Peters, G. A. (1956) 'Migraine in childhood: a preliminary report.' *American Journal of Diseases of Children*, **92**, 330-336.

Butler, S., Thomas, W. A. (1947) 'Headache: its physiological causes.' *Journal of the American Medical Association*, **135**, 967-971.

Cairo, M. S., Lazarus, K., Gilmore, R. L., Baehner, R. L. (1980) 'Intracranial hemorrhage and focal seizures secondary to use of L-asparaginase during induction therapy of acute lymphocytic leukemia. *Journal of Pediatrics*, **97**, 829-833.

Camfield, P. R., Metrakos, K., Andermann, F. (1978) Basilar migraine, seizures and severe epileptiform EEG abnormalities.' *Neurology*, **28**, 584-588.

Capildeo, R., Rose, F. C. (1982) 'Single dose pizotifen, 1.5 mgm. nocte: a new approach in the prophylaxis of migraine.' *Headache*, **22**, 272-275.

Carlson, G. A., Cantwell, D. P. (1980) 'Unmasking masked depression in children and adolescents.' *American Journal of Psychiatry*, **137**, 445-449.

Castaldo, J. E., Anderson, M., Reeves, A. G. (1982) 'Middle cerebral artery occlusion with migraine.' *Stroke*, **13**, 308-311.

Caviness, V. S., O'Brien, P. (1980) 'Cluster headache: response to chlorpromazine.' *Headache*, **20**, 128-131.

Chao, D., Davis, S. D. (1964) 'Convulsive equivalent syndrome of childhood.' *Journal of Pediatrics*, **64**, 499-508.

Chapman, L. F., Ramos, A. O., Goodell, H., Silverman, G., Wolff, H. G. (1960) 'A humoral agent implicated in vascular headache of the migraine type.' *Archives of Neurology*, **3**, 223-229.

Chapoy, P. R., Angelini, C., Brown, W. J., Stiff, J. E., Shug, A. L., Cederbaum, S. D. (1980) 'Systemic carnitine deficiency: a treatable inherited lipid-storage disease presenting as Reye's syndrome. *New England Journal of Medicine*, **303**, 1389-1394.

Chester, E. M., Agamanolis, D. P., Banker, B. Q., Victor, M. (1978) 'Hypertensive encephalopathy: a clinicopathologic study of 20 cases.' *Neurology*, **28**, 928-939.

Clarke, J. M. (1910) 'On recurrent motor paralysis in migraine, with a report in which recurrent hemiplegia accompanied the attacks.' *British Medicial Journal*, **1**, 1534-1538.

269

Cogan, D. G., Mount, H. T. J. (1963) 'Intracranial aneurysms causing ophthalmoplegia.' *Archives of Ophthalmology,* **70,** 757-771.

Cohen, M. J. (1978) 'Psychophysiological studies of headache: is there a similarity between migraine and muscle contraction headaches?' *Headache,* **19,** 189-196.

Colle, E., Ulstrom, R. A. (1964) 'Ketotic hypoglycemia.' *Pediatrics,* **64,** 632-651.

Cone, T. E., Allen, M. S., Pearson, H. A. (1957) 'Pheochromocytoma in children: report of three familial cases in two unrelated families.' *Pediatrics,* **19,** 44-56.

Congdon, P. J., Forsythe, W. I. (1979) 'Migraine in childhood: a study of 300 children.' *Developmental Medicine and Child Neurology,* **21,** 209-216.

Connor, R. C. R. (1962) 'Complicated migraine: a study of permanent neurological and visual defects caused by migraine.' *Lancet,* **2,** 1072-1075.

Conomy, J. P., Hanson, M. R., McFarling, D. (1982) 'Does migraine increase the risk of cerebral ischemic events in persons with mitral valve prolapse?' *Annals of Neurology,* **12,** 83. *(Abstract).*

Corbett, J. J., Savino, P. J., Thompson, H. S., Kansu, T., Schatz, N. J., Orr, L. S., Hopson, D. (1982) 'Visual loss in pseudotumor cerebri.' *Archives of Neurology,* **39,** 461-474.

Stroke, **13,** 308-311.

Couch, J. R., Ziegler, D. K., Hassanein, R. (1976) 'Amitriptyline in the prophylaxis of migraine.' *Neurology,* **26,** 121-127.

—— Hassanein, R. S. (1977) 'Platelet aggregability in migraine.' *Neurology,* **27,** 843-848.

—— Ziegler, D. K. (1978) 'Prednisone therapy for cluster headache.' *Headache,* **18,** 219-221.

—— Diamond, S. (1983) 'Status migrainosus: causative and therapeutic aspects.' *Headache,* **23,** 94-101.

Critchley, M., Ferguson, F. R. (1933) 'Migraine.' *Lancet,* **1,** 123-126.

Crowell, G. F., Stump, D. A., Billter, J., McHenry, C., Toole, J. F. (1984) 'The transient global amnesia-migraine connection'. *Archives of Neurology,* **41,** 75-79.

Cruse, R. P., DiMauro, S., Towfighi, J., Trevesan, C. (1984) 'Familial systemic carnitine deficiency.' *Archives of Neurology,* **41,** 301-305.

Cullen, K. J., MacDonald, W. B. (1963) 'The periodic syndrome: its nature and prevalence.' *Medical Journal of Australia,* **50,** 167-173.

Curran, D. A., Hinterberger, H., Lance, J. W. (1965) 'Total plasma serotonin 5-hydroxyindoleacetic acid and p-hydroxy-m-methoxymandelic acid excretion in normal and migrainous subjects.' *Brain,* **88,** 997-1010.

Dalessio, D. J. (1976) 'The relationship of vasoactive substances to vascular permeability, and their role in migraine.' *Research and Clinical Studies in Headache,* **4,** 76-84.

—— (Ed.) (1980) *Wolff's Headache and Other Head Pain. (4th Edn.)* Oxford and New York: Oxford University Press.

Dalsgaard-Neilsen, T. (1965) 'Migraine and heredity.' *Acta Neurologica Scandinavica,* **41,** 287-300.

—— Engberg-Pederson, H., Holm, H. E. (1970) 'Clinical and statistical investigations of the epidemiology of migraine.' *Danish Medical Bulletin,* **17,** 138-148.

Dancis, J., Hutzler, B. S., Rokkones, T. (1967) 'Intermittent branched-chain ketonuria-variant of maple-syrup urine disease.' *New England Journal of Medicine,* **276,** 84-89.

Daniels, S. R., Bates, S., Lukin, R. R., Benton, C., Third, J., Glueck, C. J. (1982) 'Cerebrovascular arteriopathy (arteriosclerosis) and ischemic childhood stroke.' *Stroke,* **13,** 360-365.

Davidoff, L. M., Dyke, C. G. (1938) 'Relapsing juvenile chronic subdural hematoma.' *Bulletin of the Neurological Institute of New York,* **7,** 95-147.

Delaney, P., Estes, M. (1980) 'Intracranial hemorrhage with amphetamine abuse.' *Neurology,* **30,** 1125-1128.

Delong, R. (1983) *Personal communication.*

Deshmukh, S. V., Meyer, J. S. (1977) 'Cyclic changes in platelet dynamics and the pathogenesis and prophylaxis of migraine.' *Headache,* **17,** 101-108.

Deubner, D. C. (1977) 'An epidemiologic study of migraine and headache in 10-20 year olds.' *Headache,* **17,** 173-180.

Dexter, J. D., Roberts, J., Byer, J. A. (1978) 'The five hour glucose tolerance test and effect of low sucrose diet in migraine.' *Headache,* **18,** 91-94.

Diamond, S. (1979) 'Biofeedback and headache.' *Headache,* **19,** 180-184.

—— (1982) 'Prolonged benign exertional headache: its clinical characteristics and response to indomethacin.' *Headache,* **22,** 96-98.

—— Kudrow, L., Stevens, J., Shapiro, D. B. (1982) 'Long-term study of propranolol in the treatment of migraine.' *Headache,* **22,** 268-271.

—— Schenbaum, H. (1983) 'Flunarizine, a calcium channel blocker, in the prophylactic treatment of migraine.' *Headache,* **23,** 39-42.

270

DiDonato, S., Rimoldi, M., Moise, A., Bertagnoglio, B., Uziel, G. (1979) 'Fatal ataxic encephalopathy and carnitine acetyltransferase deficiency.' *Neurology,* **29,** 1578-1583.
—— —— Carnelio, F., Bottacchi, E., Giunta, A. (1982) 'Evidence for autosomal recessive inheritance in systemic carnitine deficiency.' *Annals of Neurology,* **11,** 190-192.
Dillon, H., Leopold, R. L. (1961) 'Children and the post-concussion syndrome.' *Journal of the American Medical Association,* **175,** 86-92.
Di Rocco, C., McLone, D. G., Shimoji, T., Raimondi, A. J. (1975) 'Continuous intraventricular cerebrospinal fluid pressure recording in hydrocephalic children during wakefulness and sleep.' *Journal of Neurosurgery,* **42,** 683-689.
—— Caldarelli, M., Maira, G., Rossi, G. F. (1977) 'The study of CSF dynamics in apparently "arrested" hydrocephalus in children.' *Child's Brain,* **3,** 359-374.
Donat, J. R., Auger, R. (1979) 'Familial periodic ataxia.' *Archives of Neurology,* **36,** 568-569.
Dorfman, L. J., Marshall, W. H., Enzmann, D. R. (1979) 'Cerebral infarction and migraine: clinical and radiologic correlations.' *Neurology,* **29,** 317-322.
Douglas, E. F., White, P. T. (1971) 'Abdominal epilepsy—a reappraisal.' *Journal of Pediatrics,* **78,** 59-67.
Drew, J. H., Grant, F. C. (1948) 'Benign cysts of the brain.' *Journal of Neurosurgery,* **5,** 107-123.
Drummond, P. D., Lance, J. W. (1983) 'Extracranial vascular changes and the source of pain in migraine headache.' *Annals of Neurology,* **13,** 32-37.
Duffy, F. H., Burchfield, J. L., Lombroso, C. T. (1979) 'Brain electrical activity mapping (BEAM): a methód for extending the clinical utility of EEG and evoked potential data.' *Annals of Neurology,* **5,** 309-321.
Dukes, H. T., Vieth, R. G. (1964) 'Cerebral arteriography during migraine prodrome and headache.' *Neurology,* **14,** 636-639.
Dunn, D. W., Snyder, C. H. (1976) 'Benign paroxysmal vertigo of childhood.' *American Journal of Diseases of Children,* **130,** 1099-1100.
Durkan, G. P., Troost, B. T., Slamovits, T., Spoor, T. C., Kennerdell, J. S. (1981) 'Recurrent painless oculomotor palsy in children. A variant of ophthalmoplegic migraine?' *Headache,* **21,** 58-62.
Dyck, P., Gruskin, P. (1977) 'Supratentorial arachnoid cysts in adults.' *Archives of Neurology,* **34,** 276-279.
Ekbom, K. (1970) 'A clinical comparison of cluster headache and migraine.' *Acta Neurologica Scandinavica,* **46,** (Suppl. 41).
Edmeads, J. (1979) 'Vascular headache and the cranial circulation—another look.' *Headache,* **19,** 127-131.
Egger, J., Carter, C. M., Wilson, J., Turner, M. W., Soothill, J. F. (1983) 'Is migraine food allergy? A double-blind controlled trial of oligoantigenic diet treatment.' *Lancet,* **2,** 865-869.
Ehyai, A., Fenichel, G. M. (1978) 'The natural history of acute confusional migraine.' *Archives of Neurology,* **35,** 368-369.
Engel, A. G., Rebouche, C. J., Wilson, D. M., Glasgow, A. M., Romshe C. A., Cruse, R. P. (1981) 'Primary systemic carnitine deficiency. II: Renal handling of carnitine.' *Neurology,* **31,** 819-825.
Emery, C. S. (1977) 'Acute confusional state in children with migraine.' *Pediatrics,* **60,** 110-114.
Evans, O. B., Kilroy, A. W., Fenichel, G. M. (1978) 'Acetazolamide in the treatment of pyruvate dysmetabolism syndromes.' *Archives of Neurology,* **35,** 302-305.
Eviatar, L. (1981) 'Vestibular testing in basilar artery migraine.' *Annals of Neurology,* **9,** 126-130.
Farquhar, H. G. (1956) 'Abdominal migraine in children.' *British Medical Journal,* **1,** 1082-1085.
Felig, P., Cherif, A., Minigawa, A., Wahren, J. (1982) 'Hypoglycemia during prolonged exercise in normal men.' *New England Journal of Medicine,* **306,** 895-900.
Fenichel, G. M. (1967) 'Migraine as a cause of benign paroxysmal vertigo of childhood.' *Journal of Pediatrics,* **71,** 114-115.
Ferguson, K. S., Robinson, S. S. (1982) 'Life threatening migraine.' *Archives of Neurology,* **39,** 374-376.
Fernbach, D. J. (1981) 'Headache after lumbar puncture.' *Lancet,* **2,** 529.
Fishman, R. A. (1975) 'Brain edema.' *New England Journal of Medicine,* **293,** 706-711.
Frantzen, E., Jacobsen, H. H., Therkelsen, J. (1961) 'Cerebral artery occlusions in children due to trauma to the head and neck.' *Neurology,* **11,** 695-700.
Friedman, A. P., Brenner, C., Denny-Brown, D. E. (1945) 'Post-traumatic vertigo and dizziness.' *Journal of Neurosurgery,* **2,** 36-46.
—— von Storch, T. J. C., Merritt, H. H. (1954) 'Migraine and tension headaches.' *Neurology,* **4,** 773-788.
—— Finley, K. H., Graham, J. R., Kunkle, E. C., Ostfeld, A. M., Wolff, H. G. (1962*a*) 'Classification of headache.' *Archives of Neurology,* **6,** 173-176.

—— Harter, D. H., Merritt, H. H. (1962*b*) 'Ophthalmoplegic migraine.' *Archives of Neurology,* **7,** 320-327.

—— Elkind, A. H. (1963) 'Appraisal of methysergide in treatment of vascular headaches of the migraine type.' *Journal of the American Medical Association,* **184,** 125-128.

—— Harms, E. (Eds.) (1967) *Headaches in Children.* Springfield, Ill.: C. C. Thomas.

Friedman, M. W. (1951) 'Occlusion of central retinal vein in migraine.' *Archives of Ophthalmology,* **45,** 678-682.

Friedman, M. H., Agus, B., Weisberg, J. (1983) 'Neglected conditions producing preauricular and referred pain'. *Journal of Neurology, Neurosurgery and Psychiatry,* **46,** 1067-1072.

Froelich, W. A., Carter, C. C., O'Leary, J. L., Rosenbaum, H. E. (1960) 'Headache in childhood.' *Neurology,* **10,** 639-642.

Gascon, G., Barlow, C. F. (1970) 'Juvenile migraine presenting as an acute confusional state.' *Pediatrics,* **45,** 628-635.

Gee, S. (1882) 'Fitful or recurrent vomiting.' *St Bartholomew's Hospital Reports,* **18,** 1-6.

Geschwind, N., Behan, P. (1982) 'Left handedness: association with immune disease, migraine and developmental learning disorder.' *Proceedings of the National Academy of Sciences of the United States of America,* **79,** 5097-5100.

Giel, R., de Vlieger, M., van Vliet, A. G. (1966) 'Headache and the EEG.' *Electroencephalography and Clinical Neurophysiology,* **21,** 492-495.

Gjerris, F., Mellemgaard, L. (1969) 'Transitory cortical blindness in head injury.' *Acta Neurologica Scandinavica,* **45,** 623-631.

Glasgow, A. M., Kraegel, B. A., Schulman, J. D. (1978) 'Studies of the cause and treatment of hyperammonemia in females with ornithine transcarbamylase deficiency.' *Pediatrics,* **62,** 30-37.

Glista, G. G., Mellinger, J. F., Rooke, E. D. (1975) 'Familial hemiplegic migraine.' *Mayo Clinic Proceedings,* **50,** 307-311.

Golden, G. S. (1979) 'The Alice in Wonderland syndrome in juvenile migraine.' *Pediatrics,* **63,** 517-519.

—— French, J. H. (1975) 'Basilar artery migraine in young children.' *Pediatrics,* **56,** 722-726.

Goldensohn, E. S. (1976) 'Paroxysmal and other features of the electroencephalogram in migraine.' *Research and Clinical Studies in Headache,* **4,** 118-128.

Goodell, H., Lewontin, R., Wolff, H. G. (1954) 'Familial occurrence of migraine heádache.' *Archives of Neurology and Psychiatry,* **72,** 325-334.

Gormley, J. B. (1960) 'Treatment of post-spinal headache.' *Anesthesiology,* **21,** 565-566.

Graham, J. R. (1956) *Treatment of Migraine.* Boston and Toronto: Little Brown & Co.

—— (1964) 'Methysergide for the prevention of headache. Experience in 500 patients over 3 years.' *New England Journal of Medicine,* **270,** 67-72.

—— Wolff, H. G. (1938) 'Mechanism of migraine headache and action of ergotamine tartrate.' *Archives of Neurology and Psychiatry,* **39,** 737-763.

—— Suby, H. I., LeCompte, P. R., Sadovsky, N. L. (1966) 'Fibrotic disorders associated with methysergide therapy for headache.' *New England Journal of Medicine,* **274,** 359-368.

Graveson, G. S. (1949) 'Retinal arterial occlusion in migraine.' *British Medical Journal,* **2,** 838-840.

Green, M. (1967) 'Diagnosis and treatment of psychogenic, recurrent abdominal pain.' *Pediatrics,* **40,** 84-89.

Green, W. R., Hackett, E. R., Schlizinger, N. S. (1964) 'Neuro-ophthalmolgic evaluation of oculomotor nerve paralysis.' *Archives of Ophthalmology,* **72,** 154-167.

Greenblatt, S. H. (1973) 'Post-traumatic transient cerebral blindness—association with migraine and seizure diatheses.' *Journal of the American Medical Association,* **225,** 1073-1076.

Greer, M., (1962) 'Benign intracranial hypertension. I: mastoiditis and lateral sinus obstruction.' *Neurology,* **12,** 472-480.

—— (1964) 'Benign intracranial hypertension. IV: menarche.' *Neurology,* **14,** 569-573.

Griffith, J. F., Dodge, P. R. (1968) 'Transient blindness following head injury in children.' *New England Journal of Medicine,* **278,** 648-651.

Griggs, R. C., Moxley, R. T., LaFrance, R. A., McQuillen, J. (1978) 'Hereditary paroxysmal ataxia: response to acetazolamide.' *Neurology,* **28,** 1259-1264.

Guralnick, W., Kaban, L. B., Merrill, R. G. (1978) 'Temporomandibular joint afflictions.' *New England Journal of Medicine,* **299,** 123-129.

Gurdjian, E. S., Hardy, W. G., Lindner, D. W., Thomas, L. M. (1963) 'Closed cervical cranial trauma associated with involvement of carotid and vertebral arteries.' *Journal of Neurosurgery,* **20,** 418-427.

272

Haas, D. C., Sovner, R. D. (1969) 'Migraine attacks triggered by mild head trauma, and their relation to certain post-traumatic disorders of childhood.' *Journal of Neurology, Neurosurgery and Psychiatry*, **32**, 548-554.

—— Pineda, G. S., Lourie, H. (1975) 'Juvenile head trauma syndromes and their relationship to migraine.' *Archives of Neurology*, **32**, 727-730.

Halpern, L. T., Bental, E. (1958) 'Epileptic cephalea.' *Neurology*, **8**, 615-620.

Hammond, J. (1974) 'The late sequelae of recurrent vomiting of childhood.' *Developmental Medicine and Child Neurology*, **16**, 15-22.

Handa, H., Bucy, P. C. (1956) 'Benign cysts of the brain simulating brain tumor.' *Journal of Neurosurgery*, **13**, 489-499.

Hardebo, J. E., Edvinsson, L., Owman, C. H., Svendgaard, N. (1978) 'Potentiation and antagonism of serotonin effects in intracranial and extracranial vessels. Possible implications in migraine.' *Neurology*, **28**, 64-70.

Harrington, H., Heller, H. A., Dawson, D., Caplan, L., Rumbaugh, C. (1983) 'Intracerebral hemorrhage and oral amphetamine.' *Archives of Neurology*, **40**, 503-507.

Harris, P. (1957) 'Head injuries in childhood.' *Archives of Diseases of Childhood*, **32**, 488-491.

Harris, W. (1937) *The Facial Neuralgias.* London: Oxford Medical Publications.

Hayes, G. J., Creston, J. E. (1964) 'Mucocele of the sphenoid sinus.' *Archives of Otolaryngology*, **79**, 653-656.

Healy, G. B. (1982) 'Hearing loss and vertigo secondary to head injury.' *New England Journal of Medicine*, **306**, 1029-1031.

—— Friedman, J. M., Strong, M. S. (1976) 'Vestibular and auditory findings of perilymphatic fistula.' *Transactions of the American Academy of Ophthalmology and Otology*, **82**, ORL44-49.

Henderson, W. R., Raskin, N. H. (1972) '"Hot dog headache": individual susceptibility to nitrite.' *Lancet*, **2**, 1162-1163.

Herman, K., Hall, I. S. (1944) 'Sphenoidal mucocoel as a cause of the ophthalmoplegic migraine syndrome.' *Transactions of the Ophthalmological Society of the U.K.*, **44**, 154-164.

Herman, P. (1983) 'The pupil and headaches.' *Headache*, **23**, 102-105.

Herzeberg, L., Lenman, J. A. R., Victoratos, G., Fletcher, F. (1975) 'Cluster headaches associated with vascular malformations.' *Journal of Neurology, Neurosurgery and Psychiatry*, **38**, 648-649.

Herzog, D. B., Rathbun, J. (1982) 'Childhood depression: developmental considerations.' *American Journal of Diseases of Children*, **136**, 115-120.

Hilal, S. K., Solomon, G. E., Gold, A. P., Carter, S. (1971) 'Primary cerebral arterial occlusive disease in children. I: Acute acquired hemiplegia.' *Radiology*, **99**, 71-86.

Hilton, B. P., Cumings, J. N. (1972) '5-hydroxytryptamine levels and platelet aggregation responses in subjects with acute migraine headache.' *Journal of Neurology, Neurosurgery and Psychiatry*, **35**, 505-509.

Hockaday, J. M., Whitty, C. W. M. (1969) 'Factors determining the EEG in migraine.' *Brain*, **92**, 769-788.

Holguin, J., Fenichel, G. (1967) 'Migraine.' *Journal of Pediatrics*, **70**, 290-297.

Holmes, G. L., Zimmerman, A. W. (1983) 'Temporomandibular joint pain—dysfunction syndrome: a rare cause of headaches in adolescents.' *Developmental Medicine and Child Neurology*, **25**, 601-605.

Honig, P. J., Charney, E. B. (1982) 'Children with brain tumor headaches.' *American Journal of Diseases of Children*, **136**, 121-124.

Horton, B. T. (1941) 'The use of histamine in the treatment of specific types of headaches.' *Journal of the American Medical Association*, **116**, 377-383.

—— (1956) 'Histaminic cephalalgia, differential diagnosis and treatment.' *Proceedings of the Staff Meetings of the Mayo Clinic*, **31**, 325-333.

Isler, W. (1971) *Acute Hemisyndromes in Childhood. Clinics in Developmental Medicine, Nos. 41/42.* London: S.I.M.P. with Heinemann Medical; Philadelphia: Lippincott.

Jacome, D. E., Fitzgerald, R. (1982) 'Ictus emeticus.' *Neurology*, **32**, 209-212.

Jakubiak, P., Dunsmore, R. H., Beckett, R. S. (1968) 'Supratentorial brain cysts.' *Journal of Neurosurgery*, **28**, 129-136.

Jammes, J. L. (1975) 'The treatment of cluster headache with prednisone.' *Diseases of the Nervous System*, **36**, 375-376.

Jay, G. W., Tomasi, L. G. (1981) 'Pediatric headaches: a one year retrospective analysis.' *Headache*, **21**, 5-9.

Jefferson, A., Clark, J. (1976) 'The treatment of benign intracranial hypertension by dehydrating agents.' *Journal of Neurology, Neurosurgery and Psychiatry*, **39**, 627-639.

273

Jensen, T. S. (1980) 'Transient global amnesia in childhood.' *Developmental Medicine and Neurology*, **22**, 654-667.

Jensen, S., Olivarius, T. de F., Kroft, B., Hansen, H. J. (1981) 'Familial hemplegic migraine—a reappraisal and long term follow-up study.' *Cephalgia*, **1**, 33-39.

Johnson, I., Paterson, A. (1974) 'Benign intracranial hypertension. II: CSF pressure and circulation.' *Brain*, **97**, 301-312.

Jonas, A. D. (1966) 'Headaches as seizure equivalents.' *Headache*, **6**, 78-87.

Jones, H. R., Naggar, C. Z., Seljan, M. R., Downing, L. L. (1982) 'Mitral valve prolapse and cerebral ischemic events.' *Stroke*, **13**, 451-453.

Jones, R. J., Forsythe, A. M., Amess, J. A. L. (1982) 'Platelet aggregation in migraine patients during the headache-free interval.' *Advances in Neurology*, **33**, 275-278.

Kalendovsky, Z., Austin, J. H. (1975) ' "Complicated migraine": its association with increased platelet aggregability and abnormal plasma coagulation factors.' *Headache*, **15**, 18-35.

—— —— Steele, P. (1975) 'Increased platelet aggregability in young patients with stroke.' *Archives of Neurology*, **32**, 13-20.

Kangasniemi, Z., Sonninen, V., Rinne, U. K. (1972) 'Excretion of free conjugated 5-HIAA and VMA in urine and concentration of 5-HIAA and HVA in CSF during migraine attacks and free intervals.' *Headache*, **12**, 62-65.

Kanter, W. R., Eldridge, R., Fabricant, R., Allen, J. C., Koerber, T. (1980) 'Central neurofibromatosis with bilateral acoustic neuroma: genetic, clinical and biochemical distinctions from peripheral neurofibromatosis.' *Neurology*, **30**, 851-859.

Kashani, J., Simonds, J. F. (1979) 'The incidence of depression in children.' *American Journal of Psychiatry*, **136**, 1202-1205.

Kelly, J. J., Mellinger, J. F., Sundt, T. M. (1978) 'Intracranial arteriovenous malformations in childhood.' *Annals of Neurology*, **3**, 338-343.

Kempton, J. J. (1956) 'The periodic syndrome.' *British Medical Journal*, **1**, 83-86.

Kinast, M., Lenders, H., Rothner, A. D., Erenberg, G. (1982) 'Benign focal epileptiform discharges in childhood migraine.' *Neurology*, **32**, 1309.

Kjellberg, R. N., Hanamura, T., Davis, K. R., Lyons, S. L., Adams, R. D. (1983) 'Bragg-peak proton-beam therapy for arteriovenous malformation of brain.' *New England Journal of Medicine*, **309**, 269-274.

Koenigsberger, M. R., Chutorian, A. M., Gold, A. P., Schvey, M. S. (1970) 'Benign paroxysmal vertigo of childhood.' *Neurology*, **20**, 1108-1113.

Kogutt, M. S., Swischuk, L. E. (1973) 'Diagnosis of sinusitis in infants and children.' *Pediatrics*, **52**, 121-124.

Kohlenberg, R. J. (1982) 'Tyramine sensitivity in dietary migraine: a critical review.' *Headache*, **22**, 30-34.

Kudrow, L. (1980) *Cluster Headache*. New York: Oxford University Press.

Kunkle, E. C., Anderson, W. B. (1961) 'Significance of minor eye signs in headache of the migraine type.' *Archives of Ophthalmology*, **65**, 504-507.

Kuritzky, A., Toglia, U. J., Thomas, D. (1981) 'Vestibular function in migraine.' *Headache*, **21**, 110-112.

Kurtz, Z., Dilling, D., Blau, J. N., Peckham, C. (1984) 'Migraine in children: findings from the National Child Development Study.' *In:* F. Clifford Rose (Ed.) *Progress in Migraine Research, 2.* London: Pitman Books. pp. 9-17.

Lance, J. W. (1976) 'Headaches related to sexual activity.' *Journal of Neurology, Neurosurgery and Psychiatry*, **39**, 1226-1230.

—— Anthony, M. (1966) 'Some clinical aspects of migraine.' *Archives of Neurology*, **15**, 356-361.

—— —— (1971) 'Thermographic studies in vascular headache.' *Medical Journal of Australia*, **1**, 240-243.

—— Hinterberger, H. (1976) 'Symptoms of pheochromocytoma, with particular reference to headache, correlated with catecholamine production.' *Archives of Neurology*, **33**, 281-288.

Lanzi, G., Balottin, U., Ottolini, A., Burgio, F. R., Fazzi, E., Arisi, D. (1983) 'Cyclic vomiting and recurrent abdominal pains as migraine or epileptic equivalents.' *Cephalalgia*, **3**, 115-118.

Lapkin, M. L., French, J. L., Golden, J. L., Rown, A. J. (1977) 'The electroencephalogram in childhood basilar artery migraine.' *Neurology*, **27**, 580-583.

—— Golden, G. S. (1978) 'Basilar artery migraine, a review of 30 cases.' *American Journal of Diseases of Children*, **132**, 278-281.

Laplante, P., Saint-Hilaire, J. M., Bouvier, G. (1983) 'Headache as an epileptic manifestation.' *Neurology*, **33**, 1493-1495.

Lagos, J. C., Riley, H. D. (1971) 'Congenital intracranial vascular malformations in children'. *Archives of Disease in Childhood*, **46**, 285-290.

Lasater, G. M. (1970) 'Primary intracranial hypotension.' *Headache*, **10**, 63-66.

Lauritzen, M., Jorgensen, M. B., Diemer, N. H., Gjedde, A., Hansen, A. J. (1982) 'Persistent oligemia of rat cerebral cortex in the wake of spreading depression.' *Annals of Neurology*, **12**, 469-474.

—— Olsen, T. S., Lassen, N. A., Paulson, O. B. (1983*a*) 'Change in regional cerebral blood flow during the course of classic migraine attacks.' *Annals of Neurology*, **13**, 633-641.

—— —— —— —— (1983*b*) 'Regulation of regional cerebral blood flow during and between migraine attacks.' *Annals of Neurology*, **14**, 569-572.

Laxdal, T., Gomez, M. R., Reiher, J. (1969) 'Cyanotic and pallid syncopal attacks in children (breath holding spells).' *Developmental Medicine and Child Neurology*, **11**, 755-763.

Leão, A. A. P. (1944*a*) 'Spreading depression of activity in the cerebral cortex.' *Journal of Neurophysiology*, **7**, 359-390.

—— (1944*b*) 'Pial circulation of spreading depression of activity of cerebral cortex.' *Journal of Neurophysiology*, **7**, 391-396.

Lechin, F., van der Dijs, D. (1977) 'A new treatment for headache: pathophysiologic considerations.' *Headache*, **16**, 318-321.

Lee, C. H., Lance, J. W. (1977) 'Migraine stupor.' *Headache*, **17**, 32-38.

Lees, F. (1962) 'The migrainous symptoms of cerebral angiomata.' *Journal of Neurology, Neurosurgery and Psychiatry*, **25**, 45-50.

—— Watkins, S. M. (1963) 'Loss of consciousness in migraine.' *Lancet*, **2**, 647-649.

Lennox, W. G., Lennox, M. A. (1960) *Epilepsy and Related Disorders*. Boston: Little Brown & Co.

Levin, B. E. (1978) 'The clinical significance of spontaneous pulsations of the retinal vein.' *Archives of Neurology*, **35**, 37-40.

Leviton, A. (1975) 'Post carotid endarterectomy "hemicrania".' *Headache*, **15**, 13-17.

—— (1978) 'Epidemiology of headache.' *Advances in Neurology*, **19**, 341-351.

—— Malvea, B., Graham, J. R. (1974) 'Vascular diseases, mortality and migraine in the parents of migraine patients.' *Neurology*, **24**, 669-672.

—— Caplan, L., Salzman, E. (1975) 'Severe headache after carotid endarterectomy.' *Headache*, **15**, 207-209.

—— Slack, W. V., Moser, B., Bana, D., Graham, J. R. (1984) 'A computerized behavioral assessment of children with headaches.' *Headache (in press)*.

Lew, D., Southwick, F. S., Montgomery, W. W., Weber, A. L., Baker, A. S. (1983) 'Sphenoid sinusitis; a review of 30 cases. *New England Journal of Medicine*, **309**, 1149-1154.

Ling, W., Oftedal, G., Weinberg, W. (1970) 'Depressive illness in childhood presenting as severe headache.' *American Journal of Diseases of Children*, **120**, 122-124.

Lippman, C. W. (1952) 'Certain hallucinations peculiar to migraine.' *Journal of Nervous and Mental Disease*, **116**, 346-351.

Litman, G. I., Friedman, H. M. (1978) 'Migraine and the mitral valve prolapse syndrome.' *American Heart Journal*, **96**, 610-614.

Livingston, S. (1951) 'Abdominal pain as a manifestation of epilepsy (abdominal epilepsy) in children.' *Journal of Pediatrics*, **38**, 687-695.

Loewenfeld, I. E. (1980) 'Pupillary deficit in ophthalmoplegic migraine.' *In:* Glaser, J. S. (Ed.) *Neuroophthalmology, Vol. 10*. St. Louis: C. V. Mosby. Ch. 15.

Lombroso, C. T., Schwartz, I. H., Clark, D. M., Muench, H., Barry, D. (1966) 'Ctenoids in healthy youths.' *Neurology*, **16**, 1152-1158.

—— Lerman, P. (1967) 'Breath-holding spells (cyanotic and pallid infantile syncope).' *Pediatrics*, **39**, 563-581.

Ludvigsson, J. (1974) 'Propranolol used in the prophylaxis of migraine in children.' *Acta Neurologica Scandinavica*, **50**, 109-115.

McDonald, W. I., Sanders, M. D. (1971) 'Migraine complicated by ischaemic papillopathy.' *Lancet*, **2**, 521-523.

MacKenzie, I. (1953) 'The clinical presentation of the cerebral angiomata.' *Brain*, **76**, 184-214.

Mani, S., Deetor, J. (1982) 'Arteriovenous malformation of the brain presenting as cluster headache.' *Headache*, **22**, 184-185.

Maratos, J., Wilkinson, M. (1982) 'Migraine in children: a medical and psychiatric study.' *Cephalalgia*, **2**, 179-187.

Marks, R. L., Freed, M. (1973) 'Non-penetrating injuries of the neck and cerebrovascular accident.' *Archives of Neurology*, **28**, 412-414.

Masek, B. (1984) *Personal communication.*

—— Russo, D. C., Varni, J. W. (1984) 'Behavioral approaches to the management of chronic pain in children.' *Pediatric Clinics in North America (in press).*

Massey, E. W. (1982) 'Effort headache in runners.' *Headache,* **22,** 99-100.

Mathew, N. T. (1978) 'Clinical sub types of cluster headache and response to lithium therapy.' *Headache,* **18,** 27-29.

—— (1981) 'Indomethacin responsive headache syndromes.' *Headache,* **21,** 147-150.

—— Meyer, J. S., Welch, K. M. A., Neblett, C. R. (1977) 'Abnormal CT scans in migraine headache.' *Headache,* **16,** 272-279.

—— Stubits, E., Nigam, M. P. (1982) 'Transformation of episodic migraine into daily headache: analysis of factors.' *Headache,* **22,** 66-68.

Matthews, W. B. (1972) 'Footballer's migraine.' *British Medical Journal,* **2,** 326-327.

Matson, D. D. (1969) *Neurosurgery of Infancy and Childhood (2nd Edn.).* Springfield, Ill.: C. C. Thomas.

Medina, J. L., Diamond, S. (1978) 'The role of diet in migraine.' *Headache,* **18,** 31-34.

Mehegan, J. E., Masek, B. J., Harrison, R. H., Russo, D. C., Leviton, A. (1984) 'Behavioral treatment of pediatric migraine.' *Journal of Clinical and Consulting Psychology (in press).*

Menkes, J. H. (1980) *Textbook of Child Neurology (2nd Edn.).* Philadelphia: Lea & Febiger.

Mesulam, M. M., Waxman, S. G., Geschwind, N. (1976) 'Acute confusional states with right middle cerebral artery infarctions.' *Journal of Neurology, Neurosurgery and Psychiatry,* **39,** 84-88.

Mettinger, K. L., Ericson, K. L. (1982) 'Fibromuscular dysplasia and the brain. I: Observations on angiographic, clinical and genetic characteristics.' *Stroke,* **13,** 46-52.

Millichap, J. G., Lombroso, C. T., Lennox, W. G. (1955) 'Cyclic vomiting as a form of epilepsy in children.' *Pediatrics,* **15,** 705-714.

Milner, P. M. (1958) 'Note on a possible correspondence between the scotomas of migraine and spreading depression of Leao.' *Electroencephalography and Clinical Neurophysiology,* **10,** 705.

Mitchell, W. G., Greenwood, R. S., Messenheimer, J. A. (1983) 'Abdominal epilepsy—cyclic vomiting as the major symptom of simple partial seizures.' *Archives of Neurology,* **40,** 251-252.

Moffet, A. M., Swash, M., Scott, D. F. (1974) 'Effect of chocolate in migraine: a double blind study.' *Journal of Neurology, Neurosurgery and Psychiatry,* **37,** 445-448.

Mokri, B. (1982) 'Raeder's paratrigeminal syndrome—original concept and subsequent deviations.' *Archives of Neurology,* **39,** 395-399.

Montgomery, B. M., Pinner, C. A. (1964) 'Transient hypoglycemic hemiplegia.' *Archives of Internal Medicine,* **114,** 680-684.

Moretti, G., Manzoni, G. C., Caffarra, P., Parma, M. (1980) '"Benign recurrent vertigo" and its connection with migraine.' *Headache,* **20,** 344-346.

Morin, M. A., Pitts, F. W. (1970) 'Delayed apoplexy following head injury ("Traumatische Spät-Apolexis").' *Journal of Neurosurgery,* **33,** 542-547.

Moskowitz, M. (1984) 'Vascular head pain.' *Annals of Neurology (in press).*

—— Reinhard, J. F., Romero, J., Melamed, E., Pettibone, J. (1979) 'Neurotransmitters and the fifth cranial nerve: is there a relation to the headache phase of migraine?' *Lancet,* **2,** 883-885.

Mück-Seler, D., Deanovic, Z., Dupelj, M. (1979) 'Platelet serotonin (5HT) and 5HT-releasing factor in plasma of migrainous patients.' *Headache,* **19,** 14-17.

Murphy, J. P. (1955) 'Cerebral infarction in migraine.' *Neurology,* **5,** 359-361.

Murros, K., Fogelholm, R. (1983) 'Spontaneous intracranial hypotension with slit ventricles. *Journal of Neurology, Neurosurgery and Psychiatry,* **46,** 1149-1151.

Nieman, E. A., Hurwitz, L. J. (1961) 'Ocular sympathetic palsy in periodic migrainous neuralgia.' *Journal of Neurology, Neurosurgery and Psychiatry,* **24,** 369-373.

Norman, P. S., Yanagisawa, E. (1964) 'Mucocele of sphenoid sinus.' *Archives of Otolaryngology,* **79,** 646-652.

Odom, G. L., Davis, C. H., Woodhall, B. (1956) 'Brain tumors in children.' *Pediatrics,* **18,** 856-870.

Olesen, J., Larsen, B., Lauritzen, M. (1982) 'Focal hyperemia followed by spreading oligemia and impaired activation of rCBF in classic migraine.' *Annals of Neurology,* **9,** 344-352.

Olivarius, B. S., Jensen, T. S. (1979) 'Transient global amnesia in migraine.' *Headache,* **19,** 335-338.

Page, L. K., Lombroso, C. T., Matson, D. D. (1969) 'Childhood epilepsy with late detection of cerebral glioma.' *Journal of Neurosurgery,* **31,** 253-261.

Painter, M. J., Chutorian, A. M., Hilal, S. K. (1975) 'Cerebrovasculopathy following irradiation in childhood.' *Neurology,* **25,** 189-194.

Panayiotopoulos, C. P. (1980) 'Basilar migraine? Seizures and severe epileptic EEG abnormalities.' *Neurology,* **30,** 1122-1125.

276

Paterson, J. H., McKissock, W. (1956) 'A clinical survey of intracranial angiomas with special reference to their mode of progression and surgical treatment.' *Brain*, **79**, 233-266.

Patterson, R. H., Goodell, H., Dunning, H. S. (1964) 'Complications of carotid arteriography.' *Archives of Neurology*, **10**, 513-520.

Pearce, J. M. S. (1980) 'Chronic migrainous neuralgia, a variant of cluster headache.' *Brain*, **103**, 149-159.

—— Foster, J. B. (1965) 'An investigation of complicated migraine.' *Neurology*, **15**, 333-340.

Perman, J. A., Barr, R. G., Watkins, J. B. (1978) 'Sucrose malabsorption in children: non-invasive diagnosis by interval breath hydrogen determination.' *Journal of Pediatrics*, **93**, 17-22.

Peroutka, S. J., Allen, G. S. (1984) 'The calcium antagonist properties of cyproheptadine: implications for anti-migraine action.' *Neurology*, **34**, 304-309.

Phornphutkul, C., Rosenthal, A., Nadas, A. S., Berenberg, W. (1973) 'Cerebrovascular accidents in infants and children with cyanotic congenital heart disease.' *American Journal of Cardiology*, **32**, 329-334.

Pickles, W. (1949) 'Acute focal edema of the brain in children with head injuries.' *New England Journal of Medicine*, **240**, 92-95.

Pomeroy, J., Efron, M. J., Dayman, J., Hoefnagel, D. (1968) 'Hartnup disorder in a New England family.' *New England Journal of Medicine*, **278**, 1214-1216.

Portnoy, B. A., Herion, J. C. (1972) 'Neurological manifestations in sickle cell disease.' *Annals of Internal Medicine*, **76**, 643-652.

Prensky, A. L. (1976) 'Migraine and migrainous variants in pediatric patients.' *Pediatric Clinical of North America*, **23**, 461-471.

—— Sommer, D. (1979) 'Diagnosis and treatment of migraine in children.' *Neurology*, **29**, 506-510.

Prichard, J. S. (1958) 'Abdominal pain of cerebral origin in children.' *Canadian Medical Association Journal*, **78**, 665-667.

Price, R. W., Posner, J. B. (1978) 'Chronic paroxysmal hemicrania: a disabling headache syndrome responding to indomethacin.' *Annals of Neurology*, **3**, 183-184.

Priest, J. R., Ramsay, N. K. C., Steinberg, P. G., Tubergen, D. G., Cairo, M. S., Sitarz, A. L., Bishop, A. J., White, L., Trigg, M. E., Levitt, C. J., Cich, J. A., Coccia. P. F. (1982) 'A syndrome of thrombosis and hemorrhage complicating L-asparaginase therapy for childhood acute lymphoblastic leukemia.' *Journal of Pediatrics*, **100**, 984-989.

Procacci, P. M., Savran, S. V., Schreiter, S. L. (1976) 'Prevalence of clinical mitral valve prolapse in 1169 young women.' *New England Journal of Medicine*, **294**, 1086-1088.

Raeder, J. G. (1924) '"Paratrigeminal" paralysis of oculo-pupillary sympathetic.' *Brain*, **47**, 149-158.

Rahme, E. S., Green, D. (1961) 'Chronic subdural hematoma in adolescence and early adulthood. *Journal of the American Medical Association*, **176**, 424-426.

Raichle, M. E., Grubb, R. L., Phelps, M. E., Gado, M. H., Caronna, J. H. (1978) 'Cerebral hemodynamics and metabolism in pseudotumor cerebri.' *Annals of Neurology*, **4**, 104-111.

Raskin, N. H., Knittle, S. C. (1976) 'Ice cream headache and orthostatic symptoms in patients with migraine.' *Headache*, **16**, 222-225.

—— Prusiner, S. (1977) 'Carotidynia.' *Neurology*, **27**, 43-46.

—— Schwartz, R. K. (1980) 'Ice pick-like pain.' *Neurology*, **30**, 203-205.

Ravid, J. M. (1928) 'Transient insulin hypoglycemic hemiplegias.' *American Journal of Medical Sciences*, **175**, 756-769.

Reik, L., Hale, M. (1981) 'The temporomandibular joint pain-dysfunction syndrome: a frequent cause of headache.' *Headache*, **21**, 151-156.

Reinecke, R. D. (1961) 'Migrainoid symptoms associated with intracranial vascular anomalies.' *Archives of Ophthalmology*, **65**, 808-810.

Rice, G. P. A., Boughner, D. R., Stiller, C., Ebers, G. C. (1980) 'Familial stroke syndrome associated with mitral valve prolapse.' *Annals of Neurology*, **7**, 130-134.

Riley, C. M., Day, R. L., Greeley, D. M., Langford, W. S. (1949) 'Central autonomic dysfunction with defective lacrimation.' *Pediatrics*, **3**, 468-478.

Robertson, W. C., Schnitzler, E. R. (1978) 'Ophthalmoplegic migraine in infancy.' *Pediatrics*, **61**, 886-888.

Román, G., Fisher, M., Perl, D. P., Poser, C. M. (1978) 'Neurological manifestations of hereditary hemorrhagic telangiectasia.' *Annals of Neurology*, **4**, 130-144.

Rooke, E. D. (1968) 'Benign exertional headache.' *Medical Clinics of North America*, **52**, 801-808.

Rose, A., Matson, D. D. (1967) 'Benign intracranial hypertension in children.' *Pediatrics*, **39**, 227-237.

Rosen, J. A. (1983) 'Observations on the efficacy of propranolol for the prophylaxis of migraine.' *Annals of Neurology*, **13**, 92-93.

277

Rosenbaum, H. E. (1960) 'Familial hemiplegic migraine.' *Neurology,* **10,** 164-170.

Ross, R. T. (1958) 'Hemiplegic migraine.' *Canadian Medical Association Journal,* **78,** 10-16.

Rossi, L. N., Vasella, F., Baje, O., Tonz, O., Lutschg, J., Mumenthaler, M. (1984) 'Benign migraine-like syndrome with CSF pleiocytosis in children.' *Developmental Medicine and Child Neurology (in press).*

Rothner, A. D. (1978) 'Headaches in children: a review.' *Headache,* **18,** 169-175.

Rowbotham, G. F., Hay, R. K., Kirby, H. R., Tomlinson, B. E., Bousfield, M. E. (1953) 'Technique and dangers of cerebral angiography.' *Journal of Neurosurgery,* **10,** 601-607.

—— MacIver, I. N., Dickson, J., Bousfield, M. E. (1954) 'Analysis of 1400 cases of acute injury to the head.' *British Medical Journal,* **1,** 726-730.

Russell, A. (1973) 'The implications of hyperammonemia in rare and common disorders, including migraine.' *Mount Sinai Journal of Medicine,* **40,** 723-735.

—— Levin, B., Oberholzer, V. G., Sinclair, L. (1962) 'Hyperammonemia: a new instance of an inborn enzymatic defect of the biosynthesis of urea.' *Lancet,* **2,** 699-700.

Ryan, R. E., Ryan, R. E. J., Sudilovksy, A. (1983) 'Nadolol: its use in the prophylactic treatment of migraine.' *Headache,* **23,** 26-31.

Rydzewski, W. (1976) 'Serotonin (5HT) in migraine: levels in whole blood in and between attacks.' *Headache,* **16,** 16-19.

Sander, J. E., Malamud, N., Cowan, M. J., Packman, S., Amman, A. J., Wara, D. W. (1980) 'Intermittent ataxia and immunodeficiency with multiple carboxylase deficiencies: a biotin-responsive disorder.' *Annals of Neurology,* **8,** 544-547.

Saper, J. R. (1983) *Headache Disorders.* Bristol & Boston: John Wright.

Schaumburg, H. H., Byck, R., Gerstl, R. (1969) 'Monosodium L-glutamate: its pharmacologic role in Chinese Restaurant syndrome.' *Science,* **163,** 826-828.

Schneider, R. C., Lemmen, L. J. (1952) 'Traumatic internal carotid artery thrombosis secondary to non-penetrating injuries to the neck.' *Journal of Neurosurgery,* **9,** 495-507.

—— Gosch, H. H., Taren, J. A., Ferry, D. J., Jerva, M. J. (1972) 'Blood vessel trauma following head and neck injuries.' *Clinical Neurosurgery,* **19,** 312-354.

Selby, G., Lance, J. G. W. (1960) 'Observations in 500 cases of migraine and allied vascular headache.' *Journal of Neurology, Neurosurgery and Psychiatry,* **23,** 23-32.

Serdaru, M., Chiras, J., Cujas, M., Lhermitte, F. (1984) 'Isolated benign cerebral vasculitis or migrainous vasospasm?' *Journal of Neurology, Neurosurgery and Psychiatry,* **47,** 73-76.

Shinnar, S., D'Souza, B. J. (1981) 'Diagnosis and management of headaches in childhood.' *Pediatric Clinics of North America,* **29,** 79-94.

Short, E. M., Conn, H. O., Snodgrass, P. J., Campbell, A. G. M., Rosenberg, L. E. (1973) 'Evidence for X-linked dominant inheritance of ornithine transcarbamylase deficiency.' *New England Journal of Medicine,* **288,** 7-12.

Sillanpää, M. (1977) 'Clonidine prophylaxis of childhood migraine and other vascular headache—a double blind study of 57 children.' *Headache,* **17,** 28-31.

—— (1983) 'Changes in the prevalence of migraine and other headache during the first seven school years.' *Headache,* **23,** 15-19.

—— Koponen, M. (1978) 'Papaverine in the prophylaxis of migraine and other vascular headache in children.' *Acta Paediatrica Scandinavica,* **67,** 209-212.

Simons, D. J., Wolff, H. G. (1946) 'Studies on headache: mechanism of chronic post-traumatic headache.' *Psychosomatic Medicine,* **8,** 227-242.

Singleton,. G. I., Post, K. N., Karlan, M. S., Bock, D. G. (1978) 'Perilymph fistulas.' *Annals of Otology, Rhinology and Laryngology,* **87,** 797-803.

Sjaastad, O., Dale, J. (1974) 'Evidence for a new (?) treatable headache entity.' *Headache,* **14,** 105-108.

—— Dale, I. (1976) 'A new (?) clinical headache entity "chronic paroxysmal hemicrania".' *Acta Neurologica Scandinavica,* **54,** 140-159.

Snoek, J. W., Minderhoud, J. M., Wilmink, J. T. (1984) 'Delayed deterioration following mild head injury in children.' *Brain,* **107,** 15-36.

Somerville, B. W. (1971) 'The role of progesterone in menstrual migraine.' *Neurology,* **21,** 853-859.

—— (1975) 'Estrogen-withdrawal migraine.' *Neurology,* **25,** 239-244.

Spielman, F. J. (1982) 'Post-lumbar puncture headache.' *Headache,* **22,** 280-283.

Stackpole, R. H., Melicow, M. M., Uson, A. C. (1963) 'Pheochromocytoma in children.' *Journal of Pediatrics,* **63,** 315-330.

Stalon, R. D., Wilson, H., Brumback, R. A. (1981) 'Cognitive improvement associated with tricyclic antidepressant treatment of childhood major depressive illness.' *Perceptual and Motor Skills,* **53,** 219-234.

278

Starfield, B., Katz, H., Gabriel, A., Livingston, G., Benson, P., Hankin, J., Horn, S., Steinwachs, D. (1984) 'Morbidity in childhood—a longitudinal view.' *New England Journal of Medicine*, **310**, 824-829.

Strand, R. (1976) 'Cerebral acquired vascular disease in childhood'. *Progress in Pediatric Radiology*, **5**, 182-230.

Strauss, H., Selinsky, H. (1941) 'Electroencephalographic findings in patients with the migrainous syndrome.' *Transactions of the American Neurological Association*, **67**, 205-208.

Swaiman, K. F., Frank, Y. (1978) 'Seizure headaches in children.' *Developmental Medicine and Child Neurology*, **20**, 580-585.

Swanson, J. W., Vick, N. A. (1978) 'Basilar artery migraine.' *Neurology*, **28**, 782-786.

Symonds, C. P. (1931) 'Otitic hydrocephalus.' *Brain*, **54**, 55-71.

—— (1937) 'Hydrocephalus and focal cerebral symptoms in relation to thrombophlebitis of dural sinuses and cerebral veins.' *Brain*, **60**, 531-550.

—— (1956a) 'A particular variety of headache.' *Brain*, **79**, 217-232.

—— (1956b) 'Cough headache.' *Brain*, **79**, 557-568.

Theoharides, T. C. (1983) 'Mast cells and migraines.' *Perspectives in Biology and Medicine*, **26**, 673-675.

Todd, J., (1955) 'The syndrome of Alice in Wonderland.' *Canadian Medical Association Journal*, **73**, 701-704.

Towle, P. A. (1965) 'The electroencephalographic hyperventilation response in migraine.' *Electroencephalography and Clinical Neurophysiology*, **19**, 390-393.

Vahlquist, B. (1955) 'Migraine in children.' *International Archives of Allergy*, **7**, 348-355.

—— Hackzell, G. (1949) 'Migraine of early onset: a study of 31 cases in which the disease first appeared between one and four years of age.' *Acta Paediatrica*, **38**, 622-636.

Van Buren, J. M. (1963) 'The abdominal aura, a study of abdominal sensations occurring in epilepsy and produced by depth stimulation.' *Electroencephalography and Clinical Neurophysiology*, **15**, 1-19.

Van der Meche, F. G. A., Braakman, R. (1983) 'Arachnoid cysts in the middle cranial fossa: cause and treatment of progressive and non-progressive symptoms.' *Journal of Neurology, Neurosurgery and Psychiatry*, **46**, 1102-1107.

Vannucci, R. C., Solomon, G. E., Deck, M. D. F. (1974) 'Cerebral arterial occlusion and cluster headaches in neurofibromatosis.' *American Journal of Diseases of Children*, **127**, 422-424.

Van Pelt, W., Anderman, F. (1964) 'On the early onset of ophthalmoplegic migraine.' *American Journal of Diseases of Children*, **107**, 628-631.

Verret, S., Steele, J. C. (1971) 'Alternating hemiplegia in childhood: a report of eight patients with complicated migraine beginning in infancy.' *Pediatrics*, **47**, 675-680.

Victor, D. I., Welch, R. B. (1977) 'Bilateral retinal hemorrhages and disk edema in migraine.' *American Journal of Ophthalmology*, **84**, 555-558.

Vijayan, N. (1977) 'A new post-traumatic headache syndrome: clinical and therapeutic observations.' *Headache*, **17**, 19-22.

—— (1980) 'Ophthalmoplegic migraine: ischemic or compressive neuropathy.' *Headache*, **20**, 300-304.

—— Gould, S., Watson, C. (1980) 'Exposure to sun and precipitation of migraine.' *Headache*, **20**, 42-43.

Wald, E. R., Milmoe, G. J., Bowen, D., Ledesma-Medina, J., Salamon, N., Bluestone, C. D. (1981) 'Acute maxillary sinusitis in children.' *New England Journal of Medicine*, **304**, 749-754.

Walsh, F. B. (1958) *Clinical Neuro-ophthalmology (2nd Edn.)*. Baltimore: Wilkins & Wilkins.

—— Hoyt, W. F. (1969) *Clinical Neuro-ophthalmology (3rd Edn.)*. Baltimore: Wilkins & Wilkins.

Walsh, J. P., O'Doherty, D. (1960) 'A possible explanation of the mechanism of ophthalmoplegic migraine.' *Neurology*, **10**, 1079-1084.

Waters, W. E. (1970) 'Community studies of the prevalence of headache.' *Headache*, **9**, 178-186.

—— (1974) 'The Pontypridd headache survey.' *Headache*, **14**, 81-90.

—— O'Connor, P. J. (1975) 'Prevalence of migraine.' *Journal of Neurology, Neurosurgery and Psychiatry*, **38**, 613-616.

Watson, P., Steele, J. C. (1974) 'Paroxysmal dysequilibrium in the migraine syndrome of childhood.' *Archives of Otolaryngology*, **99**, 177-179.

Weil, A. A. (1952) 'EEG findings in a certain type of psychosomatic headache: dysrythmic migraine'. *Electroencephalography and Clinical Neurophysiology*, **4**, 181-186.

Weisberg, L. A., Chutorian, A. M. (1977) 'Pseudotumor cerebri in childhood.' *American Journal of Diseases of Children*, **131**, 1243-1248.

Weksler, B. B., Gillick, M., Pink, J. (1977) 'Effect of propranolol on platelet function.' *Blood*, **49**, 185-196.

279

Whitehouse, D., Pappas, J. A., Escala, P. H., Livingston, S. (1967) 'EEG changes in children with migraine.' *New England Journal of Medicine,* **276,** 23-27.

Whitty, C. W. M. (1953) 'Familial hemiplegic migraine.' *Journal of Neurology, Neurosurgery and Psychiatry,* **16,** 172-177.

—— Hockaday, J. M., Whitty, M. M. (1966) 'The effect of oral contraceptives on migraine.' *Lancet,* **1,** 856-859.

Wolberg, F. L., Zeigler, D. K. (1982) 'Olfactory hallucination in migraine.' *Archives of Neurology,* **39,** 382-384.

Wolff, H. G. (1955) 'Headache mechanisms.' *International Archives of Allergy,* **7,** 210-278.

Wong, G., Knuckey, N. W., Gubbay, S. S. (1983) 'Subarachnoid hemorrhage in children caused by cerebral tumor.' *Journal of Neurology, Neurosurgery and Psychiatry,* **46,** 449-450.

Wright, T. L., Bresnan, M. J. (1976) 'Radiation induced cerebrovascular disease in children.' *Neurology,* **26,** 540-543.

Wyllie, W. G., Schlesinger, B. (1933) 'The periodic group of disorders in childhood.' *British Journal of Childhood Diseases,* **30,** 1-21.

Zasorin, N. L., Baloh, R. W., Myers, L. B. (1983) 'Acetazolamide-responsive episodic ataxia syndrome.' *Neurology,* **33,** 1212-1214.

Ziegler, D. K. (1977) 'Genetics of migraine.' *Headache,* **16,** 330-331.

—— Wong, G. (1967) 'Migraine in children: clinical and EEG study of families.' *Epilepsia,* **8,** 171-187.

Zimmerman, A. W., Kumar, A. J., Gadoth, N., Hodges, F. J. (1978) 'Traumatic vertebrobasilar occlusive disease in childhood.' *Neurology,* **28,** 185-188.

INDEX

281

283

Thermography 22
Third cranial nerve palsy 116-17
  inflammation 117
  ischemic infarction 116
  trauma 117
  tumor 116
Thrombophlebitis, meningitis-associated 232
Tigan (trimethobenzamide HCL) 160
Tingling 49
Tissue fluid around painful vessels 22
Todd's paresis 95, 143
Tolosa Hunt syndrome 116, 117
Tomato 33
Transient global amnesia 109, 111
  case history 114-15
Traumatic carotidynia 196
Traumatic headache syndromes 44, 181-97
  acute 181-90
  case histories 194-6
  chronic 191-4
  sub-acute 191-4
Trigeminal neuralgia 57
Trimethobenzamide HCL (Tigan) 160
Truncal ataxia 207
Tyramine 24-5

U
Upper respiratory tract infection 35
  case history 36
Urea cycle disorders 105
Urticaria 20

V
Vahlquist's criteria 6, 10 (table)

Vascular headache syndrome 45
  + muscle contraction, post-traumatic, case
    history 195-6
  post-cerebral contusion, case history 194-5
Vasodilatation 22
Vasomotor instability 14, 18-20
Vertebral-basilar system 49
Vertiginous migraine 64-5
  case histories 65, 66
  clinical presentation 64-5
  management 65
  pathogenesis 65
Vertigo 4, 49, 53
  benign paroxysmal, of childhood 60, 61, 63-4
  definition 60
  differential diagnosis 61-3
  epidemiology 60-1
  management 65
Vestibular neuronitis 61, 63
Viral encephalitis 110
Vistaril (hydroxyzine pamoate) 160
Visual stimuli as precipitating factor 43-4
Vomiting 4, 53

W
Wheat 33
Wigraine 159
  suppository 160

X
x-rays of head and neck 212-13